T0299476

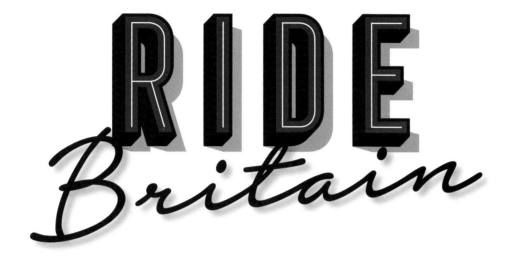

RIDE Britain

Forty inspirational cycling routes from Dartmoor to the Highlands

SIMON WARREN

With photography by Phil Hall and Andy Jones

ROBINSON

ROBINSON

First published in Great Britain in 2020 by Robinson

3 5 7 9 10 8 6 4

Text, illustrations and design © Simon Warren, 2020
Photography © Huw Fairclough, Phil Hall, Andy Jones and Simon Warren

The moral right of the author has been asserted.

All rights reserved. No part of this publication may be reproduced, stored in a retrieval system, or transmitted, in any form, or by any means, without the prior permission in writing of the publisher, nor be otherwise circulated in any form of binding or cover other than that in which it is published and without a similar condition including this condition being imposed on the subsequent purchaser.

A CIP catalogue record for this book is available from the British Library.

ISBN: 978-1-47214-454-6

Printed and bound in China by C&C Offset Printing Co., Ltd.

Papers used by Robinson are from well-managed forests and other responsible sources.

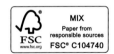

Robinson
An imprint of Little, Brown Book Group, Carmelite House, 50 Victoria Embankment, London, EC4Y 0DZ

An Hachette UK Company
www.hachette.co.uk

www.littlebrown.co.uk

Simon Warren

I'd like to thank my amazing wife Charlotte and children Lux and Ryder for their support during this mammoth project and my parents, family and friends for advice and guidance. I'd like to say a huge thank you to my wonderful photographers Phil and Andy for coping with my ruthless dawn til dusk schedules *almost* without complaint. This book could not and would not have happened without you. Thanks to Duncan Proudfoot at Little, Brown for having faith in the project and for encouraging me to spread my wings to tackle something of this magnitude, and to Dom Millar who hooked me up with Ross Matheson and Assos to dress me so fine. Also and in no particular order thanks to Peter Walker at www.tourofpembrokeshire.com, Dan Evans, Nick Burton, James Ward, Ben Lowe at veloviewer.com, Matt and Jess at ridethestruggle.com, everyone at Humanrace.co.uk and all cyclists out there for following me on this crazy adventure. I'll see you in the hills.

Phil Hall

To my wife Lisa and my girls Ada and Emmie, thank you for your love and support.

INTRODUCTION

Right, here we go, I have shaken myself free from the shackles of my pocket guides and for the first time linked the dots between the hills to present you with 40 awesome routes. They are of course all PACKED with hills: would you expect anything else? All set in the most beautiful scenery mainland Britain has to offer. After years of travelling up and down the island on adventures to tackle hideous gradients I've seen a myriad of roads which I've been desperate to share and now I can. Although I have ridden just about every road covered in the book, some many times, I can't claim to have ridden every route in its entirety. The inspiration for them came from parts of famous sportive courses, from research trips, family holidays, races I have competed in, each ride an amalgamation of a collective set of memories. There are a couple of real monsters within the pages with the longest standing at 274 kilometres but the vast majority are more modest. Although they all offer a hearty challenge they should be well within the capabilities of most riders.

During the production of my previous books I have always been a one-man band taking a pocket camera with me up all the climbs and although this approach was perfect for a small format this project needed proper photography and proper photographers. The images within needed to inspire and lure you into the hills, to show off the landscape in glorious CinemaScope so I enlisted the services of two good friends, Andy Jones and Phil Hall. Anyone who has been reading *Cycling Weekly* for the past 20 years will be aware of Andy's work shooting riders from Mont Ventoux to Monsal Head, and I worked with Phil for close to ten years on photography magazines so knew he would be perfect for the job. With both being cyclists they instantly saw what I was after, although Phil I suspect will be having nightmares about riding up Great Dun Fell and Bealach-na-Ba for many years to come!

As you will see in the photography they not only captured the best of the British scenery but also the best of the British weather. Of course it would have been nice to see wall-to-wall blue sky – it would have certainly made the rides easier – but that would not be a fair reflection of our often inclement climate. We hardly saw the sun on our 'summer' trip to Scotland, it was utterly dire weather – likewise in County Durham and Wales

– but we were blessed with a few decent days and were especially lucky to capture some snow.

The format of the book is pretty straightforward. Each route is essentially a chapter with a description of the ride followed by a map, a simple profile and the low-down on three key climbs. You'll get an idea from the distance and the amount of elevation gain as to how hard each ride is but to help I have also rated them all out of 10. As the book is too large to take on rides you can visit **www.100climbs.co.uk/ride-britain-gpx** to download the gpx. files to your computer, or if you prefer you can go old school take paper maps out with you.

I have indicated places where supplies can be obtained but I have not listed individual cafés or shops so I'll leave you to do that bit of research if needed. When, where and for how long you choose to rest is up to you but where there is a water symbol you know there will be at least a garage where you can grab the essentials. So whether it's a long summer's evening or a weekend away here are 40 challenges, 40 adventures through 40 remarkable areas of natural beauty for you to tackle. Take care out there and enjoy riding Britain.

Simon

GPX. ROUTE FILES
All the routes in the book are available to download as gpx. files for you to transfer to your computer from the following web address. www.100climbs. co.uk/ride-britain-gpx

MAPS
Most of the maps are pretty straightforward but some will need a closer look especially where the same road is used more than once. Just follow the direction arrows and distance numbers though and you will work them out.

THE RIDES

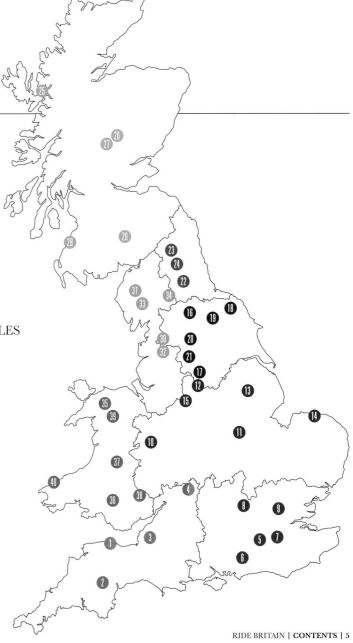

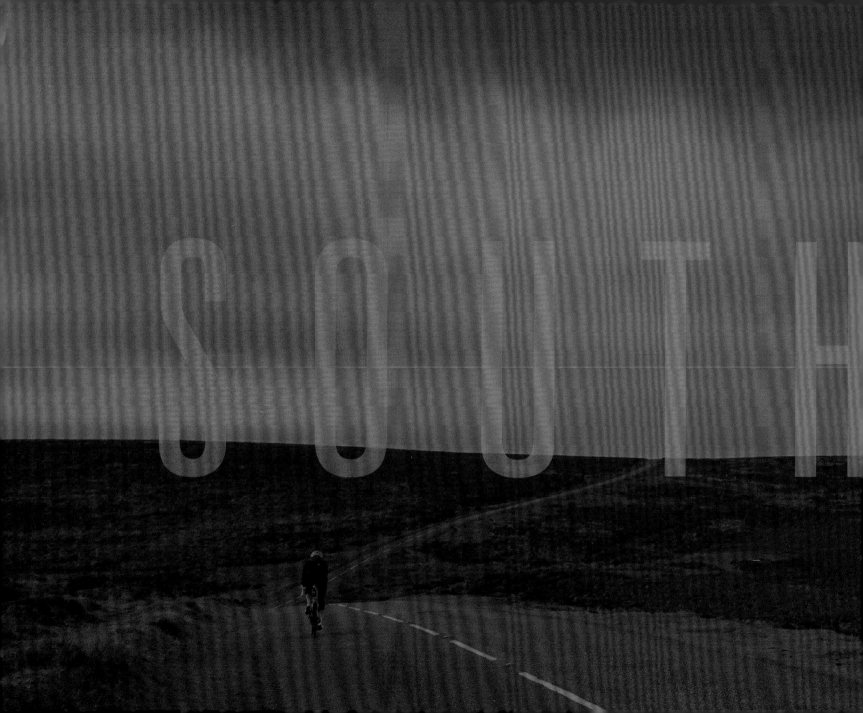

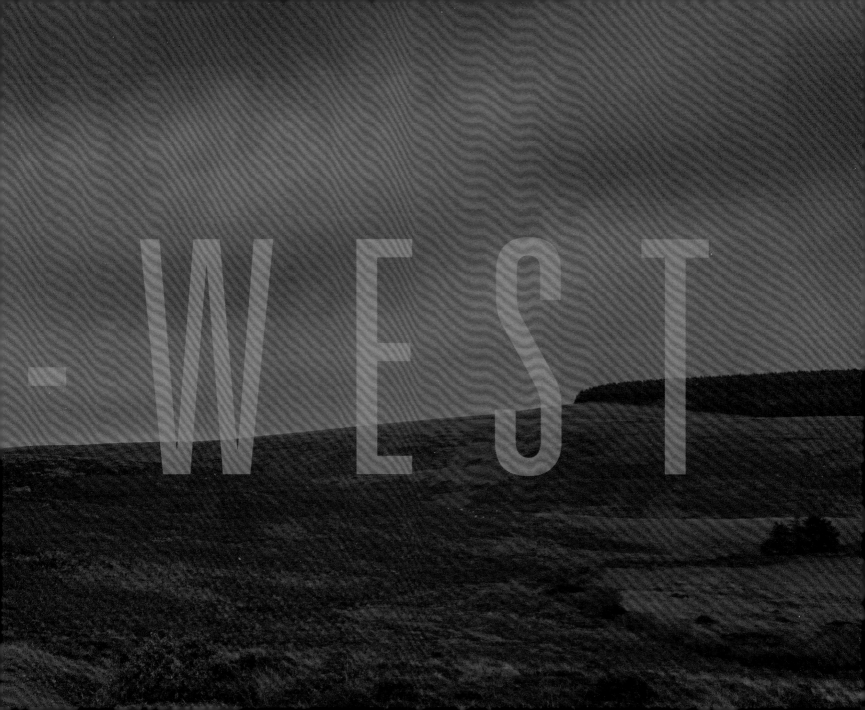

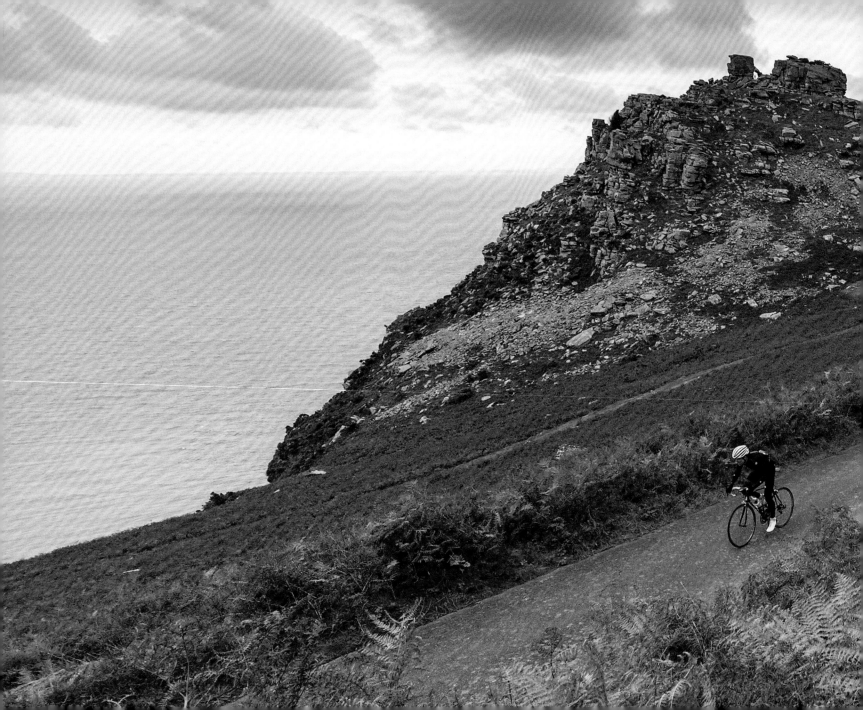

IT GETS NO TOUGHER

DISTANCE 121KM | **CLIMBING** +3,231M

PHOTOGRAPHY ANDY JONES

Relentless climbing and relentless beauty across the hills of Exmoor National Park

PREVIOUS PAGE
*Passing through the rather
extravagantly named
Valley of Rocks.*

Statistically, for every kilometre travelled divided by every metre climbed this is the toughest ride in the book. Tougher than the Lakes, tougher than the North York Moors, tougher even than North Wales. Riding and photographing it on the first day of the 2019 'off season', the morning after the National Hill Climb Championship, I had to summon up a bucketload of motivation, not to mention energy, for one last big hit out before a much-needed end-of-year break. Starting and finishing in Porlock and set entirely within the realms of Exmoor National Park, it has a profile like a bed of nails and is about as comfortable, as it climbs over 3,200 metres in just 120 kilometres!

Heading west, there are two ways out of Porlock: the A39, 'Porlock Hill', famous for snaring caravans on its 25% hairpins, or the far more pleasant Porlock Toll Road. As much as I love Porlock Hill, and even though it's one of the most notorious pieces of savage gradient in England, I've chosen the Toll Road, because no one really wants to begin a ride on a 25% slope. The younger me would have never considered taking the easy route, of course, and he would also never have considered paying the £1 toll all cyclists must cough up for the privilege of using this beautiful road. I can tell you, though, it's the best £1 you can spend on a bike. Comprised of seven perfect, snaking kilometres, all but devoid of traffic, it's a mini-Alpinesque ascent complete with hairpins that, once conquered, rewards you with simply stunning views out across the Bristol Channel.

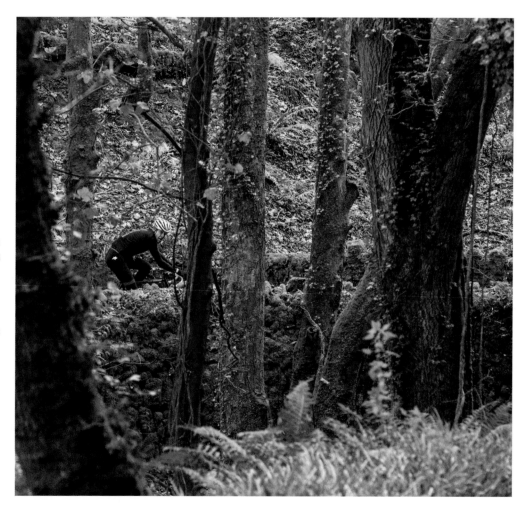

ABOVE *Winding through the
thick woods on the lower slopes
of Porlock Toll Road.*

With the summit crested it is time to enjoy the fast run to Lynmouth which, although predominantly downhill, does squeeze in a couple of short kicks up as you cross the tops of the cliffs before reaching Countisbury. Plummeting down to sea level, passing the 20% gradient sign that advises cyclists to walk (no need for that, just keep your fingers near the brakes), you fly into Lynmouth, bridge the river and hit the base of Lynmouth Hill. Coming to an immediate halt, you'll go from one end of the gear spectrum to the other in an instant, and legs that had been smashing it along at 60kph will now be reduced to grinding up the 25% incline at 10kph. Once you've made the adjustment to your new 'speed', pull yourself up away from the seafront, then turn right and continue climbing into Lynton.

Passing through the popular tourist village, which seems to have a café for each day of the year, you exit to drop back down towards the coast once more and into the Valley of Rocks. Although the dramatic name slightly oversells it – the 'valley' is only about a kilometre across, and there aren't really that many rocks – it is still a breathtaking spot to ride through. Brushing the rugged coastline and crossing the bracken-covered hillside, you roll through the hollow, then out the other side, to reach the second toll road of the day. This one, though, is free for cyclists – *bonus*!

Progressing westwards, it's time for the next of the countless inclines that populate the entire length of this route. Hugging the coast, you

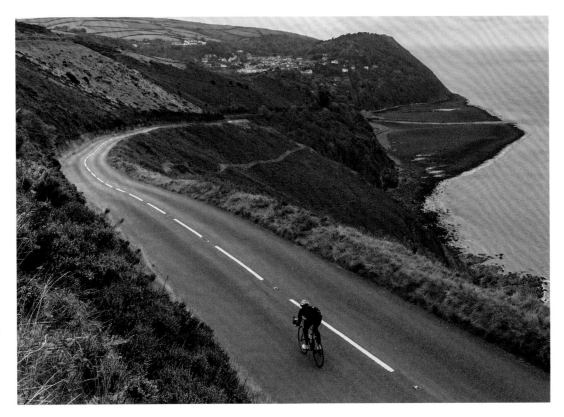

climb past Lee Bay and Woody Bay, cutting through Croscombe Wood via inclines of 20% and tight switchback bends, to emerge once more high above the sea below. You've a few minutes to admire the view again, then it's time to delve back into the hills, starting with the perilous descent of King's Lane to Hunter's Inn. Take care here on these steep, narrow and debris-strewn lanes.

A brief hiatus comes as you spend a fleeting moment on the valley floor, before taking on

one of the most beautiful climbs I know up to Trentishoe Down. Winding through the woods under an arched canopy of twisted trees you are simply enveloped in nature, the road beneath your wheels a single path of grey in an ocean of green. Every rock, branch, twig and stone is smothered with a thick layer of vibrant moss so complete and perfect it could have been plucked straight from a Hollywood fantasy. Once you've emerged from this tunnel of flora, the next treat this amazing climb serves up is

ABOVE *The descent into Lynmouth just gets faster and faster and faster.*

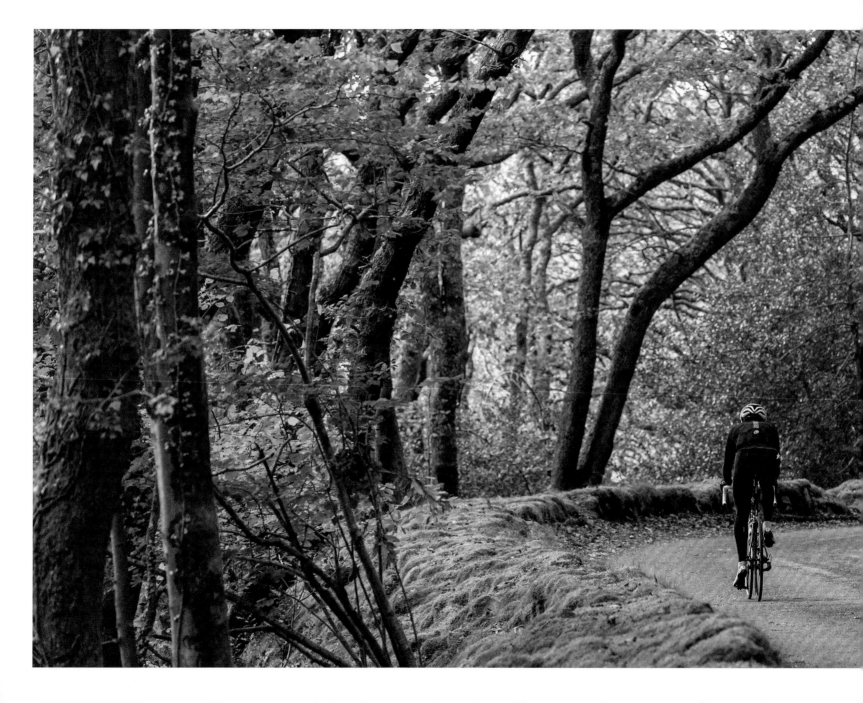

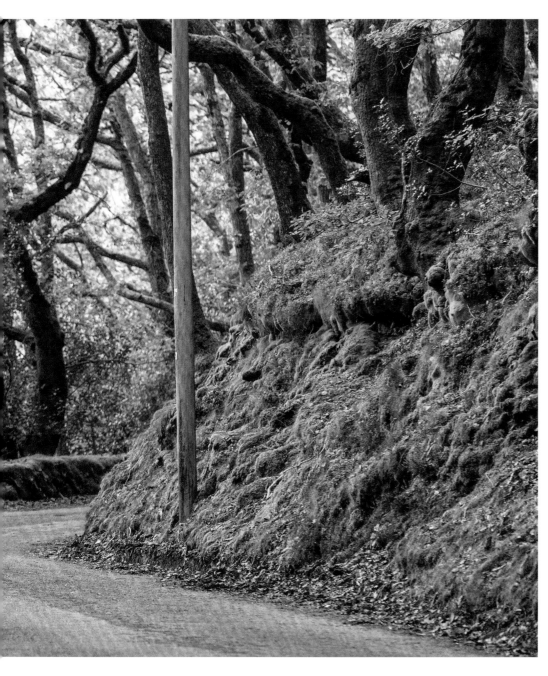

LEFT *Enveloped by nature, the climb up to Trentishoe Down.*

the view to the left over the interlocking valleys, before it arrives under huge skies at its grand finale. Keeping straight on at the junction, with the summit in sight, yet still a long way off on the horizon, you can now take in the stunning vista out over the sea below.

The climb finds its summit bisecting Trentishoe Down and Holdstone Hill, and shortly afterwards you reach the western apex of the loop and it is time to head south. First you follow the A399 along the edge of the National Park, then shortly after Blackmoor Gate you turn east through Barton Town to the southernmost point before heading north-east up Beara Hill. The previous 20 kilometres, in the context of this ride, have been pretty benign – a few sharp up-and-downs – but this period of relative rest is shattered at the base of this hill, which rises on various degrees of gradient for close to 5 kilometres.

Still heading north-east, drop down, then climb out of Simonsbath before crossing the quietest, emptiest part of Exmoor, heading due north towards Lynmouth. If it's big skies and vast open spaces you have come for, then this is what you'll find, and all set on the long gentle run-in back towards the coast. It will be close to 8 kilometres before you are required to apply any real pressure to the pedals where, leaving the B3223, you head east back into the tangled lanes.

Dropping down to the banks of the East Lyn river, trace its course through the base of the valley and, following another period of calm,

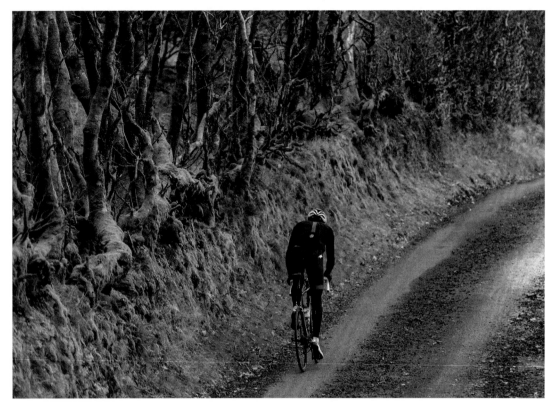

Porlock to Allerford, so the maximum gradient can be climbed by starting the ascent on Chisland Lane, but these early slopes aren't the climb proper: they are just intended to further weaken the limbs. The climb truly starts at the crossroads as you enter Horner Wood, where the road ramps up skywards.

The gradient is immediately formidable, and if there's not a point on this climb where you don't want to stop, get off the bike and cry, then you're not human. It just never relents. Once out of the trees there is a slight cessation in punishment, but each false brow offers only false salvation from the continual torture. High above the coast below, the views are naturally spectacular in all directions, as are the surrounding moors, but this may be of scant consolation. A climb like this would be great as a finale, a brutal end to a giant ride, but, alas, there are still *three more* hills to cross.

Drop down to Luckwell Bridge, head west and rise out of the valley on the B3224 to Exford. One down, two to go. Heading north from Exford you must overcome 3.5 kilometres of harsh gradient to the top of Exford Common, followed by the rapid descent to the final challenge. Crossing Pool Bridge at the apex of this perfect valley hairpin, throw whatever you have left at this vicious little incline, because once over the top, you're almost there. The final two kilometres of fast descent back to Porlock will allow you time to reflect on the highs and more highs of the day, and of course turn your attention to all the food you can now eat as a reward.

arrive in Brendon to turn right and take on Cross Lane all the way back up the valley side. A beautiful climb with a couple of nice bends, it delivers you to Easter Lane, where you turn left to drop down and cross the first of a series of three fords, all of which are perfectly rideable if you take care. If you've negotiated them safely it's time for yet another wicked ascent: the climb from Robber's Bridge back up to the A39 on Hookway Hill. Hitting a brace of seriously steep corners with your now sore legs you will most

likely see your speed drop to walking pace as just preserving traction becomes your best hope in the quest for the end. Your reward for making it is the exhilarating, lightning-fast descent into Porlock, via the aforementioned notorious 25% hairpins, back to the start point, but not the end of the ride – oh, no. *Far from it. . .*

Everything up to this point has been the warm-up. Now it's time to tackle the big one: a genuine 10/10 climb, the mighty Dunkery Beacon. I have taken the route away from

ABOVE *Keep up the pace on the relentless climbs or you too may end up covered in moss.*

RIDE 1

SOUTH-WEST

EXMOOR

DISTANCE	121KM
CLIMBING	+3,231M
DIFFICULTY	10/10

FOOD & WATER | LYNMOUTH / SIMONSBATH / PORLOCK

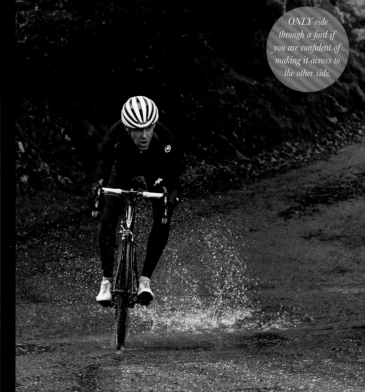

ONLY ride through a ford if you are confident of making it across to the other side.

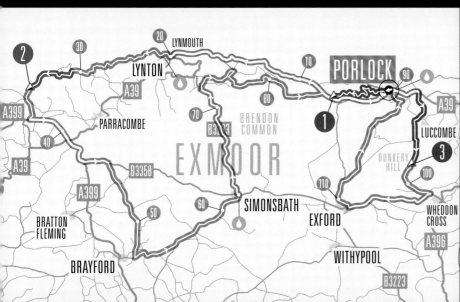

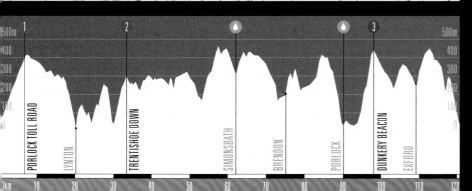

KEY CLIMBS

1 PORLOCK TOLL ROAD

6,573m +357m

A perfect ribbon of tarmac that swirls through Worthy Wood from the edge of Porlock heading for the cliff tops. Set on an almost consistent slope which peaks at 9% and averages 5% it is all but unique in Britain, just don't forget your £1 for the toll

2 TRENTISHOE DOWN

3,307m +258m

Submerged in an ocean of moss the climb up to Trentishoe Down starts by twisting through the thick woods then emerges to reveal stunning views out to sea. With a 7% average and a 16% maximum it may be beautiful but it's no walk in the park

3 DUNKERY BEACON

3,111m +319m

Averaging 10% and maxing out at 17% for almost all of the last half this climb is a bona fide 10/10 beast. The first part is sheltered in the woods then following a slight levelling at half way the push to the summit across the empty moor is relentlessly tough

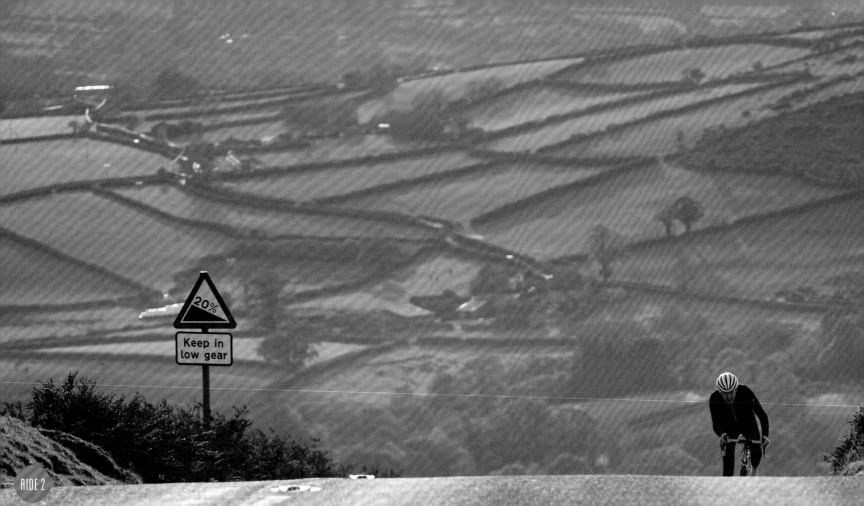

20%

Keep in
low gear

IF YOU WANT HILLS...

DISTANCE 137KM | **CLIMBING** +3,424M

PHOTOGRAPHY ANDY JONES

*Up and down all the way on Dartmoor's
vicious climbs and hidden lanes*

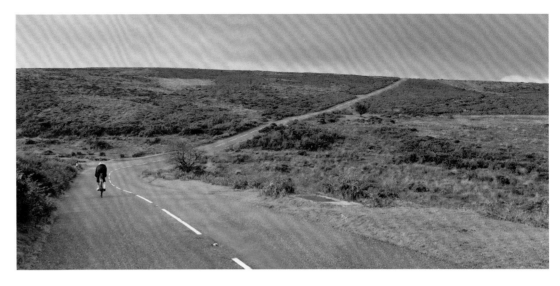

Just as the first route on Exmoor is ranked the hardest in terms of climbing per kilometre, so this ride through Dartmoor is, coincidentally, ranked the second toughest. (The rest of the book will not proceed in this fashion.) This will come as no surprise to the locals: as you will soon discover, the wonderful Dartmoor National Park is packed with climbs of every persuasion, from glorious long drags over empty moors to wicked 25% slopes, two of which have been the venues for past National Hill Climbs.

From the start in Moretonhampstead, the ride describes a giant figure of eight, set almost entirely within the boundaries of the Park and climbing close to 3,500 metres along its modest 139-kilometre length. That's the sort of altitude gain you'd expect from a ride in the Alps or Pyrenees – we are talking proper Tour de France numbers here, so I'd recommend an extra Weetabix (or two) before you hit the road.

As you head off south-west there is no easing yourself in: the climbing starts almost from the gun, as you begin to pound up the B3212 into the heart of the Park. The initial elevation gain isn't constant, as your upward progress is interrupted by a number of short descents on the 9-kilometre journey to the first significant summit of the day, in line with the top of Birch Tor. The further west you ride, the more beautiful the scenery, many of the hills topped by the granite tors for which Dartmoor is famed.

Leaving the wilderness briefly, the route passes through Postbridge on the East Dart river, then continues its relentless progress south-west to the centre of the figure of eight at the road junction in Princetown. Home to the famous Dartmoor Prison, constructed in 1806-09 to hold French prisoners during the Napoleonic Wars, this imposing granite building (now Grade II-listed) has the appearance of some sort of English Alcatraz. Isolated on the moor, seemingly impossible to escape from and, by the looks of it, home to the worst of the worst offenders, it is in fact, somewhat disappointingly, now used to house mostly low-level criminals. Still, it looks like a scary place, and I wouldn't want to be locked up in it.

Past the prison and, after close to 15 kilometres of bumbling along the undulations across the top of the moors, it's time to drop down the other side of the plateau via Walkhampton into Horrabridge. Heading north-west, follow Whitchurch Road into Whitchurch, then carry on to the centre of Tavistock to reach the 40-kilometre mark. A bit early for a stop (although there is plenty here if you fancy one), the town marks the most westerly point of the route and the base of the climb of Rundelstone which takes you all the way back to Princetown. Close to 10 kilometres long, but with a kilometre's descent in the middle, this huge climb passes through Merrivale to peak near the base of the giant radio transmitter. As a carrot to chase, this landmark will help you keep those pedals ticking over as you close in on the top. Once past it, drop down the other side and get ready for a flurry of vicious climbs that will show you the true meaning of Dartmoor.

First on the menu is my favourite, Dartmeet. Starting where the East and West Dart rivers 'meet', the B3357 loses its classification and, as it narrows, crosses the bridge then ramps directly up the hillside. Snaking through the bracken-

LEFT *Cresting the brow after climbing out of Widecombe in the Moor.*

ABOVE *Take speed to the base and the climb will be easier, in theory.*

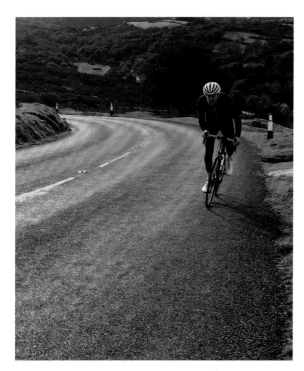

LEFT *Climbing the steep slope of Yartor Down from Dartmeet.*

covered slopes, this short rise across Yartor Down is just so perfect in length and gradient as a challenge that doesn't make the legs sting too much. Once over the top you begin the precipitous drop down through Poundsgate into the jumble of roads that fill the valleys and link the climbs to the north of Ashburton. It's easy to lose your bearings here on the narrow tree-lined lanes that rise and fall, crossing streams and rivers as they navigate the series of steep banks. Falling all the way to Hele Cross, you turn immediately left to rise once more, up past Ausewell Rocks and over into Buckland in the Moor and after that Widecombe in the Moor.

Here, at the 80-kilometre mark, is the perfect place to stop and, since Widecombe has more cafés and indeed gift shops per capita than anywhere else I have visited, you'll not struggle to find refreshment or, for that matter, a souvenir.

The only souvenirs you really need from your day, though, are sore legs and fun memories, and the next climb will make sure you have those. Venue for the 1990 National Hill Climb Championship, where Chris Boardman won the third of his five titles, Widecombe is an unrelenting ramp set on a constant double-digit gradient between 10% and 18%! In an all but arrow-straight line up the hillside that makes no attempt to lessen the impact of the slope, the 1,400-metre road rises to Top Tor to reveal just perfect views stretching out behind you. With one hallowed slope conquered, it's time to head via a short loop north through Manton to the next: the climb up to the ever-popular Haytor Rocks. Playing host to the 2019 National Championship, and also having welcomed a summit finish of the Tour of Britain, the road to the summit is a far from straightforward challenge. It packs in a multitude of gradients, rises, falls, goes on and on and then, when you emerge from the protection of trees lower down, the wind at the top can hit you like a hammer. Often busy with people on sunny weekends who don't ride bikes, this climb has a reputation of being a little congested at the top, and you'll soon see why: it's a simply magnificent place.

Over the summit, there are still five more climbs left, of varying shapes and sizes, but you have a nice long descent before you hit the first one, the easiest of those remaining, the short ramp up from Sigford into Ilsington. From here there's another, followed by a brief excursion outside the boundary of the Park to pass through the centre of Bovey Tracey, then out the other side up a crazy little road I found while researching this route. Furzeleigh Lane, or Hospital Hill as the locals call it, is just over a kilometre, set on an average gradient of 12.5%, with plenty in excess of 20%! This, the narrowest of roads framed by towering hedges, is just so Dartmoor, and so perfect, you'll want to ride it again and again. (No? OK, just me, then.)

Once over the top, there's another short spike past Tottiford Reservoir, then another smaller one into Bridford, before the plunge to the base of your final challenge. Making your way to the B3193, then turning onto the B3212, you'll find the ride ends with the perfectly pitched climb of Doccombe Hill rising up through Bridford Wood. Neither exposed moor nor vicious ramp, it's 5 kilometres of 4% gradient that will allow you to climb with efficiency and ease (if you have anything left in the tank, that is) as you flow round the contours of the valley, rising through Doccombe to close in on the finish. The end comes in the shape of a very welcome descent, followed by an equally unwelcome kick up into the centre of Moretonhampstead, to round off a truly challenging day across the South-West's finest hills.

RIDE 2 SOUTH-WEST

DARTMOOR

DISTANCE	137KM
CLIMBING	+3,424M
DIFFICULTY	10/10

FOOD & WATER | TAVISTOCK / WIDECOMBE / BOVEY TRACEY

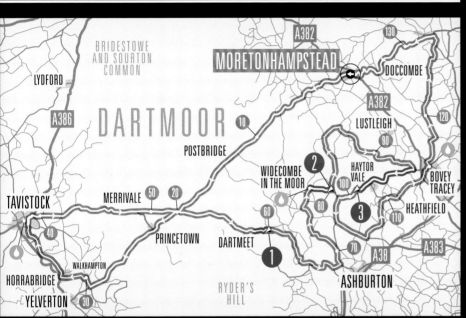

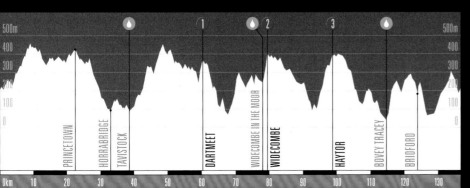

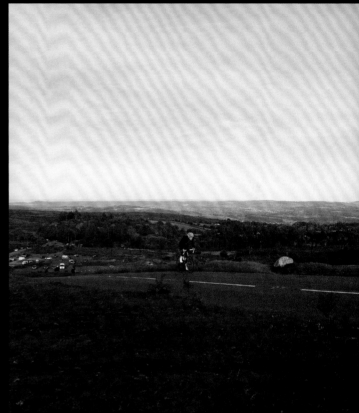

KEY CLIMBS

1 DARTMEET
1,072m +123m

With an average gradient of 11% you just know this climb is going to pack a punch at some point or another and in this case it's right at the base. As soon as you cross the East Dart river you hit the 20% slopes which although short put you on the back foot for the rest of the ascent.

2 WIDECOMBE
1,381m +159m

With only slight deviations in its course to the summit Widecombe is a mind killer as well as a leg killer as every time you look up you see how far you still have to climb. Set on a 12% average with spikes around the 16% mark, just focus on the ground before your front wheel and grind it out.

3 HAYTOR
5,378m +339m

At over 5 kilometres long and with a multitude of varying gradients the climb to Haytor Rocks is notoriously difficult to pace. At its steepest it reaches 12% and for a significant stretch it's flat so knowing where to apply the gas and when to hold back in order to set a good time takes a lot of practice.

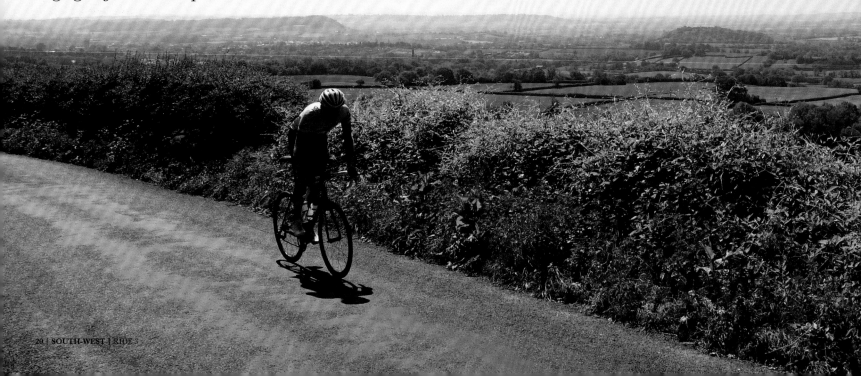

SOUTHERN DISCOMFORT

DISTANCE 104KM | **CLIMBING** +1,683M

PHOTOGRAPHY ANDY JONES

Linking the climbs and gorges of the Mendips

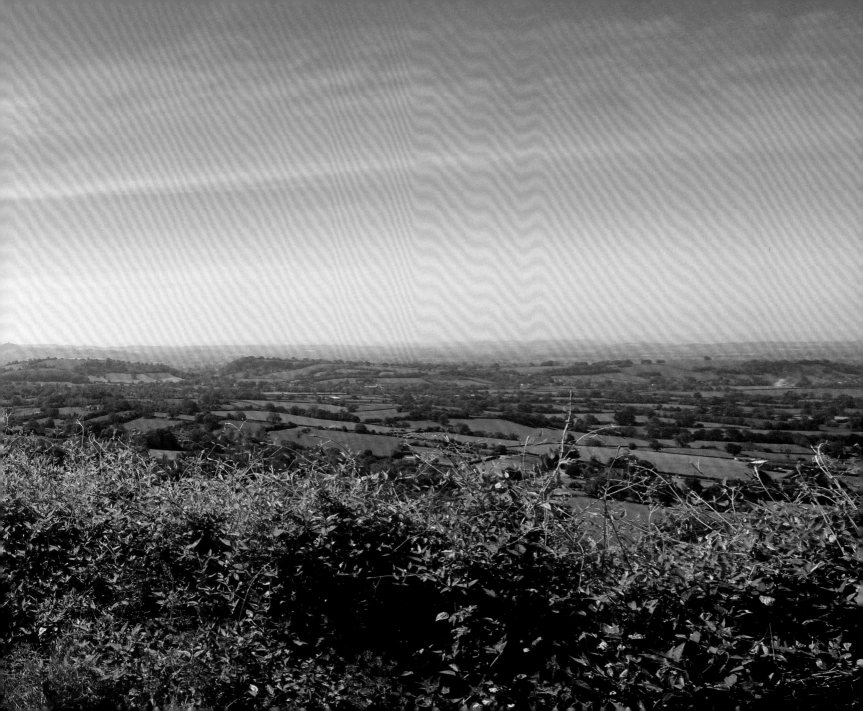

RIGHT *Heading into the
jaws of the Canyon, dwarfed by
its towering spires.*

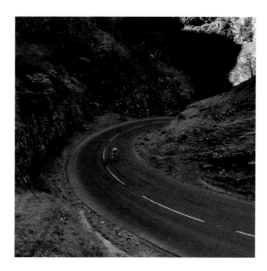

Unless you've been living on Mars I assume you are all aware of the Cheddar Gorge. It's pretty much Britain's answer to the Grand Canyon (albeit on a comparatively microscopic scale), and the star attraction in the Mendip Hills. Running west-to-east between Weston-super-Mare and Frome, this limestone ridge sits high above the Somerset Levels and the Chew Valley, an elevated plateau punctuated with caves and gorges. An attraction for cavers, walkers and pretty much anyone with a love for the outdoors, they are also a great place to ride your bike. And if you're looking for a ride that ticks off just about every climb, and squeezes every last drop of beauty out of this quiet corner of the island, look no further.

The start and finish lie in Cheddar, at the base of the famous gorge, but I leave that climb for later, to build the anticipation. To begin with, the ride heads south for ten absolutely pan-flat kilometres on the lowlands, leaving Cheddar on Station Road to link up with the B3151. Travelling through Hythe you cross the Levels, then turn back east via Cocklake, round the base of Nyland Hill (which, out of interest, is the 19,346th-highest peak in the British Isles), and up to the A371 at Draycott. Warm-up over, it's time to start climbing, and first up is the toughest climb of the day, the aptly named Draycott Steep.

Turn right on the A371, then, in the village, take the second left onto New Road, to immediately head upwards. Gaining the same altitude as Cheddar Gorge, but in half the

distance, tells you all you need to know about this fearsome road. Averaging 11% over its 2-kilometre length, this hill does not muck about, especially on the 20% slopes at around half way. Meeting up with the B3135, you follow this east to the B3134, where you turn left. At the next split, take the Old Bristol Road down into West Harptree and, after 10 kilometres crossing the high plateau, you will now be back almost at sea level once more, to join the A368 heading to the Chew Valley Lake.

Although you are never far from the water's edge, views out over the reservoir are all but permanently obscured by hedgerows and trees as you ride into Bishop Sutton. Turn left as you exit the village, heading on to Bonhill Road, then Walley Lane. You follow this all the way into Chew Stoke where, just before you reach the village, you get the sight out over the water you have until then been denied. It's well worth the wait. Cross the dam wall and pause to soak in the tranquillity

before getting stuck into some more hills.

At the T-junction in Chew Stoke turn right. Being a little cheeky, I've thrown in a climb just to liven the legs up before you return to bigger ascents further south. Heading north on the B3114, reach the B3130 and turn right into Chew Magna. Then, from the centre of the village, head north to tackle Chew Hill which, with 1.2 kilometres at an average gradient of 7%, will get you back in the mood for climbing. As soon as you reach the top you take the first left, back down Limeburn Hill, to cross the B3130, then instantly ramp up again.

Now you head south on Pagans Hill and, before entering Chew Stoke again, turn right, to keep rising gently for a further 5 kilometres, heading due west. As you thread your way through the tiny lanes trapped between high hedgerows, you are looking for the turn to Butcombe, to head due south in the direction of Blagdon Lake. Crossing your second dam wall of the day, this one even more spectacular and worthy of a pause, you are now almost in place to begin the next big climb, Burrington Combe.

After passing over the dam wall, continue to Blagdon, and then turn right onto the A368. After just a few metres take the right turn onto Bourne Lane, to then re-join the A368 for a short while, before taking the second left into Burrington Combe. Often overlooked due to its proximity to its more dramatic neighbour in Cheddar, Burrington Combe is still plenty dramatic, and in many other parts of the country would get top billing.

ABOVE *Roads don't come
much more spectacular in
Britain than Cheddar Gorge.*

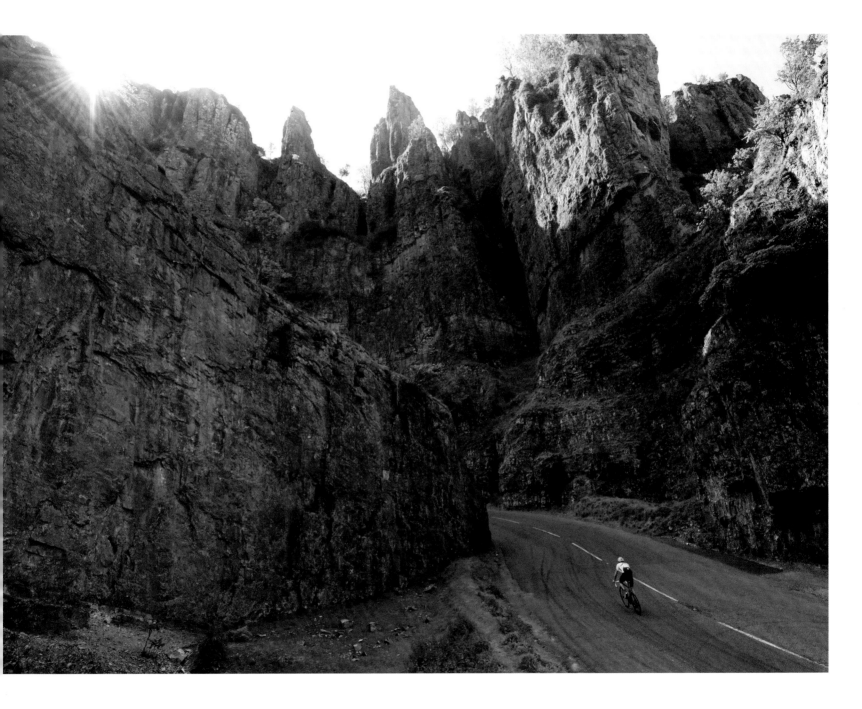

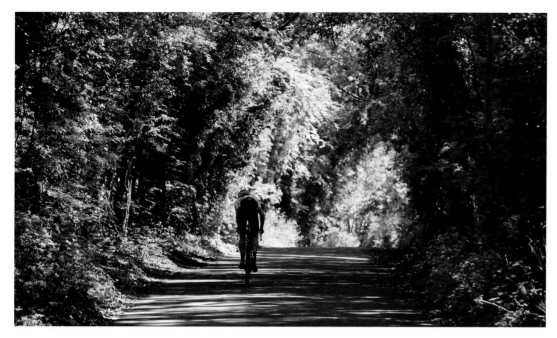

The climb doesn't start right away: you've a few minutes to gather yourself. Then, once you cross a cattle grid, the slope tilts up. The modestly pitched incline winds through the gully, at first framed by towering rocks, then, as the height of the gorge walls diminishes, by tall trees. At 4 kilometres this is a proper climb and, even though it only has a maximum gradient of 10%, is not to be misjudged.

With the warm-up act ticked off, it's time for the main event. Turn off the B3134 to Charterhouse, then follow the road west along the tops to meet the summit of Cuck Hill, where it's time to descend into Cheddar. As soon as you meet the A371, take the first left at the roundabout onto Axbridge Road into the heart of town, and you'll arrive at the base.

Packed with garish gift shops and cafés, over-run with tourists pouring off coaches like rats leaving sinking ships, the base of Cheddar Gorge is a carbuncle of tat and consumerism (too harsh?) but, once past the large coach parks, everything changes. Dwarfed by the giant limestone cliffs either side, the slopes hit their toughest gradients, approaching 16%. Snaking through a series of tight bends in the shadows of the surrounding slabs of rock, the first kilometre is a struggle, then the climb begins to get easier and easier. The further you ride, the faster you will climb, clicking up the gears as the gorge walls recede. Cheddar Gorge is a unique British road that never ever disappoints.

Once you've completed its 4 kilometres of

ascent there's just one more climb left to finish the ride. Just to squeeze that little bit more out of the area, I had to cram in one more, so, once on the level at the top, carry on all the way to the B3134, then turn right to drop down Old Bristol Road all the way into Wells. As you hit the A39 turn right, then right again, onto the A371, then head right off this onto Titlands Lane towards Wookey Hole (no, not Wookie), home to the famous caves.

The last climb up through Ebbor Gorge boasts arguably the best views of the day, as the steep and narrow road heading west out of Wookey Hole rapidly gains altitude. Casting your eyes left, you'll see forever over the Somerset Levels, which will partially distract you from the severity of the gradient. Averaging 8% over its 2.5 kilometres, this climb is no pushover, and will punish tired legs as they seek out the summit. Bending right and turning your back on the huge vista, you pass the Deerleap Standing Stones and continue all the way to the village of Priddy, which you cut through to meet the B3135.

Now, it would be a shame to visit the Mendips and only see Cheddar Gorge from the one perspective, so the route, sticking to the B3135, allows you to enjoy the thrilling descent through its luscious curves back to the finish point. With the gorge sides this time increasing in height, and the pitch of the slope too, the final kilometre is both adrenaline rush and geological spectacle, that delivers you back into the clutches of the town, where you'll certainly have no trouble finding a café.

ABOVE *Grinding up the slopes of Draycott Steep, which are, you guessed it, very steep.*

RIDE 3

SOUTH-WEST

MENDIPS

DISTANCE 104KM

CLIMBING +1,683M

DIFFICULTY 3/10

FOOD & WATER | BLAGDON / WELLS / CHEDDAR

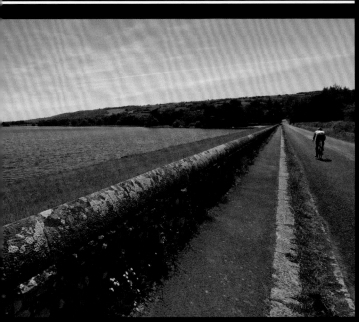

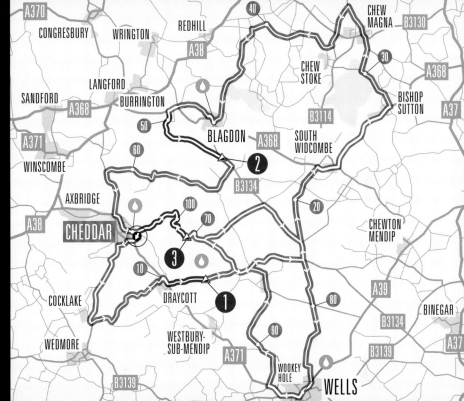

KEY CLIMBS

1 DRAYCOTT STEEP

1,930m +214m

With an 11% average this climb is a real beauty that will hit the legs hard at the start of the ride. Ramping up out of Draycott it wastes little time before arriving at its harsh 20% middle section which will need some grunt to get through before the easier final stretch to the summit.

2 BURRINGTON COMBE

4,100m +193m

At its steepest the gradient on this climb reaches 10% and across its distance it averages just over 4% but that isn't to say it's all easy going. There are sections which require a sustained effort but it's an effort that can be done in the saddle at a nice even pace.

3 CHEDDAR GORGE

3,540m +150m

The toughest slopes on this climb come just after the start where it ramps up to 16%. Once you round the initial tight steep bends it gets easier and easier until you can click into the big ring and cross the top like you are heading for the finish line on the Champs-Élysées

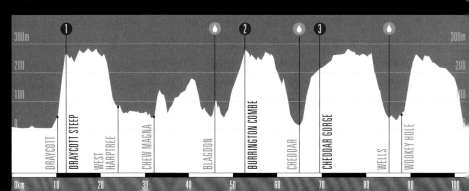

I HAVE A BAD FEELING ABOUT THIS

DISTANCE 168KM | **CLIMBING** +3,347M

PHOTOGRAPHY ANDY JONES

A brutal, but oh so beautiful route through the Cotswolds

LEFT *The long steady slopes of Forcester Hill where the views getter better the higher you climb.*

Ah, the beautiful Cotswolds: a magnet for tourists from around the globe, all coming to see the classic vision of sleepy England. Villages and towns untouched by the ravages of time and technology, immaculate stone buildings, manicured gardens and the picture-perfect rolling countryside. Underneath this façade, though, behind the chocolate-box image of serenity that fills the travel brochures lie hidden horrors. Like the subtext of a David Lynch movie, if you scratch away the beautiful surface you'll find the Cotswolds are home to countless savage hills. This is the Cotswolds we cyclists want. This is what we have come for: not the faux veneer but the torturous underbelly. One look at the profile is enough to turn you white with fear – it has more spikes than an upturned rake. But fear not: they are all small spikes – it's just that some are brutally steep.

The base for the day is Winchcombe and, to kick things off, the route travels north out of town on the B4632 for 3 gentle kilometres where you can get comfy on your saddle before the climbing begins. Taking the first right turn south towards Hailes, you hit the slopes of Salter's Hill, which take you to the high point of the day's ride. This climb ramps up pretty steeply towards the end, after you've traversed its exposed middle section – in fact, the geography of this climb is quite unique, as all other hills on the route are far more sheltered.

Once over the summit, turn left, then immediately right, to head due south on the

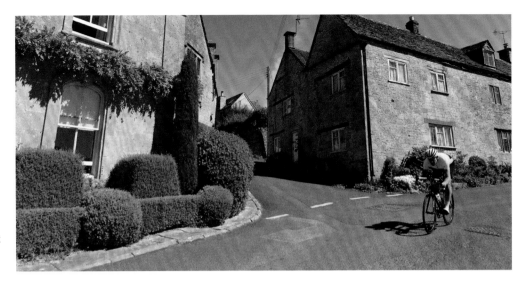

Salt Way, which follows the path of an ancient track that was used to transport – yes, you guessed it, salt – from the mines in Cheshire to the head of the River Thames. Taking a right turn before the village of Hawling, ride through Brockhampton, Sevenhampton and Whittington to descend down Ham Road all the way into Cheltenham. Entering the outskirts of the town on Ryeworth Road, cross the A40 and A435 and keep heading south-west until you eventually hit the A46. By now you'll be begging for another climb and, after a slight foray on the A46 around the roundabout at the A417 (take care here), and then coming up to the next junction, you'll find one.

Turning left on the Ermin Way, you're about to be treated to the delights of Birdlip Hill. Famous for its inclusion of the now-defunct Tour of the Cotswolds bike race, this is a feisty road that ramps up the ridge through the woods, getting harder and harder until it peaks in the village of Birdlip. With legs on fire and eyes blurred, make sure you take the first right turn, after which you can recover for a while. Roll along the B4070 for a short distance, then take the right onto Buckholt Road to join the A46 once more to the village of Paradise. Via the B4073 and Sevenleaze Lane ride through Edge and then Harescombe into Haresfield for climb three of the day, Haresfield Beacon.

Very similar in character to Birdlip Hill, but a little more direct in its course to the summit, it also hides a wicked section of 20% towards the top, so be warned. Once over the brow you rocket down the other side through Randwick, skirting the edge of Stroud, to cross the A419 towards King's Stanley and Leonard Stanley. The next climb is one of my favourites – indeed, when my good friend Nick Burton got to the top, he proclaimed that it was 'the perfect hill'. The views are delightful (this is the Cotswolds), and the gradient is pitched right on that sweet spot between shallow to the point of being too easy and not steep enough to be too hard. It flows between the hedgerows through sweeping corners, and there is a bit of a ramp towards the top, before it ends at the junction with the B4066. Not all gradients in the Cotswolds are so accommodating, so savour this climb as you ascend the B4066 road towards Uley, then take the left turn to Owlpen.

For the next 50 kilometres the climbs come thick and fast with relentless regularity, each one appearing like a needle on the profile: straight up, then straight down, over and over again. First of this barrage of 'fun' is Owlpen Hill. Maxing out at 25%, it will really burn. At the top turn right, fall down Lampern Hill back to the B4066, then head west all the way into Dursley. At 77 kilometres I'd say this would be a good spot for a break, before you rise rapidly from the small town onto the 20% slopes of The Broadway.

This gem of a climb, trapped in the woods, rises above the gully below, snaking skywards on a punishing slope, yet it's just short enough not to do any real damage. At the top take the hard left to keep rising for a while, before heading south to North Nibley and then, via a series of smaller spikes in gradient, on the B4060 to Wotton-under-Edge. Once you've passed through the town it's time for serious climb number (I am already losing count) seven, Hillmill Lane.

This quiet, narrow road has an abrupt

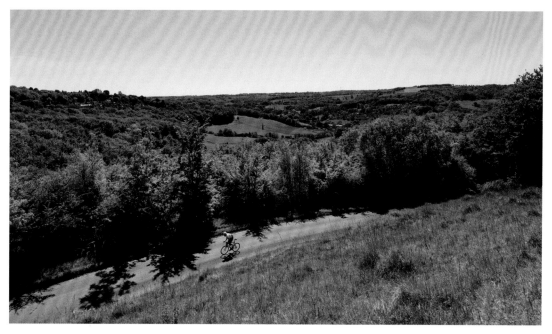

follow the River Frome on the A419, before turning off to Chalford to the base of climb 12, Oakridge Lynch. Boasting yet more double-digit gradient, this ramp rises into the village, through it, and then continues to rise all the way to Bisley.

Now here is where you are allowed a rest. I know, I've gone soft, but take time to relax as you roll along the tops, in and out of the beautiful villages, past the meandering tourists, along Calf Way to meet the B4070. Leaving it shortly afterwards, turn right, to make your way through Brimpsfield and Cowley, all the way down Leckhampton Road and into Cheltenham.

By now you may be starting to feel uneasy at the lack of hills. As in a scary movie when it's been far too quiet for far too long, you just know something is going to jump out of the shadows, and you're right. Something certainly is, and I've saved the best for last (evil laugh), *ha ha ha. . .*

Navigating through Cheltenham, make your way to Prestbury, turn off the B4632 and into Woodmancote. Just 6 kilometres from home now, and you can see the finish, you can taste the cake – but in front of you lies the brutal Bushcombe Lane. A true 10/10, complete with a 30% left-hand corner towards the top, Bushcombe Lane is the toughest climb in the Cotswolds and, if you get over this without dismounting, you've done bloody well. Curse me all you like at the top, and you will, but I can take it – hell, I deserve it – then relish the fast run into Winchcombe, where you can then ponder selling your bike on eBay, because you never want to ride it again.

90-degree corner at about two-thirds distance, and a seriously stiff finale through the bends to Park Lane, where you turn left and drop right away back down into Wotton-under-Edge. Ride all the way to the B4058, then, turning right, follow that road through the sweeping bends of Coombe Hill to the Old London Road, where you head left before dropping down through Laycombe Ditch Wood to Watery Bottom.

Up next is a killer: Breakheart Hill (don't you just love the name?), which is a short ramp with a 20% finale through its hairpin that leads you back into Dursley, where you'll be tempted, I'm sure, to stop for a second time. Head north from the town, and the next climb on the horizon is the not-so-comfortable way up Frocester Hill,

and its evil twin Lever's Hill. The views are just as good – no, I'd say better: it's just that, instead of sedate 7% slopes, you're treated to something approaching 15%, as it gains the same altitude over far less of a distance.

Joining Frocester Hill just as it gets steep, you continue to the B4066, where this time you head left. Ride all the way to North Woodchester, crossing the A46, and it's time for another of my favourites, Bear Hill. All twists and turns, this fabulous road kicks up out of the valley, flanked by beautiful grassy banks, into the woods at the top. Once crossed, it leaves you with only three hills left. (You'll not know whether to cry with joy or sadness.)

Descend Butterrow Hill, then, turning right,

ABOVE *The top of Bear Hill offers an excellent vantage point to survey the rolling hills.*

RIDE 4 SOUTH-WEST

COTSWOLDS

DISTANCE	168KM
CLIMBING	+3,347M
DIFFICULTY	10/10

FOOD & WATER | STROUD / DURSLEY

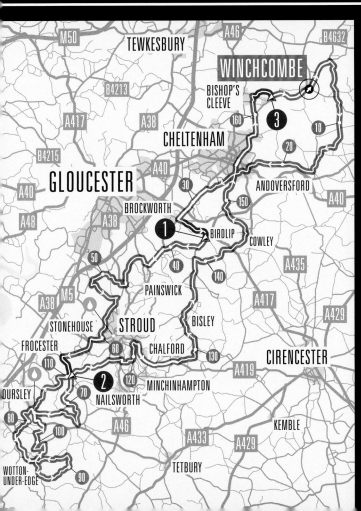

KEY CLIMBS

1 BIRDLIP HILL
2,910m +219m

Following a gentle start the first half of this climb settles into a 10% gradient with great views out over your right shoulder. When it bends into the woods though, here the real fun starts as the slope increases to 15% all the way to the top. The

2 FROCESTER HILL
3,100m +203m

A wonderful road to climb set on a sublime pitch that although steep in places is never unpleasant. The

average is 6.5% for the whole climb and it's only really right at the end that you'll have to dig deep.

3 BUSHCOMBE LANE
1,540m +167m

A monster. Leaving Woodmancote you pass not one but two 25% warning signs, just to make double sure you know what lies ahead. As the road rises it gets harder and harder until, peaking at far beyond the advertised 25%, it climbs round its final corner then eases to the summit.

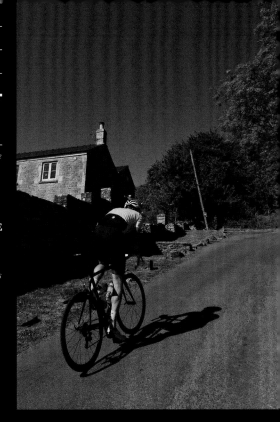

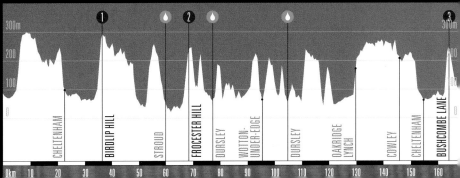

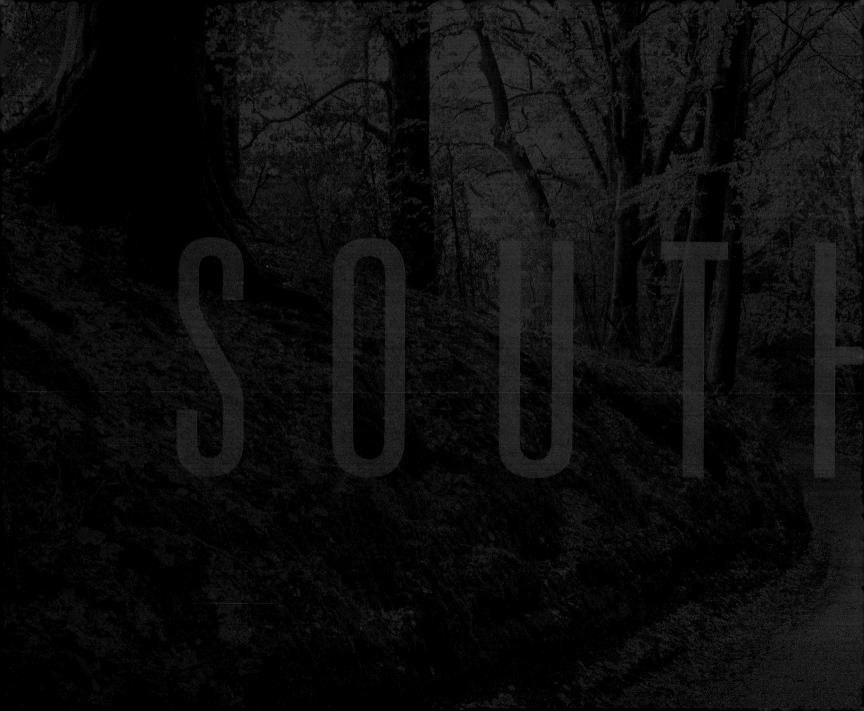

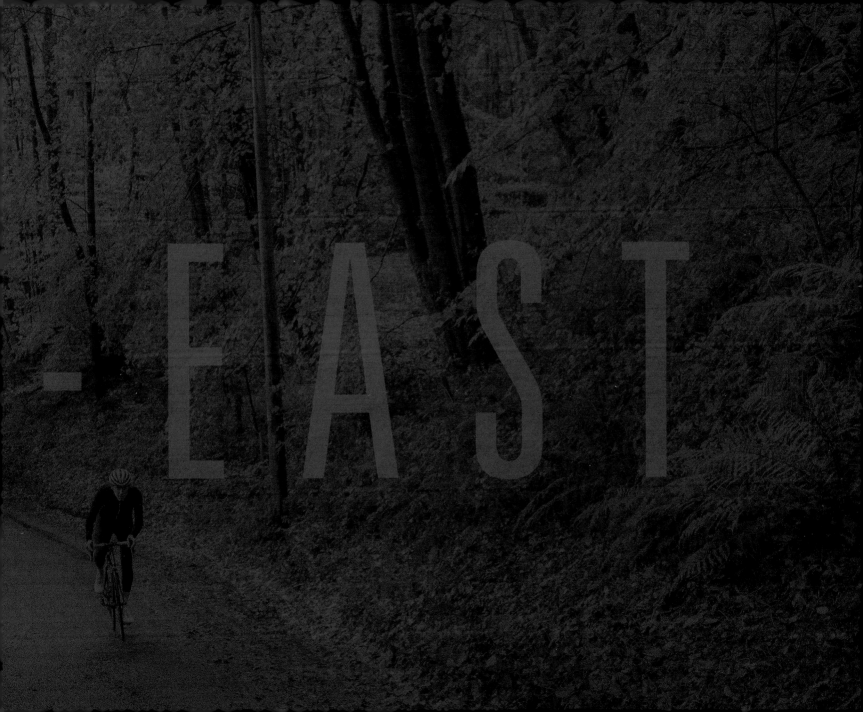

EAST

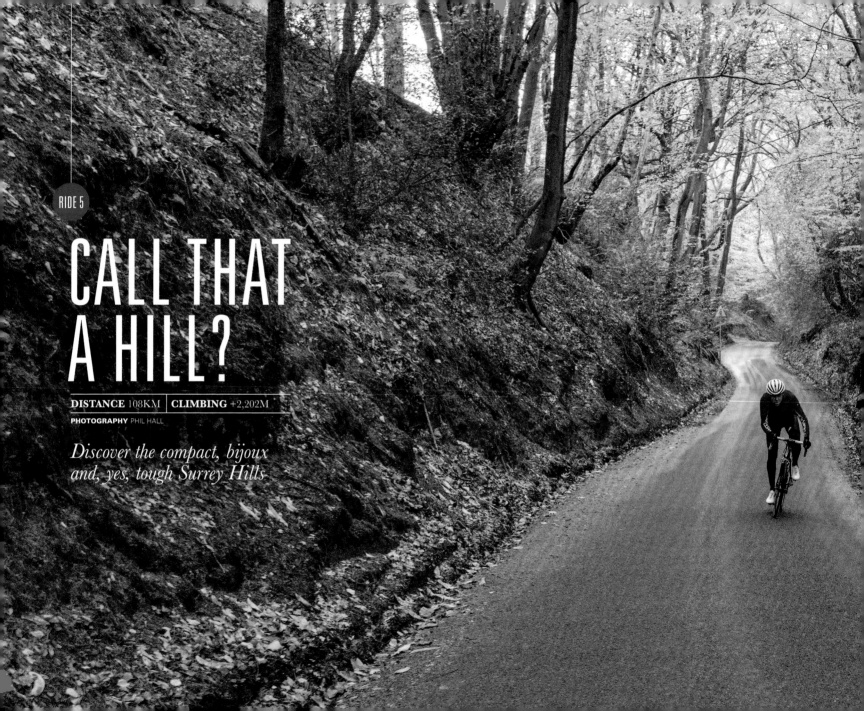

RIDE 5

CALL THAT A HILL?

DISTANCE 108KM | **CLIMBING** +2,202M

PHOTOGRAPHY PHIL HALL

Discover the compact, bijoux and, yes, tough Surrey Hills

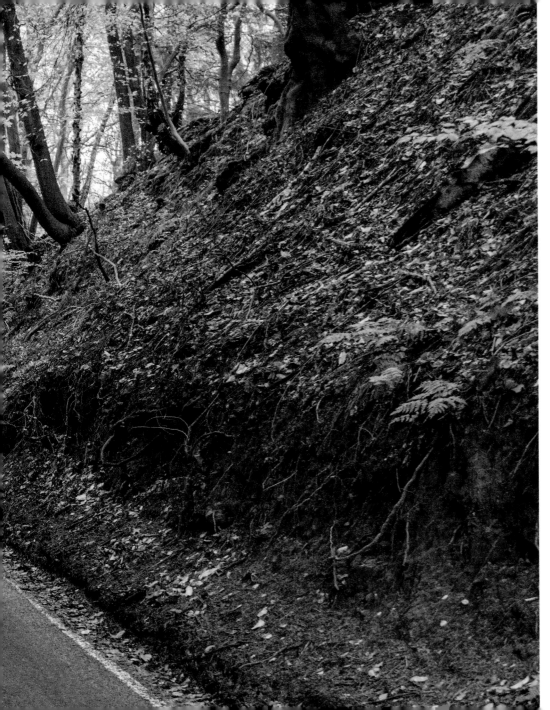

LEFT *Climbing through the deep trench of Coldharbour Lane.*

I spent longer deciding the make-up of this route than any other in the book. To get it just right I had to include all my favourite climbs, ridden in their 'correct' orientation. I also wanted to preserve some sort of order, a degree of logic, in the route, to try and prevent those who follow it from getting desperately lost in the tangle of roads that populate the treasured Surrey Hills. These diminutive yet numerous climbs are a playground for cyclists of all persuasions, no matter what the width of their tyres is or how tightly their clothes fit. On any day you'll see every type of rider and machine, on-road, off-road, clean and covered in mud, all here to escape the metropolis and get their kicks on the myriad of lanes and tracks. Taking my inspiration from events such as the CTC Hilly 50, the Tour of the Surrey Hills Audax and the Leith Hill Octopus, not to mention the countless hours I spent pounding these roads while I lived in London, this is my homage to this designated Area of Outstanding Natural Beauty (AONB). I hope you enjoy it.

The ride starts in the centre of Dorking, which has plenty of cafés, restaurants and bike shops, so all your needs are catered for before you leave town heading south on Coldharbour Lane. There's little chance for a warm-up, because as soon as you turn off South Street to cross Falkland Street you are heading uphill. This is just a bump, though, a prelude to the first big climb, which lies a few hundred metres the other side. Coldharbour Lane, or Boar Lane as it is also known, is a thug

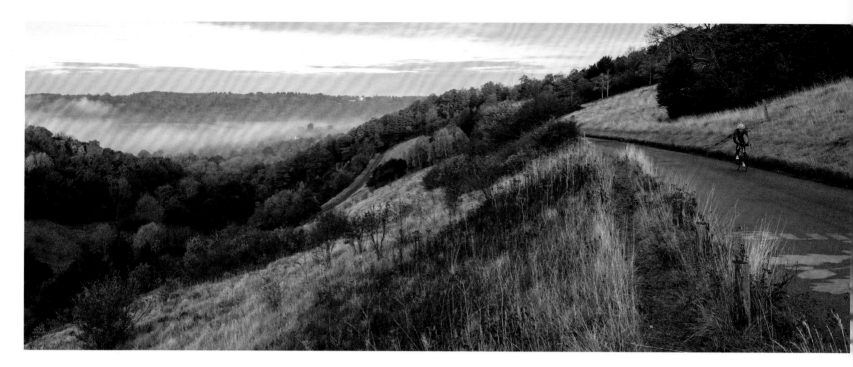

of a road, and if you ever find yourself trying to hold the wheel of a stronger companion in front it will have your legs beaten black and blue by the time you reach the top.

The climbing comes in waves of intense bursts with tiny patches of respite between them and, as you reach deeper into the forest, the sides of the road rise up to form a twisting canyon with you stranded at its base. Even on the brightest sunny day it's dark in these mini-ravines, with all light blocked by the towering canopy overhead and the trenches of mud either side. Rising all the way into Coldharbour, across three false summits, the slope does get progressively easier the higher it climbs. Before entering the sylvan

village, take the first left to exit the forest by descending the tight bends of Anstie Lane. Dropping to meet the A29 you turn right, continue to Ellen's Green, then turn right again and make your way to the notorious Leith Hill.

Arguably the secondmost 'famous' climb on the route (after Box Hill), it features on the Ride London race and sportive route, and has also been immortalised on the online riding platform Zwift. Many years ago, before it was famous, I rode a couple of very minor races that climaxed at the top, which gave us amateurs a taste of a punishing hilltop finish. The course was composed of five laps on the flatlands below, then a final lap that reared up for a summit

finale at Surrey's highest point. Those five laps were essentially nothing but biding time, waiting to pounce, because it was all about the finish. As our ramshackle peloton approached the base of the hill we all, in true pro style, jettisoned our water bottles into the hedgerows to save weight for the climb.

Thing is, once the race was over, unlike the pros on TV we then went back into the bushes, getting stung by nettles, our Lycra torn by brambles, to retrieve them, because we couldn't afford to be throwing bottles away every week! Leith is a tough climb: starts steady, ramps up hard, eases a bit and then, when you see the tall brick wall on the left, kicks up once more. Entering the trees, you arrive

ABOVE *You've got to get out early to find the curves of Box Hill as quiet as this.*

at a junction of roads which you will hope is the summit, but oh no, and it's always the next part that hurts the most.

With two big climbs ticked off, it's time to make your way to the toughest of the lot, hopefully without getting lost, as I have plenty of times around here. On your way down the other side, pay attention so you take the turn onto Pasture Wood Road once you've descended Leith Hill Road. Follow this onto Holmbury Hill Road, round the foot of the hill, then all the way to meet Ewhurst Road in Peaslake. There's a shop and café here if you feel like a stop, but with only 25km covered you're more than likely to press on, heading south to Ewhurst, then west to Cranleigh and the foot of the big one: Barhatch Lane.

In my opinion this is the hardest climb in the South-East, and one of the very few to have anything near a 20% gradient. Barhatch Lane hits you hard, and keeps hitting you harder and harder all the way to the top, where you descend straight away to Hound House Lane, then turn left to the beautiful village of Shere. Carefully cross the A25 and line up to climb Combe Lane. Not as tough as some others, but with a wonderful 90-degree bend towards the top, Combe Lane climbs up the ridge and marks the start of your journey back east, and your date with the one and only Box Hill.

Crossing Ranmore Common and dropping down to the A24 via Westhumble, you start to climb what may be the most famous hill in England. Passing Rykers Café, there is a short ascent on Old London Road, then you turn right

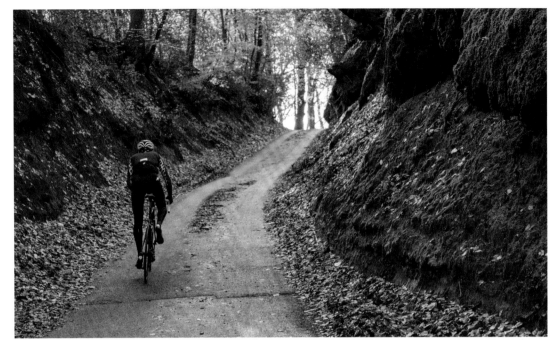

onto the perfectly named Zig Zag Road, and it's here you begin your real effort – if you plan to log a serious time to post on social media, that is. This is one of the most popular roads in the world, and also the one that derives the most jeers and laughs from those up north, who scoff at its credentials. No, it's not Hardknott Pass or Rosedale Chimney but, as I always say, any hill ridden hard has the ability to hurt and, with its wonderful hairpins set in the beautiful hillside, Box Hill is not only stunning to look at, but it can also certainly hurt.

Once at the top (if you are planning a KOM* attempt you must ride past the café first), you reach the halfway point of the ride, so this is the perfect

place for a break – but be warned: on a warm Sunday morning this café is as busy as Oxford Street on the last weekend before Christmas. Great if you like looking at other people's expensive bikes, but terrible for getting served.

Pressing on, you could drop back down the hill, but I prefer to keep the flow of the ride in one direction where possible, so head into Box Hill village, turn left on Headley Common Road, then left again on Lodge Bottom Road to loop back round to Rykers. Cross the A25 once more and head to the base of Ranmore Common. Another climb used by Ride London, and the venue for my club Norwood Paragon's annual hill climb, Ranmore is no killer, but watch

ABOVE *Have the roads sunk or the banks risen? The deep gully of Sheephouse Lane.*

* The KOM (King of the Mountain) is given to the rider with the fastest time up a hill.

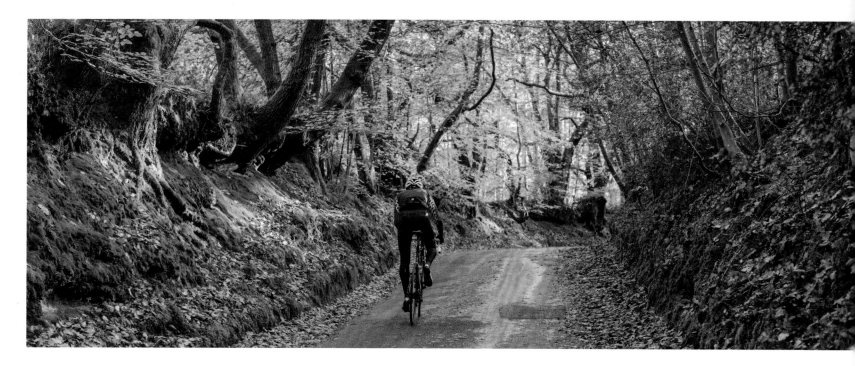

yourself on the final 90-degree bend: this will bite if you're not in the right gear.

Heading back once more into the Surrey Hills instead of routeing through Dorking, turn right at the top of Ranmore, then after undulating across the ridge turn left to next climb the easier side of White Downs Hill (more on this later). After the fast descent take the A25 east to the base of my favourite of Surrey's little ramps, Sheephouse Lane. Like a mini version of Coldharbour Lane which started the ride, this is a perfect little road, reaching 20% at the top where its asphalt, enclosed within another of the Surrey Hills' typical dirt trenches, really stings the legs.

There are now just two big climbs left: Tanhurst Lane and the one all the locals hate, the dreaded White Downs. Turn onto Leith Hill Road to descend the side of the hill you bagged earlier, head right at the bottom, then right and right again to start the first, Tanhurst Lane. Very narrow and often covered in debris from the trees above, this twisting road brings you via 16% slopes back to the junction on Leith Hill, where you turn left. Keep climbing, then drop all the way down through Abinger to the A25 and gather yourself. All local killer rides, from club runs to sportives and Audaxes, seem cruelly to feature this climb towards their finish. It has laid waste to more egos, broken more legs and severed more friendships than any other road south of London. It's not simply sadistic organisers wishing suffering on riders' legs, more that, as the only passage north between Shere and Dorking, it is just convenient, and avoids sending people down the A25, which would be even worse.

Even the knowledge that this is the last hurdle before home never seems to help, as its ever-steepening slope chews riders up and spits them out as they empty their legs in an effort to get one up on their mates. You will beat it eventually, though, and once you roll over the summit all that is left to do is head back along Ranmore Common once more and drop down into Dorking, to complete one hell of a ride through the small but perfectly formed Surrey Hills.

ABOVE *It's easy to get lost in the maze of roads that criss-crosses the Surrey Hills.*

RIDE 5

SOUTH-EAST

SURREY HILLS

DISTANCE 108KM

CLIMBING +2,202M

DIFFICULTY 6/10

FOOD & WATER | PEASLAKE / SHERE / BOX HILL

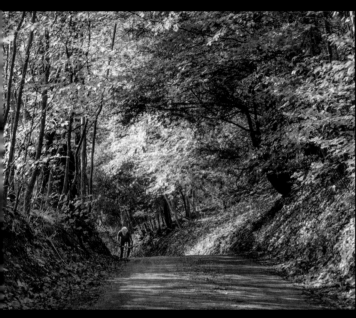

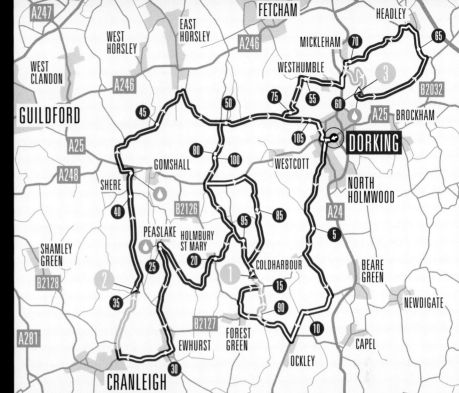

KEY CLIMBS

1 LEITH HILL

2,004m +140m

Leith Hill hits you with multiple tough ramps, each separated by a brief lull to allow you a recovery. With 7% average and 16% maximum it's no killer but the 2-kilometre length means you must measure your effort out if you are to arrive at the top in

2 BARHATCH LANE

2,448m +154m

In my opinion the toughest climb in the South-East and one of the very few roads in the area to boast a 20% plus gradient. Although pretty hard all the way up the steepest slopes which reach 23% are saved for the very end, just to make sure your legs are tired when you reach them.

3 BOX HILL

2,496m +133m

Compared to many on the route Box Hill is a pussy cat, but that means you just have to ride it faster. Everyone has a 'PB' on this climb so if you are feeling frisky and the wind is coming from the north-west then why not empty your bottles and give it a proper go.

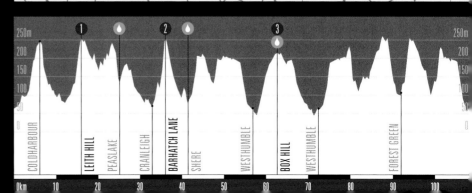

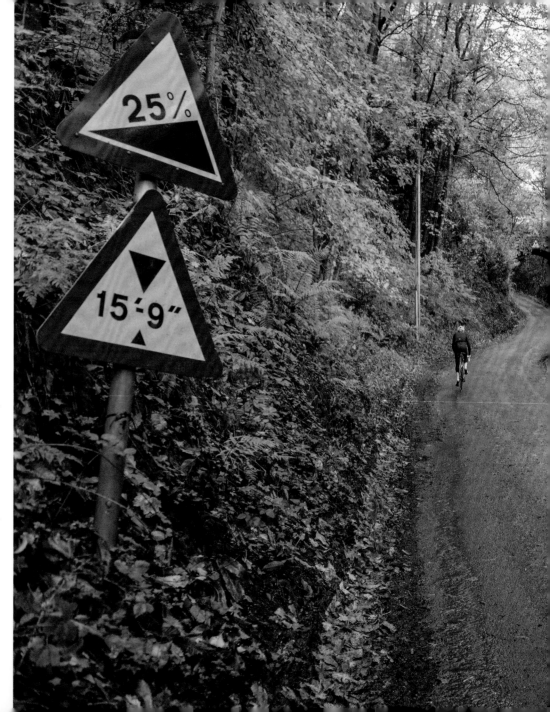

I toiled over this route for ages, and it was one of the last I put to paper, because at first I was simply trying to squeeze in too many hills. Not that that's normally a problem (it hasn't stopped me on other rides in this book), but in this case there was an unavoidable obstacle that ruined all the routes.

Brighton.

The majority of the course was always going to lie to the west of the seaside town, but I was determined to include at least one of the big climbs further east – either Ditchling Beacon, Steyning Bostal or even, further east, Firle Bostal. The thing is, as you approach from the west, the only routes there and back are horrid: either on busy A-roads or trapped in the urban sprawl along the coast. The dilemma was therefore whether to stomach the traffic and dodge tourists with ice creams, or forgo the big climbs and keep the ride rural. The latter option won. There's still plenty of elevation to be gained, and wonderful roads to experience, though.

Using Midhurst as the base, I start the ride heading west on the A272, before turning right onto Woolbeding Lane. The first objective of the day is Milland Hill and, to reach it, head north into Woolbeding, take the left onto Stedham Lane. Then it's right onto Iping Lane, all the way to the village of Milland. Over the crossroads, and the hill is just the other side of the village.

It's one I've raced up a number of times. On paper it suited me perfectly, as it's steep enough for long enough to ensure the heavy powerful riders

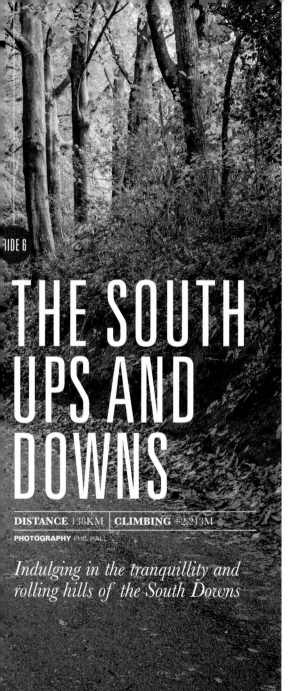

THE SOUTH UPS AND DOWNS

DISTANCE 138KM | **CLIMBING** +2,213M

PHOTOGRAPHY PHIL HALL

Indulging in the tranquillity and rolling hills of the South Downs

LEFT *To start the ride a little bit of 25% gradient on Milland Hill.*

ran out of steam, and because of this I'd always be one of the first over the crest. On the last lap, however, the finish line was placed about 500 metres beyond the summit, so some of said heavier riders, the sprinters who could also climb a bit, were then able to come back into contention, and would swamp me, because I had zero sprint. The incline twists a little entering the woods, and rises dramatically between the high banks either side, with the arch of the bridge overhead. Kicking up more steeply still, the road reaches its maximum 25% gradient before bending left to the crown, then fading onto the plateau.

After getting your breath back, take a left turn at the end of the road for a brief passage on the B2070, then turn right in Rake onto St Patrick's Lane. Follow this to Liss, then, crossing the A3 on Hawkley Road, carry on down Mill Lane into the village of Steep to reach the base of Stoner Hill. The first time I rode this climb it had just been resurfaced, and I swear I must have been the very first person up it: the tarmac was immaculate. Regardless of surface, it's a gorgeous road, with sumptuous curves set on a steady gradient that weave up through the woods. At the top, turn left onto High Cross Lane, then, dropping south across the A272, make your way to East Meon, for what is arguably the standout climb of the day: Butser Hill. Heading south from the village, then turning left onto Oxenhope Lane, you are soon at the base, and face 2.5 kilometres of ascent which, although steady to begin with, get

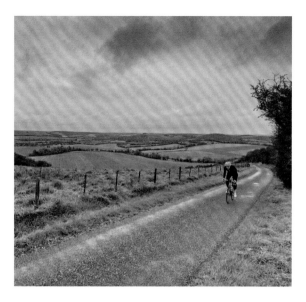

tougher as they rise. From the higher slopes the views are, as to be expected, worth all the effort. Look behind you and the South Downs roll gently away into the distance.

At the summit turn right, then next left. Descend to cross the A3, then head east through Chalton to Idsworth. Turn left here and, deep in these impossibly quiet lanes, begin your undulating journey north to South Harting. Joining up with the B2146, follow this up and then down to the heart of the small village, where refreshments could be taken. Turn east onto Elsted Road, and the next climb comes in the shape of Harting Downs, which takes you immediately back up the ridge you have just descended, but on a much smaller road.

A twisting, narrow ascent with a maximum of 12% gradient, it picks its way through the woods to join the B2141, then, turning left,

ABOVE *Climbing Butser Hill to reveal the best view in the South Downs.*

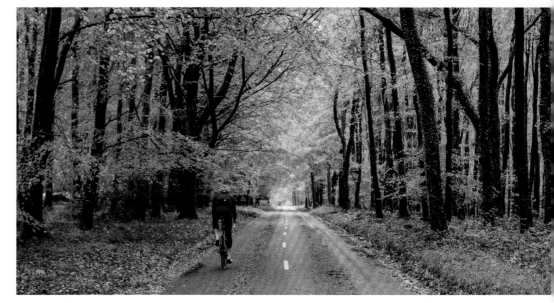

keeps climbing all the way to the top of North Marden Down. Sticking on this road for a while, you gradually descend into the wide valley, between the elevated ground on your right and the gently sloping hills to your left. This tranquillity is ended at the junction with Binderton Lane, where you turn left up a short, sharp hill towards West Dean and Singleton: perfect for a little dig if the wind is on your back. Give it full gas all the way to join the A286, where you turn left into West Dean, then begin to climb gently through Singleton and East Dean and Upwaltham.

Here in the heart of the Downs the scenery isn't dramatic: it's not shock and awe – it's just nice. Very nice. It's calming, serene; the hills roll gently as you pass from village to village between neat hedgerows and small woods. Not exposed, not savage or hostile, just perfectly placid: the South Downs have a feel to them that I've found in very few other places in Britain.

Upon reaching the A285 turn north, to continue to climb all the way to Ducton Down, then navigate round the high ground to head east through Barlavington, then south to Sutton, Bignor and West Burton. This next part of the ride takes you onto the plains surrounding the River Arun, where you can enjoy a rest from the continual undulations and gather yourself for the tougher climbs that lie ahead. Crossing the B2138, join the A29 into Coldwaltham, then turn right on Brook Lane across the river to the A283. Heading north, follow the road round west into

Pulborough, then carry on through to Stopham, where life on the flat ends and the hills return.

Ride the A283 into Petworth, then out of the town on the A272. The road crests and dips with increasing frequency and sharpness until, after you've turned right in Tillington, what has been a flurry of minor ascents comes to the top on Upperton Common. None of these blips on the profile are anything to worry about; however, with a good distance in your legs already, what follows might be.

Heading north to Lurgashall and Dial Green, you turn right through Windfallwood Common to find the bottom of Quell Lane. Although not quite as steep as Milland Hill which opened the ride, this snaking journey through the thick woods is arguably the toughest test on the whole route. Ramping up as soon as it begins, the climb

sticks to a stiff gradient which peaks at over 20%, before reaching its summit on Fernden Lane. Your adventure is now nearly at an end, and there is just one more climb to make sure it's not just memories of peaceful lanes and sleepy villages you take home with you.

Taking the A286, descend through Fenshurst, then, escaping the somewhat claustrophobic main road, take the left turn at the small triangular junction to follow the direct route up through Henley Copse. Gaining the same altitude as the main road you have just left, but covering half the distance, this will, you don't need to be a mathematician to realise, hurt some. Ramping up with a real kick into Henley that should assure you finish on empty tanks, you re-join the A286 and complete the ride by descending all the way back into Midhurst.

ABOVE *A cyclist took a ride through the deep dark wood…*

RIDE 6 SOUTH-EAST

SOUTH DOWNS

DISTANCE	138KM
CLIMBING	+2,213M
DIFFICULTY	4/10

FOOD & WATER | SOUTH HARTING / PETWORTH

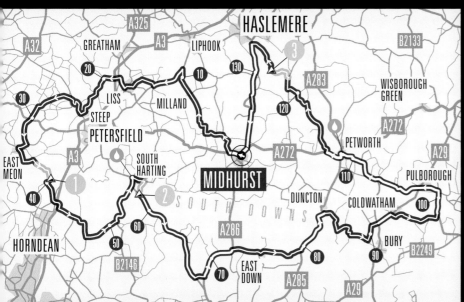

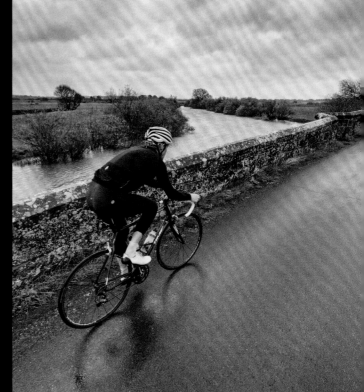

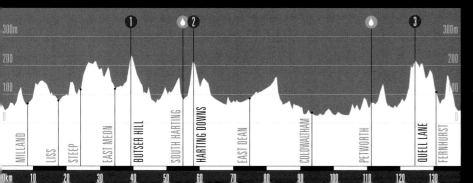

KEY CLIMBS

1 BUTSER HILL
2,540m +119m

Climbing to reveal my favourite view in the South Downs, Butser Hill is pretty long at over 2.5 kilometres and reasonably stiff with a 4.7% average gradient. There's no steep bits on it though so just sit back and enjoy the vista which improves with each and every pedal rev

2 HARTING DOWNS
1,400m +113m

With an 8% average this is a tough climb but there are no real killer steep ramps. The gradient does stick close to the 10% mark for most of it as the narrow road weaves up through the woods towards the T-junction where, turning left, you continue to climb on the B road to the eventual summit

3 QUELL LANE
1,050m +88m

Hidden and rough, Quell Lane starts as it means to go on with an immediately tough kick up away from the main road. Featuring many twists and turns, not to mention a serious amount of stiff double-digit gradient this is a proper little climb and one not to be underestimated

One of my old training routes, this is etched on my memory, road by road. Some I'd like to have surgically removed, but most are filled with fond memories. This ride will be congested at times, and is a little complicated, but that's the South-East for you: it's a busy and congested place. But trust me: there are quiet lanes out there, and even some wide open spaces, when you get to the top of the High Weald.

Base for the day is Westerham on the A25, and it's uphill from the gun as you leave on Hosey Common Road into Hosey Hill. Once over the brow, take the left turn to drop down Mapleton Road to the B269, then turn left into Four Elms. At the crossroads head straight over, before taking the second right to Hever, then left on Uckfield Lane to climb into Markbeech. This part of the ride is all up and down, in and out of the saddle, changes of gear and direction – the whole day is, for that matter. From Markbeech you continue heading south to meet the B2026. Turn left to follow the Hartfield Road to the A264, then left again, before taking the second right onto Beech Green Lane to Balls Green. If you have managed not to get lost you will now have reached the edge of your first destination of the day, the Ashdown Forest.

Although a mere pinprick in size compared to the vast swathes of open land that bless the less populated parts of the country, Ashdown Forest is no less a prized sanctuary for people looking for some peace and quiet. It's also home to a handful of great climbs, starting with the long ascent from its north-east corner to its centre. When you hit

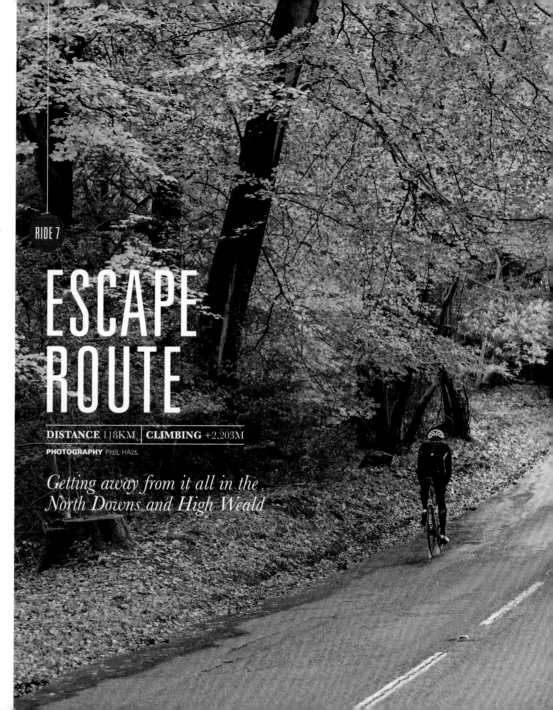

ESCAPE ROUTE

DISTANCE 118KM | **CLIMBING** +2,203M
PHOTOGRAPHY PHIL HALL

Getting away from it all in the North Downs and High Weald

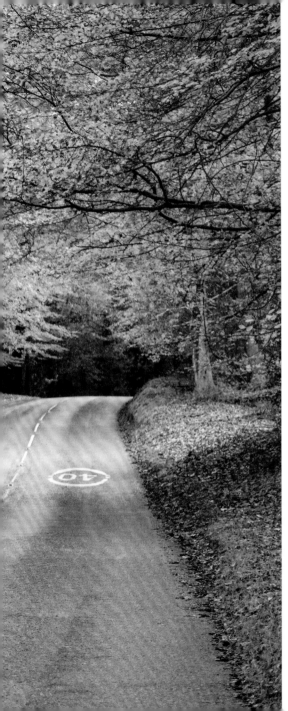

LEFT *Just one of many false summits on the long climb through Five Hundred Acre Wood.*

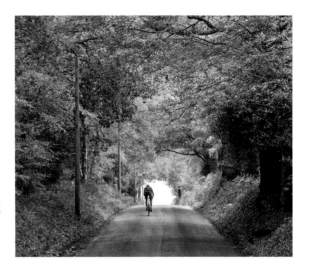

the B2110 just east of Withyham turn left, then right onto Ladies Mile, which you follow all the way to the crossroads with the B2188. Here you head south and, after a short descent, begin to climb up past Lye Green and Friar's Gate through Five Hundred Acre Wood.

Back in the day, when I'd ride the local early-season training rides, this is when the action would kick off. Arriving at the base we would generally be a large group, but everyone knew the drill here, and it was a case of hitting it hard to the top, with everyone wanting to be the last man, or woman, standing. It would still be a while until the first race of the year, but this was always a good test of form or to see how strong your peers were. Then at the summit we would regroup and return to a more civilised pace again.

You can give it some beans if you so desire, or take it steady – either way, once you've climbed to the junction at the summit turn left. Descend a little, then take the right onto Crowborough Road to ride through the gorse-covered landscape to cross the A22 and continue through Chelwood Gate to the A275. Turn right up to Wych Cross, then, after a few metres on the A22, right again to Coleman's Hatch.

Up next is the fantastic little climb up Kidd's Hill or, to use its more popular name, 'The Wall'. I'm not sure who named it or when, but this is what I've always known it as, and when you get to the bottom you'll see why. Turning right in Coleman's Hatch and riding through Newbridge, you reach the base and, in front of you, rising

dead straight into the trees, is, yes, you guessed it, what looks like a wall of asphalt. Converging to a hole in the trees at the summit, this killer little road offers nowhere to hide, until you break out into the light to return to the open, gorse-covered plateau. Roll to the junction, then head left to enjoy the last of the Ashdown Forest, before setting your sights on the smörgåsbord of climbs that run up and over the North Downs.

Head first to Hartfield, then turning right on the B2110, ride to Groombridge. What follows is the climb up Groombridge Hill (a bit of a lump), before you turn left onto the A264, then right onto the B2188. Make your way to Fordcombe, then take Chafford Lane and Bradley Road to Chiddingstone Hoath, heading due north all the way to meet the B2027. Turning left here, then first right, you'll find yourself, unless something has gone terribly wrong, approaching the shores of the Bough Beech Reservoir. Take a moment here to enjoy the flat land, shake your legs, maybe

ABOVE *Striving to reach the light at the end of the tunnel and the summit of The Wall.*

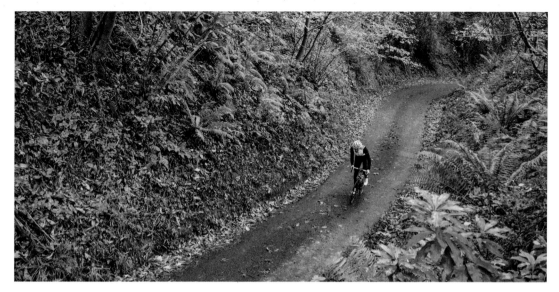

eat a gel – because you're about to hit a barrage of hills, starting with the famed York's Hill.

Home to the annual Catford CC hill climb (the oldest continually running bike race in the world), York's Hill has witnessed more pain and screams than a dentist's chair. I'll forever have flashbacks of waiting at the bottom to race up it, palms sweating, pulse racing, looking ahead at the road as it kicks up into the trees and questioning my sanity. Its cruel 25% slope cuts its way between the steep, canyon-like dirt walls, forming a tortuous, meandering passage to the summit. If you ever do get the inclination to race a hill climb then, if I haven't put you off, this is the event to enter, as the atmosphere among the cheering crowds at the top is second to none.

Having hit York's Hill hard with burning legs, turn left, then join the B2042 to drop back down the ridge to the base of the next test. Making sure you take the second of two right turns from the junction where the B2042 road heads south, you turn north in the direction of Toy's Hill. Longer than York's, but not quite as steep, with the joy of a hiatus in the climbing at half way, Toy's Hill will hurt, not quite as much as York's but, yes, it will hurt. Over the top, drop down to Brasted, and right away it's up again. Yes, you'll be getting sore now, but stick with it.

Up next is Brasted Hill, the venue for the very first National Hill Climb Championship in 1944, contested on bikes that weighed as much as a small car ridden by men in tweed shorts and flat caps. At the top turn left, and left again onto Grays Road, then left once more to drop down the A233 for a short while, before taking the right turn onto the Pilgrims' Way. Follow this – once part of the pilgrims' path between Winchester and Canterbury – along the side of the ridge to Titsey. Here, turn left down into Oxted and take the first right onto Bluehouse Lane, which you follow east until you hit the base of my favourite climb on this loop: Chalkpit Lane. It's not the prettiest, longest or steepest, but it has everything in just perfect proportions, including a fabulous hairpin bend on its way through the hillside trees to the top.

Now there is just one climb to come, and more hallowed ground to visit. Every October on the same day as the Catford CC hill climb on York's Hill in the morning, the Bec Cycling Club hold their event in the afternoon, here on White Lane. It is etiquette to ride both in the same day – in fact, turning up to the Bec CC in the afternoon with fresh legs, having not ridden the Catford event should simply not be allowed!

You need a keen eye to find the base as dropping down Titsey Hill it's easy to miss the junction on the left, so keep your eyes peeled. Then, once you've made the turn, the climb begins. An insignificant little hill it may be, but one laced with history, and in 2005 even Britain's first Tour de France winner Bradley Wiggins raced up it (I beat him that year, not that I ever mention it, and no, I don't care if he wasn't trying: it's there in the official results in black and white!).

Once at the top, a place I've never been without seeing stars and coughing up my lungs, you turn right, and all that's left of the journey is the drop down into Westerham, where you can rest your battered legs after a great day on the North Downs.

ABOVE *The brutal 25% amphitheatre of York's Hill, perfect for spectators, evil for riders.*

RIDE 7

SOUTH-EAST

NORTH DOWNS

DISTANCE	118KM
CLIMBING	+2,203M
DIFFICULTY	5/10

FOOD & WATER | GROOMBRIDGE / BRASTED

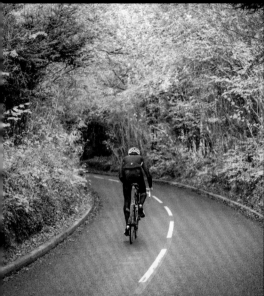

KEY CLIMBS

1 THE WALL
1,440m +125m

A single straight line of arduous gradient that offers little if any distraction for the mind. Staring ahead the summit is always in sight, the ever-so-slowly growing hole in the trees which taunts you as you grind up the 15% slopes.

2 TOY'S HILL
2,650m +176m

First of all to tick off the 'Official' segment make sure you start the climb from the left fork at the bottom. The first part into the village is reasonably steady, however after a short interlude at half way the second half is anything but.

3 CHALKPIT LANE
2,420m +144m

My favourite of the North Down climbs Chalkpit Lane boasts an average gradient of just 6% but it's a whole lot steeper towards the top. Creeping gradually away from Limpsfield it's once you spy the perfect right-hand bend that the real gradient kicks in.

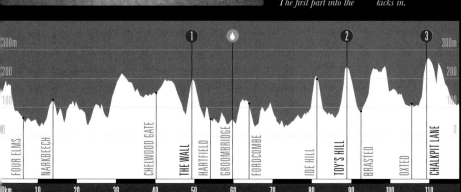

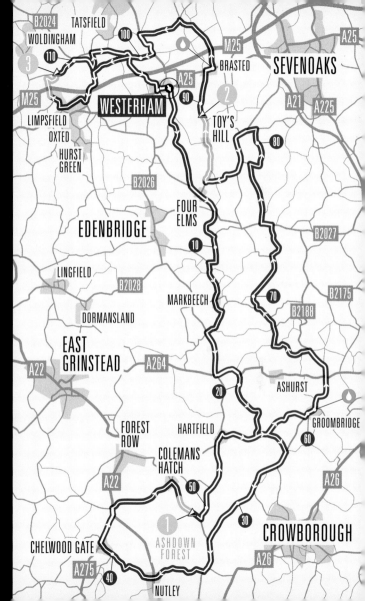

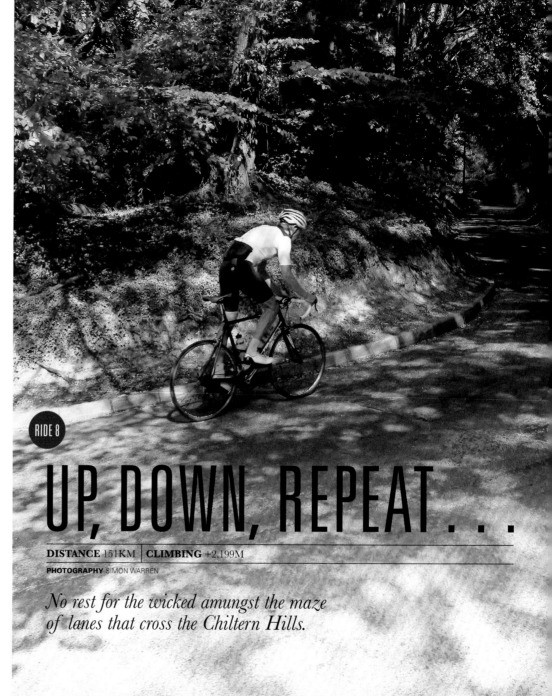

The Chilterns, like the Surrey Hills to the south of the capital, are a compact oasis of tightly packed climbs that make a perfect location for a day's escape from the metropolis. Set on a 45-degree angle, they run roughly from Luton in the north to Reading in the south, fading out towards London in the east, but ending abruptly to the west. This diminutive ridge of peaks and troughs, populated by sleepy villages and beautiful market towns, makes for a splendid day on the bike getting lost, or hopefully not, in its labyrinth of lanes. I've taken Great Missenden, almost slap-bang in the middle, as the start point. It's quieter than Chesham, Amersham or High Wycombe, but still has enough shops for you to grab anything you need pre- or post-ride.

The profile, resembling a bandsaw blade, wastes no time heading upwards as, right after crossing the A413, you climb up the B485 on Frith Hill. Nothing too serious, but certainly enough to get you out of the saddle breathing hard. Rolling over into Chesham, turn left into town, then, after a couple of roundabouts on the A416, climb out via the stiff slopes of Eskdale Avenue. Nine kilometres in, and two punchy climbs already ridden, which has set the tone well for the day ahead.

Turning left at the top, head to Lye Green and then, after a short time on the B4505, north to Ashley Green, where you head right onto the A416 to drop down into Berkhamsted. After crossing the A41, turn left at the roundabout, then first right onto King's Road, which you

RIDE 8

UP, DOWN, REPEAT...

DISTANCE 151KM | **CLIMBING** +2,199M

PHOTOGRAPHY SIMON WARREN

No rest for the wicked amungst the maze of lanes that cross the Chiltern Hills.

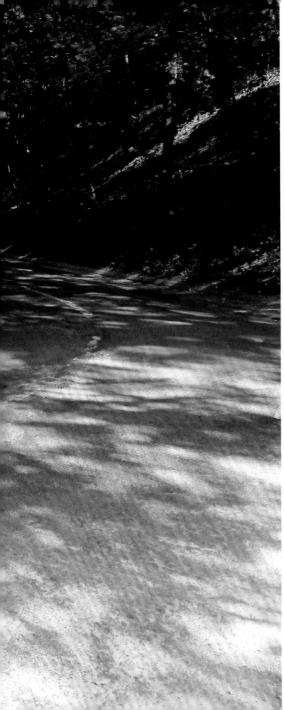

LEFT *Winding curves and endless gradient.*

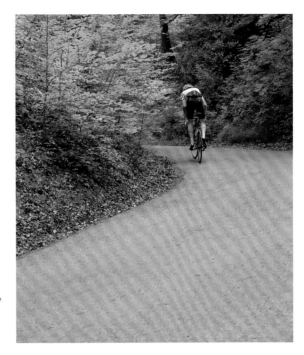

follow through the town, across the High Street and over the Grand Union Canal to run parallel with the railway lines. Taking the second left under the railway arches, turn right onto White Hill for a nasty little kick up to Nettleden Road, which you follow to Nettleden. Then turn right to ride Pipers Hill. A vicious little beast, trapped between tall muddy banks topped with a dark canopy of trees, it rises directly up and over to join the B440, where you head left.

Upon reaching Hudnall Corner, head left and bang: another climb. The frequency with which the constant fluctuations in gradient hit you is intense at times, so just take each one as it comes, and don't go too deep into your reserves just yet. Once over the summit, make your way to the most northerly point of the route, via Little Gaddesden and Ringshall then, heading back south, descend through Aldbury to Wigginton. On this ride there's no scenery you could call open: quiet lanes, yes – but you're never far from a village, farm or town, which is to be expected in the South-East.

Climbing out of Wigginton, turn right, then right again, drop down into Tring, then head left, and take another left to Dancers End. To say this route is complicated is an understatement, so I do hope you can follow the map, because there are endless left and right turns and I simply can't include them all.

The next climb on the route is my favourite, and one that had passed under my radar for many years until I first rode a Sportive on these roads.

The wonderfully named Crong arrives shortly after passing through Dancers End, and features what is in my opinion the 'Best Hairpin in the South-East'. A wonderfully steep left-hand bend through the gorge-like banks either side, it kicks up to a 20% gradient as it arcs through the thick woods searching for daylight at the summit. Back and forth, up and down, ride to St Leonards, then double back to the B4009, then, descending all the way through Wendover, cross the A413 to climb into the woods and drop down to the outskirts of Princes Risborough, and the base of the most famous road on the route: Whiteleaf.

For over fifty years the Archer Grand Prix cycle race was held on these roads, and its killer

ABOVE *The seriously steep slopes of The Crong are just waiting to hurt your legs.*

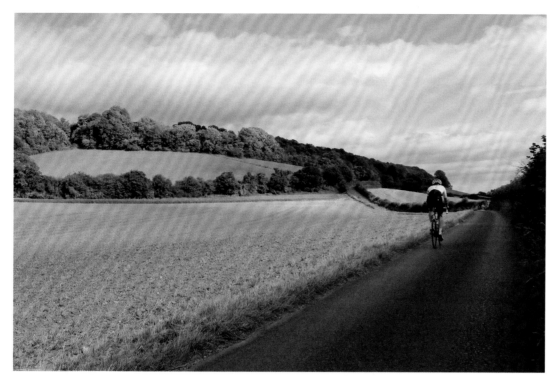

beaut of a corner that transfers you from one tough ramp into the next. Drop down through Radnage, climb into Stokenchurch, then, looping clockwise, head over the M40, then through Turville over the long climb to Christmas Common (mandatory selfie spot next to the village sign), then down to the sanctuary of the plains for the last time to reach Watlington. Now we're entering the final phase of the ride.

Turn right, back over the M40, then right again for the climb of Kingston Hill. Good enough to make it onto my second list of Britain's Greatest Climbs, and the last big challenge for your legs, it ramps up through Grove Wood then, at the top, turns left back to Stokenchurch for the long descent to the foot of the last two lumps on the profile.

By now you should, if you have paced the ride correctly, be in survival mode, not quite picking berries off bushes and eyeing up roadkill, but broken enough to beg passing strangers for food and shelter. As you make your way back east, the first of the final hurdles is Small Dean Lane, and ouch! it bites at the top. A local club hill-climb venue, this small, gnarly road really sticks the knife in at the top where, turning right, you have the briefest of recoveries before the final climb.

Turning left in Walter's Ash, then left again, drag yourself up Speen Hill into Speen, and you've done it. There are just 5 kilometres left to roll down back to base in Great Missenden, where you can comfortably say, if anyone asks, you have completed the Chiltern Hills.

hill, the climb that made the race, was Whiteleaf. Feared by most, avoided by some, but respected by all, Whiteleaf heads south from the A4010 in a series of demanding ramps which get steeper as they come. Many a time I have seen people go full gas from the bottom, only to catch sight of the stiffer gradients ahead and fall to pieces, so don't under any circumstances throw the kitchen sink at this climb until you get through the 90-degree right turn at half way. After this bend you may spy what you believe to be the top, but it's not: it's a fake summit, and only after crossing this is the end in sight. Once at the top, take the immediate right to rocket down Kop Hill, turn left at the base, keep falling, then rise up Wardrobes Hill before heading back to the base of the escarpment for a period of relaxation.

If you haven't stopped already, the village of Chinnor makes a good stopping point just after half way, especially as directly after is the next beast on the route, Chinnor Hill. If your legs are starting to ache, don't worry: there are only six climbs left and, unlike the first half of the ride, they are a little more spaced out, with a modicum of downtime between them. Chinnor Hill features a tight left turn midway, a real

ABOVE *A rare moment of calm between climbs.*

RIDE 8 | SOUTH-EAST
CHILTERNS

DISTANCE 151KM

CLIMBING +2,199M

DIFFICULTY 5/10

FOOD & WATER | WENDOVER / CHINNOR

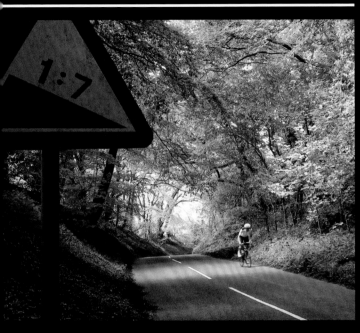

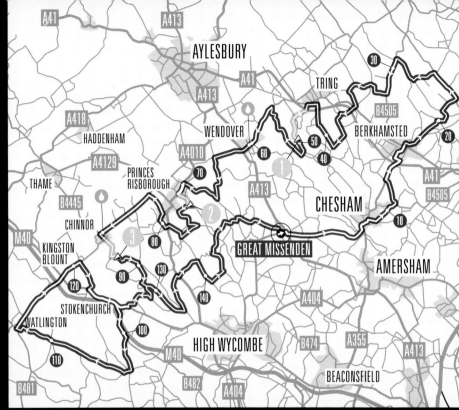

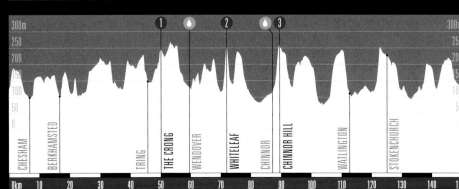

KEY CLIMBS

1 THE CRONG
520m +53m

Featuring the best corner in the Chilterns the wonderfully named Crong may be short but it packs a serious punch. Rising gently at first it's when you see the fearsome corner that the gradient kicks in. Reaching 20% it's steep round the bend in and out of it before easing to the transmitter at the summit

2 WHITELEAF
1,420m +127m

The toughest climb in the Chilterns, the gradient on Whiteleaf is packed with fluctuations, each one putting you further into the red. With an average gradient of 9% and slopes as steep as 16% make sure you measure your effort across its length to avoid blowing before the top.

3 CHINNOR HILL
2,050m +129m

One of the longer Chiltern ascents, Chinnor Hill eases away from the village then kicks up violently once it enters the woods. The average gradient of 6% only tells half the story because up to and beyond the climb's tight hairpin, the slope is consistently over 10% before it eases towards the top.

I spent close to fifteen years pounding these lanes while I lived in London, and have a more intimate knowledge of them than anywhere else in the country. For riders in East London this is where they head to break out of the city, and every weekend the Lea Bridge Road, the main artery that punctures this part of the capital, is thick with riders all taking the most direct route to quiet lanes and fresh air. I won't start the ride in the middle of the city, though, to spare you the torture of the Lea Bridge Road, but just outside the North Circular in Woodford, on the edge of Epping Forest.

From Woodford Green head north-east on Monkham's Lane to Buckhurst Way, then turn left to ride up to the B170. At this junction turn right, drop down and across the River Roding, then start the first climb of the day. Yes, climb. Everything that goes uphill around here, no matter how slight, is designated a climb of some description. As the saying goes, beggars can't be choosers. Ascending as you cross the M11, take the first left, then, as the road bends right, go up the now more imposing gradient of Roding Lane into Chigwell. Turning left at the junction, then right at the roundabout, drop down a short, fast descent before it's time to climb again. Take as much momentum into the base as you can, then push it hard through the bends all the way to join the B173.

The city is well behind you now and, heading east, you pass through Chigwell Row and Lambourne End into Stapleford Abbotts via a

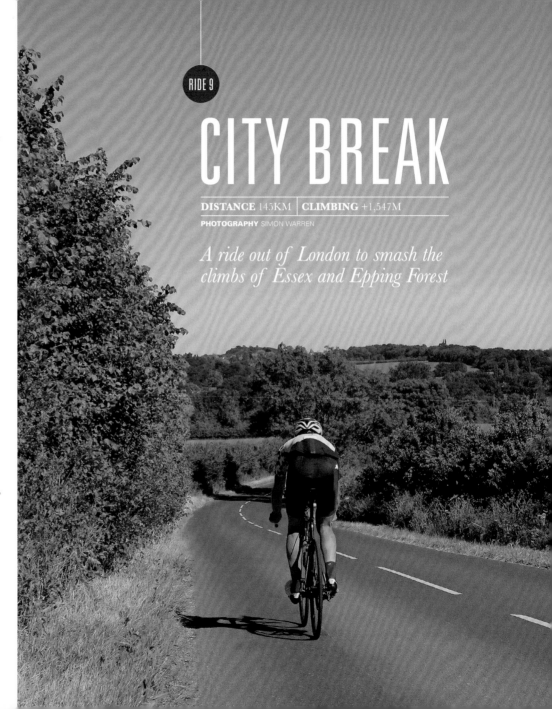

CITY BREAK

DISTANCE 145KM | **CLIMBING** +1,547M

PHOTOGRAPHY SIMON WARREN

A ride out of London to smash the climbs of Essex and Epping Forest

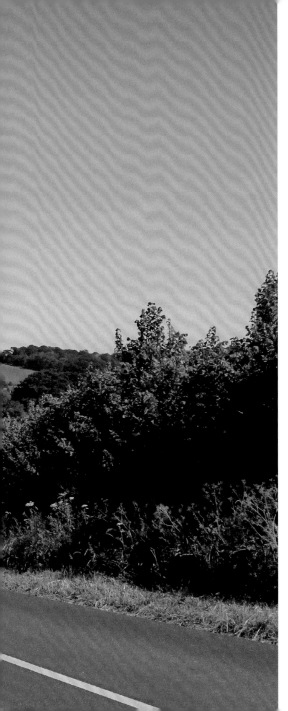

constant stream of ups and downs – anything but flat. Turning right on the B175, climb Oak Hill Road, then turn left onto Tysea Hill, then right onto Horseman Side. Here you can blow the dust off the big chain ring and get some proper speed up, as the route travels across the M25, through Navestock Side, to Kelvedon Hatch. Joining the A128, turn left, take the first right into the village, and then proceed out to Wyatts Green.

There you take the left turn onto Wyatts Green Road, then keep heading east to Mountnessing to cross over the A12. It's all lumpy, and for a while there is nothing that really constitutes a hill – at least nothing you'd be tempted to build a Strava segment on unless you were really desperate. After passing through Padham's Green and taking the left turn, go right on Ingatestone Road onto the B1007, where you turn left, and here there is a bit of a hill ascending into Stock. It's no beast, but will get the heart pumping harder. In the middle of the village turn right onto Mill Road, before taking a left onto Mill Lane to keep progressing east, always east, through West Hanningfield, across the A130 to East Hanningfield, until you turn north towards Bicknacre.

OK, now we are nearly there. Where? I hear you ask. Oh, only the biggest, baddest hill in Essex: a road so fearsome it has its own Twitter feed. Yes, it's the one and only North Hill. What, you've never heard of it? Well, it's time to introduce you. Passing through Bicknacre onto the B1418, take this road to briefly join the

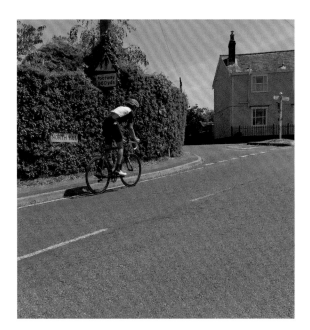

A414 at Woodham Mortimer, before leaving it on Tom Tit Lane to head north to Woodham Walter. Descending all the way to the River Chelmer, ride through Ulting, then take the left on Bumfords Lane to Mowden Hall Lane, where you turn left again onto Baddow Road.

And here you are, on the approach to North Hill. Now, although it's no Monte Zoncolan, it does manage to pack a punch lower down and, if ridden at pace, will certainly hurt. Commencing as soon as it leaves the River Chelmer, the gradient momentarily reaches double figures, then eases back as the road bisects Little Baddow. Many believe the top of the climb to be here, where the more testing gradient disappears, but I disagree. I believe the top lies where the elevation gain is complete – all the way into Danbury and

LEFT *Free of the metropolis and into the rolling hills.*

ABOVE *The mighty North Hill always feels longer than you remember.*

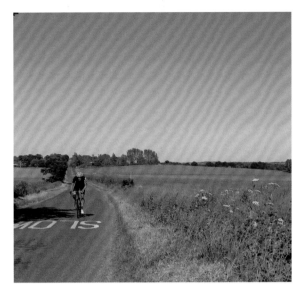

the junction with the A414 – so if you want to, put a time down on the Full Monty, then press on all the way to there.

With that mountain scaled, it's time to head home, and the route back is packed with delights – in fact, I saved all my favourite Essex hills for the return journey. Passing over the A414 the first job is to negotiate the outskirts of Chelmsford, by heading west into Sandon, then continuing to pick your way to Galleywood, and going over the A12 into Margaretting. Take Ivy Barns Lane to Fryerning, then Blackmore Road via Wedlocks Lane into Hook End, before turning right to take Ongar Road through Stondon Massey on the ever-undulating path into Chipping Ongar.

The next target on the horizon is Toot Hill, a small village that sits on top of a small mound with four roads that climb 'all the way' up to it. A bit like Mont Ventoux in France. (Well, actually,

nothing like it.) The route I favour is from the north, via Greensted Green, and turning onto Toot Hill Road you see the hill outlined ahead of you all the way to the twin bends at the top. Passing right through the village, drop down the other side of the mound, past the golf course, then take the right up Berwick Lane through Knightsland Wood. With a testing ramp at its start, the climb of Berwick Lane takes you to the A113, which you follow south, until the first right turn at Passingford Bridge.

Up next is one of my favourite roads in Essex, described by someone as a 'mini-Flanders'. The narrow, undulating Tawney Lane climbs gradually in stages between fields devoid of hedgerows, open and exposed much like the famous lanes of Belgium. Arriving in Woodhatch via yet more undulations, make your way onto Mount Road to pass under the M11 and come into Fiddlers Hamlet. Take the route into town, and it's time for the climb through Ivy Chimneys, skirting the lower edge of Epping: a nasty ramp, which kicks up to almost 20% under the railway bridge, then presses on after a brief lull at half way to join Theydon Road.

The climbs come thick and fast now as we approach the much-loved Epping forest. After all the hours, days, months I spent on these hills I know every one like the back of my hand. I tried and tried to bag the Strava KOM on them all over the years, succeeded briefly on some, but never quite managed a few.

Before we get into the forest, drop down

Piercing Hill into Theydon Bois, then turn right up the slog of a climb that is Coppice Row. Once over the summit, push on to cross the roundabout, then take the first left onto Wade Road. At the end, drop down Claypit Hill, turn left onto Pynest Green Lane, and follow this to Avey Lane to head right all the way to the A112. Turning left, then at the next junction left again, you'll be on Mott Street. Included in *100 Greatest Cycling Climbs*, Mott Street is the toughest of the Epping climbs, and the one everyone wants to be king of.

Heading east from the main road, you'll find the gradient creeps up on you like a ninja. Then, just as the legs start to feel the pinch, you reach the junction with Lippitts Hill, where it really ramps up. Coming in waves of 12% slopes, Mott Street can just about be tackled in one full-gas effort but, if not, there is a nice flat bit in the middle where you can rest. You can't leave Epping Forest without doing a couple more climbs, so, at the top, head left down Avey Lane, turn right, then right again, to climb Wellington Hill and, at the top, turn right and head back down Mott Street, and at the junction turn left up Lippitts Hill.

Once you've come back, via Church Road, to the top of Mott Street, that will do. You could of course spend a couple of hours here, but your legs will likely have had enough for now, so head to the A104 for the run-in back to Woodford, tracing the route of Stage 3 of the 2014 Tour de France to the finish of your Essex adventure.

ABOVE *The view looking down from Toot Hill!*

RIDE 9

SOUTH-EAST
ESSEX AND EPPING FOREST

DISTANCE 145KM

CLIMBING +1,547M

DIFFICULTY 2/10

FOOD & WATER | DANBURY / CHIPPING ONGAR

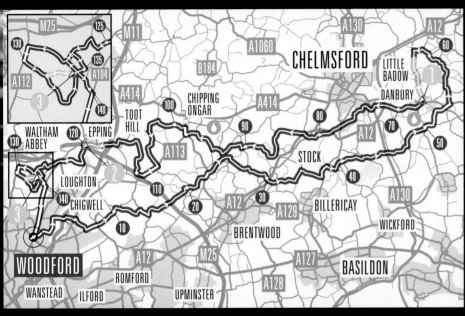

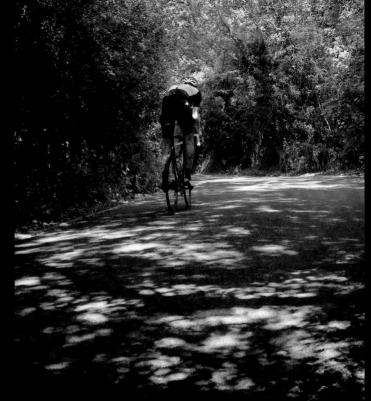

KEY CLIMBS

1 NORTH HILL
3,783m +94m

A long hill for Essex but with an average of 2% it's no killer. Still, all hills are hard if ridden fast and everyone wants to post a good time on North Hill. The steepest part comes shortly after the start where the slope does reach 10% then once through Little Baddow it fades to the flat finish.

2 IVY CHIMNEYS
1,034m +43m

The start to this climb is wickedly steep but if you carry enough momentum to its base you can usually romp up it no bother. There is a lull at midway through the village and then it kicks up hard again to hit the legs for a second time as it bends round to meet the junction at the top.

3 MOTT STREET
1,503m +77m

The climb all East Londoners love, Mott Street is the venue for many a club hill climb and is a great hill to ride. With the steep gradient split into two distinct sectors of 12% separated with a rest between them pacing your effort and getting your gear changes right are key on this one.

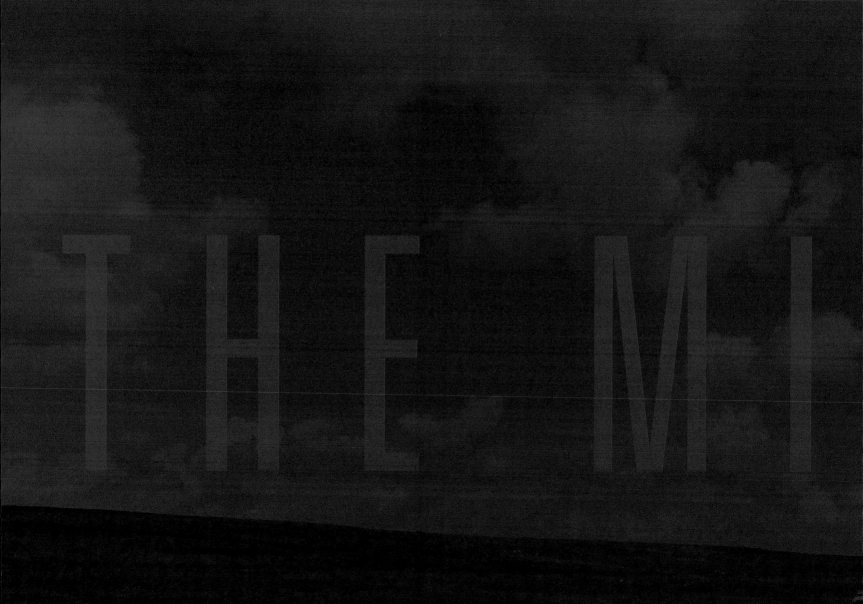

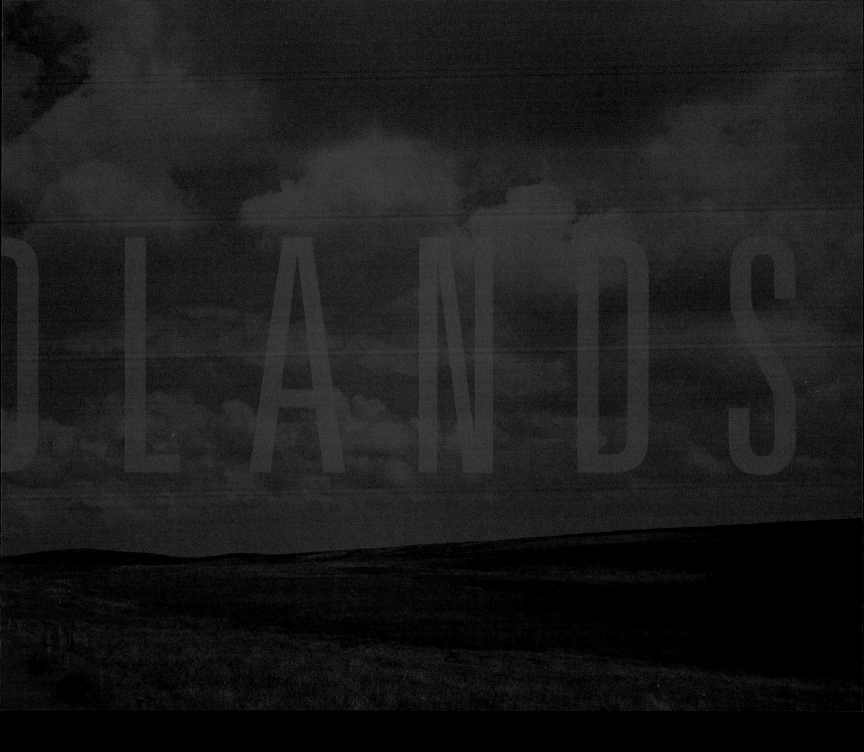

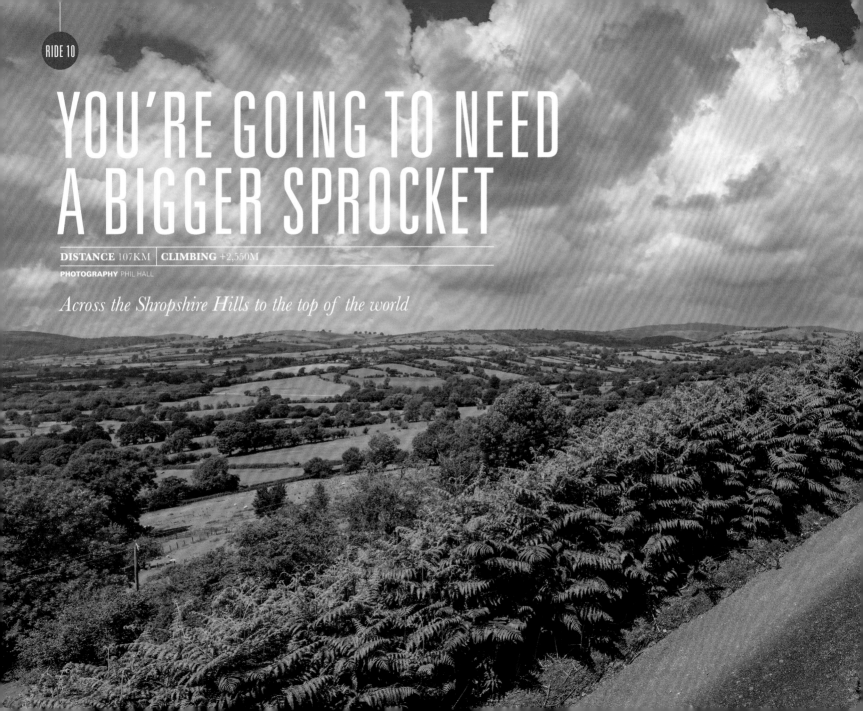

YOU'RE GOING TO NEED A BIGGER SPROCKET

DISTANCE 107KM | **CLIMBING** +2,550M

PHOTOGRAPHY PHIL HALL

Across the Shropshire Hills to the top of the world

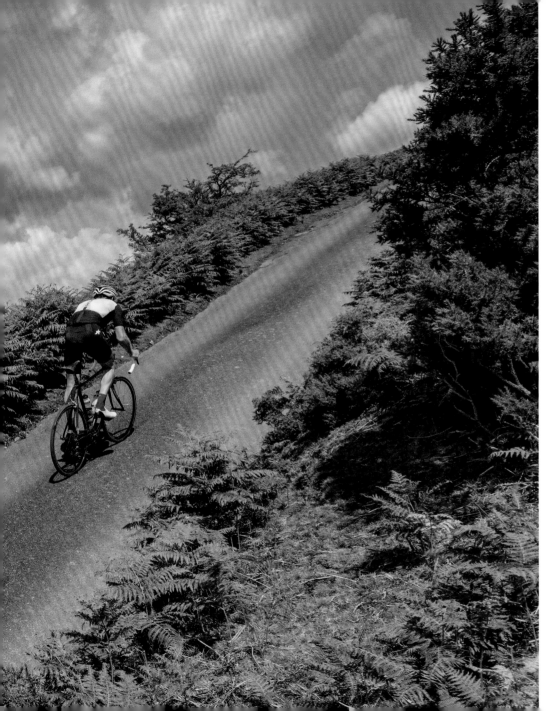

I met a man once who had commuted up and down the A49 through Church Stretton for ten years with no idea the Long Mynd even existed. One day, by chance, he decided to divert west, and simply could not believe what he saw – the beauty that had been under his nose all those years! The name Long Mynd means 'long mountain', but it's not to be confused with *the* Long Mountain a few miles further north near Welshpool. This 11-kilometre-long, 5-kilometre-wide plateau is a true wonder of the British landscape, but to get up onto its high plains you've got to put in some serious work, no matter what direction you arrive from.

There are three absolutely belting climbs on this route and, to be kind (you can thank me later), I've placed them at regular intervals so you'll be able to attack each with fresh(ish) legs. First of the three, and it's a real bone-crusher, is the outrageous Asterton Bank, one of the most feared roads in England. The first time I encountered it was descending in a car with the family after a trip to The Burway. Barely wide enough for even a modest-sized vehicle, and perched precariously on the edge of the cliff, it had my wife and daughter both screaming in panic. All I could think about, of course, was getting the bike out and heading back up.

Before we get there, the route starts by climbing a more pleasant way over the Long Mynd, heading north out of Church Stretton on the B5477, then turning west after All Stretton onto Plush Hill. Turning left at the next

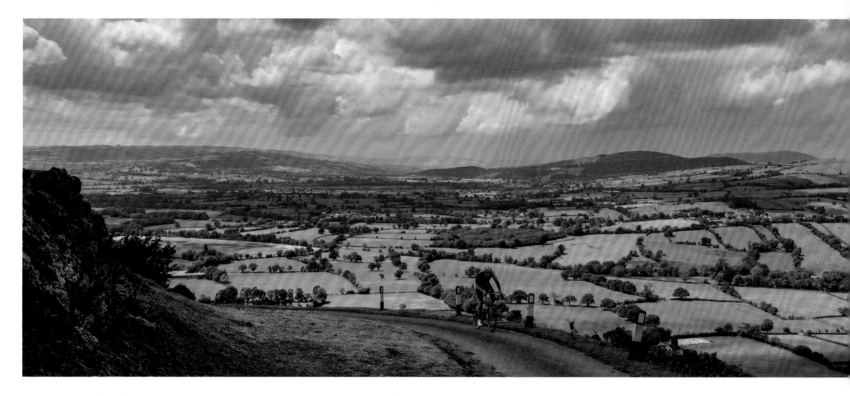

crossroads, then continuing to ascend onto the moorland, you will have gained over 200 metres of elevation before you reach the crest, and then get settled into 10 solid kilometres of descent. Falling through Ratlinghope and Bridges, then following the course of the River East Onny, you lose altitude all the way, until you turn back east towards the village of Wentnor. There's a tiny blip in the profile here – a pocket-sized hill to reawaken the legs – then another kilometre on the flat before you reach Asterton.

Leaving the tiny village beyond the red phone box, Asterton Bank kicks up viciously right from the off, bends left, then sticks remorselessly to the same, uniformly brutal gradient its entire length. Looking up, you'll not know whether to laugh or cry, and if you're not suitably equipped with a small-enough gear there's a good chance you'll be grinding to a halt at some point. The views out to the left become more spectacular the higher you climb, until this infernal road ends almost abruptly as it starts by bending right to level out at the Midland Gliding Club. You're well within your rights to take a moment here and get a few breaths, as Asterton Bank is more than worthy of its 10/10 ranking. Amazingly, though, it's not the toughest climb on this route: that's coming next (cue evil laugh). . .

Take your time to enjoy the journey across the tops of the Long Mynd. Then, as you approach the descent back to Church Stretton, you are treated to the world-famous views east over the whole of the Shropshire Hills. From the Wrekin in the north to Clee Hill in the south, the horizon is dotted with smooth green mounds, all emerging from the patchwork of fields. There in the middle is tallest of them all, Brown Clee Hill, which, reaching its peak at Abdon Burf, is – yes, you guessed it – where you are headed: right to the very top.

ABOVE *The view from the top of Asterton Bank looking out over Wales.*

First, ride east out of Church Stretton to Hope Bowdler, then leave the B4371 to Rushbury and take on the small climb up and over Wenlock Edge. Falling down the other side into Corve Dale, cross the B4368, turn left onto Sandy Lane, then head to Holdgate, Stanton Long and, ultimately, the village of Ditton Priors, sitting firmly in the shadow of Brown Clee Hill. The moment you leave the village you are climbing. What lies ahead is a total monster. Standing at 540 metres above sea level, Abdon Burf is one of the best challenges there is for a cyclist in England and, on top of that, boasts some of the greatest views the country has to offer.

Once out of Ditton Priors the climb starts on Bent Lane, nice and civilised at first. At the end of this road turn left, then, at the next right turn, you'll have to stop, as the road to the summit is blocked by a gate. Closed to traffic, this service road for the antennae at the top is open to walkers and cyclists and, once you have negotiated the obstacle, the 'fun' begins. After about three pedal revolutions the gradient tilts up like the sinking *Titanic*, and almost instantly assumes its 20% pitch. Not for a few metres: all the way to the horizon.

The first time I attempted this climb I had to stop and walk, three times. It was simply too much for my winter bike, and of course my legs, to cope with. Slippy under the trees, and with not an inch of respite, the journey to the brow at the end of this infernal ramp takes an eternity. In any civilised country a series of bends would

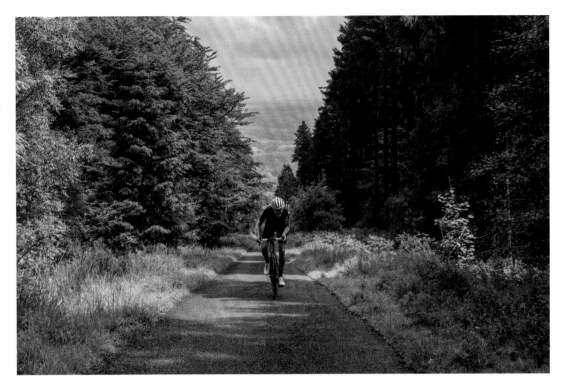

have been installed to reduce the impact of the gradient, but no, not in England. Stick with it, though, because what lies past the cattle grid is some kind of paradise. Home to the remains of an old Iron Age fort and crumbling quarry buildings, devoid of all traffic, the road continues to climb across the lofty plateau past rocky outcrops, making its way to the radio towers at the summit. Boasting a jaw-dropping 360-degree panorama, Abdon Burf is indeed a special place, and worth all the effort needed to get there.

After taking as much time as you can afford at the top, it's time for the descent, which must be

treated with as much respect as the climb. Then it's back through the gate to turn left to start the return journey to Church Stretton. Routing through Abdon and Tugford, you continue to descend all the way to Diddlebury at the crossing of the B4368. Climbing back over Wenlock Edge into Ticklerton, and then up to Hope Bowdler, you turn left to cross the A49 and line up for the final of the day's three big climbs. You have already descended this road following the climb of Asterton Bank, so you'll have a good idea of what lies ahead.

A degree easier than its nasty neighbour, but

ABOVE *The utter madness of Abdon Burf, enough to make you weep.*

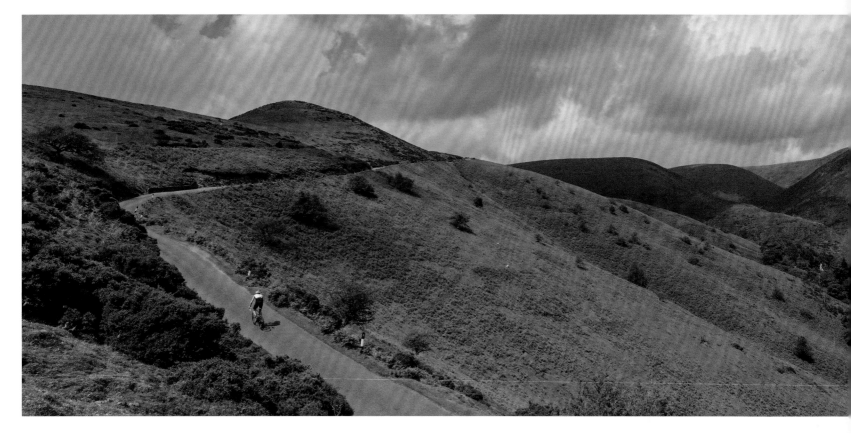

still bloody hard, The Burway is a legendary hill in the world of cycling. Home to the 1989 National Hill Climb Championship – the second won by Chris Boardman – this hill is the epitome of Beauty and the Beast. Following its contours on a punishing gradient that winds into the heart of the Long Mynd, its narrow path hugs the side of the hill with, at times, nothing between you and a drop to certain death. With peaks above and valley below it's impossible not to love this

road: just don't look up how fast Boardman rode up it – it defies comprehension. Once you reach the top that's the last of the three real killers in the bag, but there is still one ascent of the Long Mynd we've not ticked off yet, so it would be sacrilege to leave without tackling that too.

Head back down Asterton Bank, making sure to keep a check on your speed. Retrace your steps back through Wentnor to Ratlinghope, then, just before arriving in the village, turn

right, following the signs to Church Stretton. There's nothing particularly easy about this climb, but it is a degree kinder than its peers as it winds up through the barren moors between the interlocking hills. You can never spend too long on the Long Mynd, but now the ride is almost at an end. Drop back down The Burway once more, take one last look out over those glorious hills, then ride into Church Stretton to consume your own weight in food.

ABOVE *Not much beats The Burway on a sunny day.*

DISTANCE	107KM
CLIMBING	+2,550M
DIFFICULTY	8/10

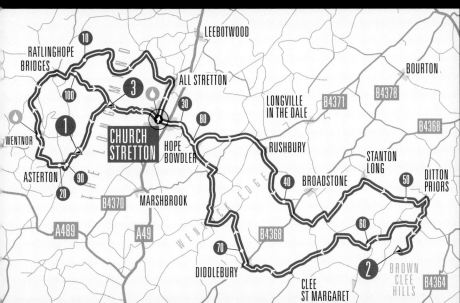

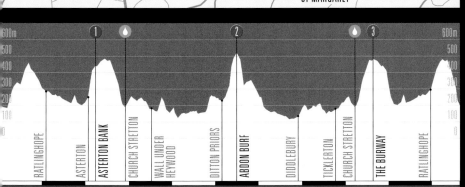

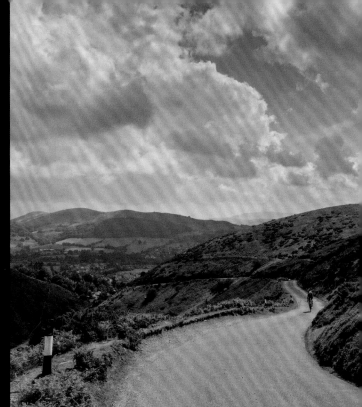

KEY CLIMBS

1 ASTERTON BANK
960m +163m

I can hear the groans from here, yes Asterton Bank. Home to more horror stories, feet going down, minds and bodies broken than almost any other climb. Its wicked slopes which AVERAGE 17% are a proper challenge, but the views are more than worth the effort when you do get to the top.

2 ABDON BURF
1,850m +208m

The first part of this climb is pure madness: it defies all road-building logic which is also why it's so amazing. Drag yourself up the 800 metres of 20% gradient and you'll be transported to a secret world with unparalleled 360-degree views out over the whole of the Shropshire Hills.

3 THE BURWAY
3,060m +290m

A contender for most beautiful climb in England, certainly the Midlands, The Burway is also one of the hardest. It kicks up violently out of Church Stretton and before long is hugging the hillside on a 20% slope with a vertical bank one side and a precipitous drop the other.

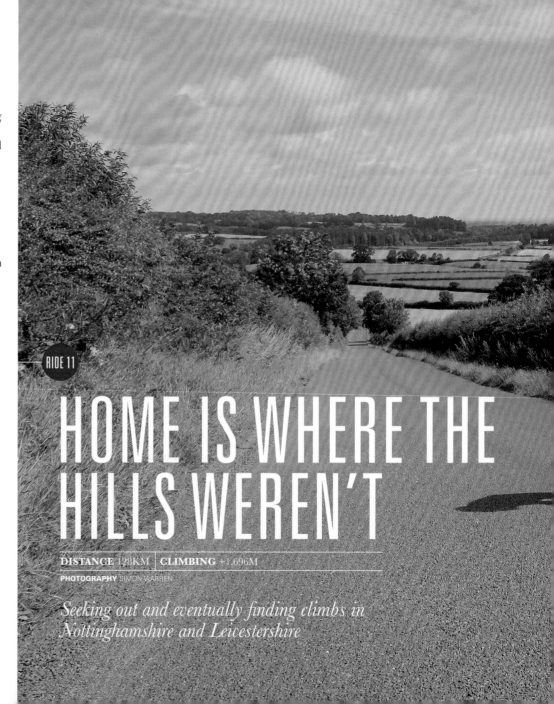

My early years as a cyclist were spent seeking out hills wherever I could find them, with each ride a quest to check out a road I had spotted on the map, to see if it lived up to expectation. Unfortunately, growing up on the border of Nottinghamshire and Lincolnshire, I really didn't find much on offer – until, that is, I discovered the Vale of Belvoir, or, to be more accurate, the hills that lie just south of it. Following my Uncle David's advice, I headed south one weekend with my mate Nick on a then galaxy-spanning 25-kilometre trek, and what we found would become our Disneyland. There were hills, loads of them! and over the coming months we rode them all. We would always take the same route there, for it was not the journey we were bothered with but the destination, and the chance to tackle this alien terrain. As a tribute to those rides, and to throw in a whole host of treats from that part of the world, I've put together this route around the town of Oakham in the heart of Rutland.

Without delay the course makes a beeline for the hills, heading due north and passing through the villages of Ashwell, Teigh and Edmondthorpe before arriving, after roughly 11 kilometres, at Wymondham Windmill. Home to a café and, believe it or not, a bike shop, this would make an excellent alternative start–finish point if so desired, and is definitely worth considering before you make your plans.

Moving on from the windmill and continuing north, the rolling course gradually gains altitude

RIDE 11

HOME IS WHERE THE HILLS WEREN'T

DISTANCE 128KM | **CLIMBING** +1,696M

PHOTOGRAPHY SIMON WARREN

Seeking out and eventually finding climbs in Nottinghamshire and Leicestershire

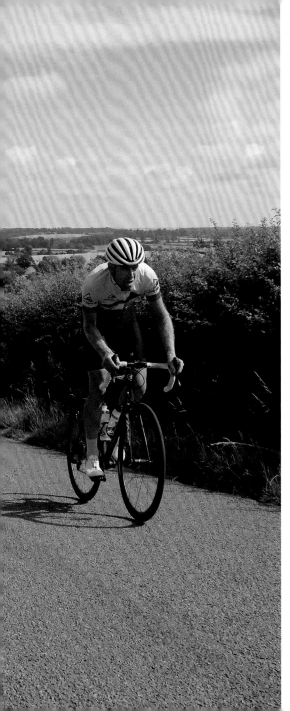

LEFT *Lings Hill out of Branston, we only used to climb it to race back down.*

until you reach Croxton Banks, where the more pronounced undulations begin, with a rapid drop down through Harston to Woolsthorpe By Belvoir. Turning left at the crossroads, you head up the sublime rise between the grand avenue of trees that line the road on the approach to Belvoir Castle. Having occupied the hill on your left since Norman times, the current incarnation was completed in 1832 and is a spectacular sight to come upon via the gently arcing road. When you reach the junction at the entrance to the castle grounds, home to the wonderful Café Allez, the views to the north stretch out over the River Trent and on to Nottingham. With just 30 kilometres covered it may be too early for a stop, but extra fuel before the flurry of hills ahead may help you defeat them.

A typical ride out to Belvoir 'back in the day' would include a choice of at least two, ideally three, little climbs, but would always, without fail, include Terrace Hill. This pint-sized beast is not only the first 'proper' hill I ever rode, but was also the setting for the first bike race I won (I haven't won many). Terrace Hill had and still does have a fearsome reputation in the surrounding counties as the toughest test available, and is therefore the default venue for cycling clubs' annual hill-climb competition. On race day, and at the end of a boisterous ride out, as we turned onto the long, straight road perpendicular to the imposing ridge, everyone would go quiet, their nerves starting to jangle in anticipation of the torment ahead.

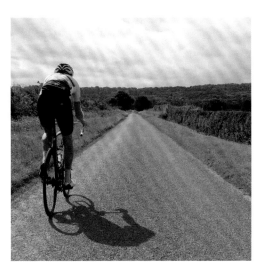

As the asphalt vanishes into the darkness of the wood there is only one way out the other side and, like a long slow walk to the gallows, the prolonged approach gives you plenty of time to contemplate your impending fate.

Of course, I've climbed far worse roads over the years, and for this reason I only awarded Terrace a 1/10 in *100 Greatest Cycling Climbs*, but it's still a decent challenge. And once you've ticked it off, it's time to tackle a couple more in the same area. Dropping back down the ridge through Stathern, you turn left to Harby, then head back up the ridge via Harby Hills. At the northern edge of the Leicestershire Wolds, this is another local hill-climb venue, which boasts

ABOVE *The long and agonising approach to the base of Terrace Hill.*

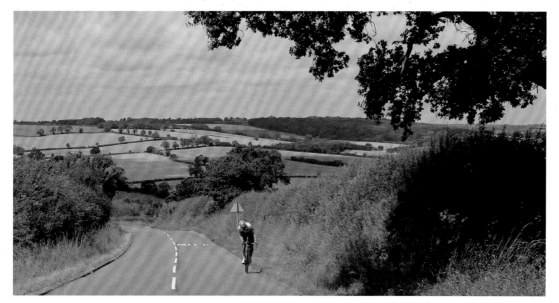

LEFT *King's Hill, the last 'big' lump before home.*

a tasty right-left S-bend towards the top, after which it climbs steeply before easing to the summit. Once over the crest, drop down into Eaton and head towards Branston.

Then, after turning south, you reach the base of one final Belvoir climb, Lings Hill. Straight as an arrow and uniformly steep, this road was where we would go to try and beat our top speed on the way back down. Timed with our old Avocet computers, the magic target was always 50 mph, which we'd aim for, naturally, without a helmet or a care in the world. As this is the last test for the legs for a while give it some welly and, if you fancy yourself as a speed demon, by all means head back down, but remember you'll have to climb it all over again.

With the delights of Belvoir behind you and four decent, albeit modest, climbs in the legs, it's time to pick your way south to tackle more treats hidden in the Leicestershire lanes. Unfortunately, you must first put up with a couple of kilometres on the busy A607 through the beautiful village of Waltham on the Wolds, but you are soon back on the quiet roads to continue through Stapleford, Somerby and Owston on the way to Launde Abbey.

With the majority of the route sandwiched between high hedgerows, the landscape around the Elizabethan manor makes for a dramatic change, as the scenery opens up to reveal the small grass-covered basin. Winding through this clearing, populated by marauding sheep and giant trees, the narrow road leads you to the base of the next pint-sized hill, which transports you from the calm oasis back to normality. Continuing further south, it's now on to the final

two targets of the day, Nevill Holt Road and, to finish off the ride, the wonderful King's Hill. Before you reach them, there's a whole slew of tiny ramps to contend with, most notably those into the village of Belton-in-Rutland and, following that, Hallaton Road, rising out of Allexton after the crossing of the A47. Passing through Hallaton, then Medbourne, the route reaches its southernmost tip in the village of Drayton before turning hard left.

Having just navigated the base of the mound you are about to cross, you will have had plenty of time to size it up before you head north for the summit outside the gates of Nevill Holt Hall. This grand building has sat proudly on top of the hill above the surrounding landscape since the 1300s, in one guise or another, but after sharing its commanding view for a few seconds it's time to rocket back down the other side. Joining the B664, make your way via Stockerston, and then get ready to throw whatever you have left in your legs at the final challenge of the day, King's Hill. With its pair of 90-degree bends towards the top, the first boasting some pretty stiff gradients, you climb for over 1,500 metres in total before the road levels on the run in to Uppingham. Although that was the final 'big' hill, there are still three more slightly trivial peaks to cross via Ridlington and Brooke.

The ride ends, as all good rides should, with a long, fast descent, which takes you home to Oakham with proof that, if you look, and are maybe given some help, you'll find hills wherever you live.

RIDE 11 — MIDLANDS

BELVOIR AND RUTLAND

DISTANCE	128KM
CLIMBING	+1,696M
DIFFICULTY	1/10

FOOD & WATER | BELVOIR CASTLE / WALTHAM ON THE WOLDS / SOMERBY

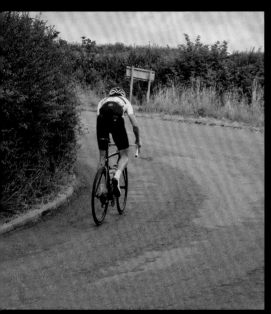

KEY CLIMBS

1 TERRACE HILL

1,083m +83m

Following the long approach the climb rises when you enter the woods. Increasing gradually to its maximum 15% gradient it then bends right then left. Not easing enough to allow you any recovery, the summit arrives as you exit the trees.

2 HARBY HILL

1,200m +76m

A slightly longer ascent than Terrace Hill the key feature of Harby Hill is its twin 15% bends. Bisecting the ascent you want to put the power down here then try and hold your effort until the slope fades to meet the junction at the summit.

3 KING'S HILL

1,950m +90m

As you cross the brook at the base you see the slope rising gradually in front of you increasing in severity as it climbs through a long sweeping bend. Following this is the tight left-hand corner which very briefly hits 20% at its apex before easing all the way to the summit.

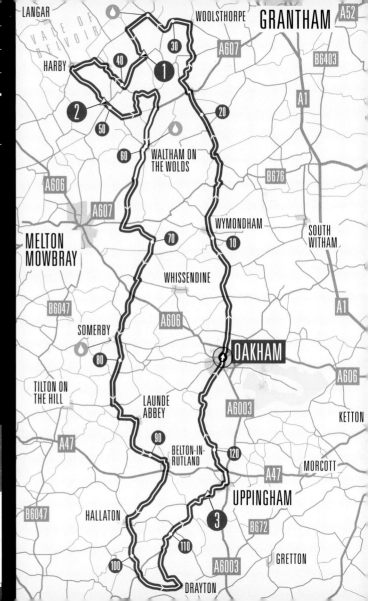

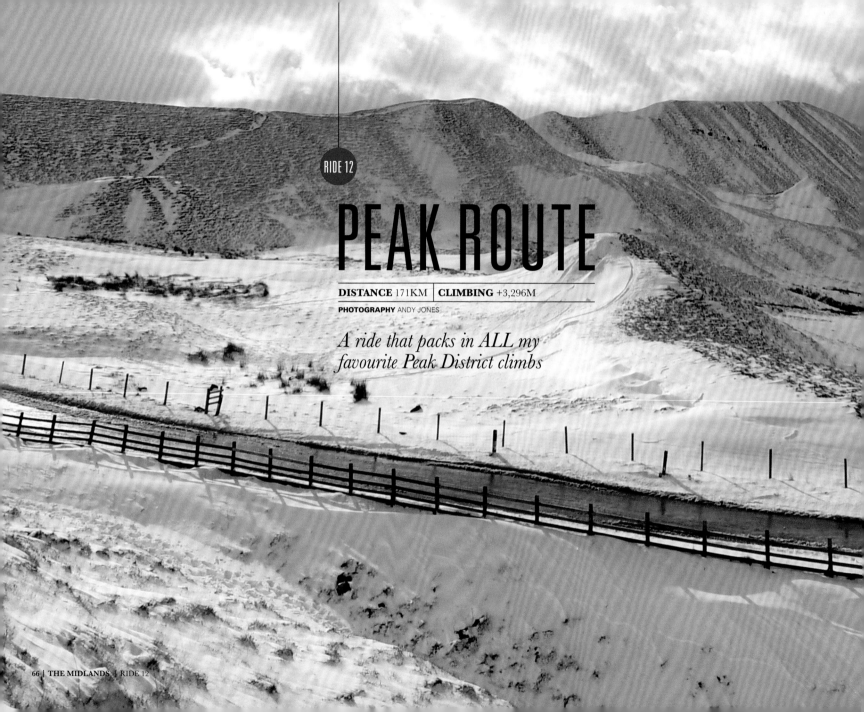

PEAK ROUTE

DISTANCE 171KM | **CLIMBING** +3,296M

PHOTOGRAPHY ANDY JONES

A ride that packs in ALL my favourite Peak District climbs

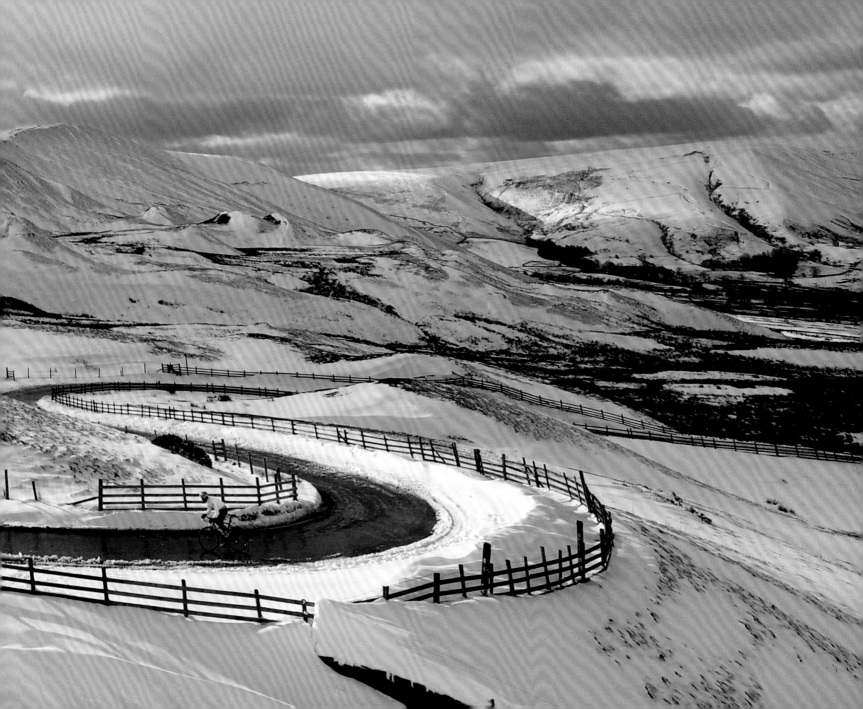

PREVIOUS PAGE
*The curves of Mam Nick are
beautiful in all weathers.*

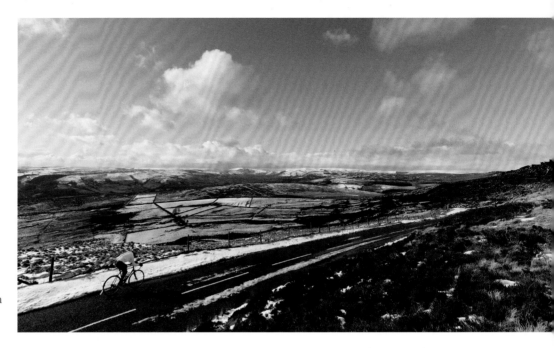

This is a big one. I didn't hold back, cut any corners or leave anything out. It is a proper Tour of the Peak District because there is so much I want to showcase. Before I moved to Sheffield I'd ridden many times in the Peaks and raced up its famous climbs for years, but it was only once I had it on my doorstep that I really got to know it properly, and now I pass that knowledge on to you.

Starting and finishing in Sheffield and, like all rides that head west out of the city, it starts with a huge climb. Like death and taxes there is simply no avoiding this. (Oh, and nine times out of ten it will be into the wind.) I have also chosen the toughest exit route of them all: not for any malicious reasons – it's just practical and direct so we can get right into the heart of the action.

Leaving the Hunters Bar roundabout, head out on the A625, Ecclesall Road, through three sets of lights, then, at a small plateau, turn right onto Knowle Lane. Follow this road to where it becomes Ringinglow Road, and this will take you to the countryside. Climbing in steps in a dead-straight line past the Norfolk Arms pub, you will soon pass the familiar millstone sign announcing the Peak District and emerge on top of Burbage Moor. For the first year I lived in Sheffield I couldn't pass this point without stopping to take a photo. I simply couldn't believe that, just a few minutes away from the bustling city, I could be surrounded by such simple, stunning beauty. Why did I not move here earlier! Traversing the top of the exposed moor takes you into

Derbyshire, then, beyond Higger Tor, descend the road known as 'Fiddler's Elbow' to join the A6187 into Hathersage.

Once you're out of town again you'll find yourself in the most bizarre of Peak District places: a flat road. It runs the length of the Hope Valley and, by my reckoning, is the only one. You want to follow it all the way into the village of Hope, where you turn right into Edale. The Edale Road takes you on a steady upward trajectory through the quiet valley to the town of Barber Booth, and the base of the first killer climb of the day: the amazing Mam Nick. A series of sweeping bends beneath the towering hills, Mam Nick is set amid some of the best scenery the Peaks have to offer, but if

your journey through the Edale Valley has to this point been calm and gentle, now you have to escape it, and you'll need to work very hard.

Once through the 'Nick', at the top drop down, then turn right onto Sheffield Road for the long fast descent along Rushup Edge, and bypass Chapel-en-le-Frith by riding through Wash to join the A624 to Glossop. There are three stinging peaks to cross in the next 14 kilometres, all of which will weaken your legs slightly, but take it easy, as you want to save your best for bigger battles ahead. In Glossop, turn right at the crossroads, and it's time for the Snake Pass.

Now, this is easily one of the most beautiful and dramatic roads in England. The trouble is, it can get a bit busy, and many people see its luscious

ABOVE *Heading down from
Burbage Moor towards the
snow-covered High Peak.*

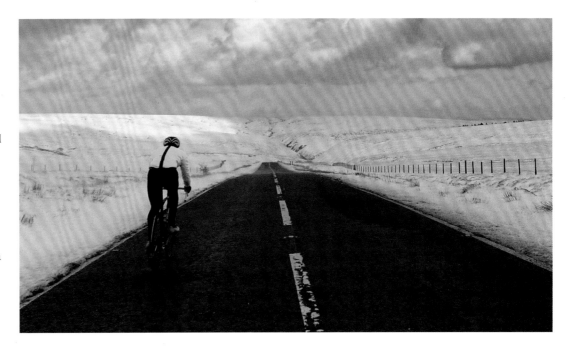

curves not as a thing of beauty but as a challenge for their driving skills (or lack of), so keep your eyes and ears open for idiots. Always the first road to be closed if it snows, this major link between Manchester and Sheffield literally snakes across the moors, tops out at over 500 metres altitude, then rockets back down the other side to the shores of the Ladybower reservoir. This descent through the conifers is, in my opinion, as close as you can get to an Alpine descent in England: twisting, fast and 16 kilometres long, it will leave a smile on your face for hours afterwards.

At the bottom, turn south over the reservoir and follow the A6013 through Bamford back to the Hope Valley once more. Turning west, you'll again arrive in Hope, but this time press on straight through to Castleton – either village would be ideal for a stop at about half distance. I warn you, though: don't take on too much ballast, as up next is the hardest climb on the route, and one of the toughest in Britain. Yes, it's time for Winnats Pass.

Nothing compares to the drama of Winnats. No other road in England can hold a torch to its sheer in-your-face wow factor, as the narrow path soars through the towering limestone cleft. Starting to climb the moment the route leaves the main road, and shooting up ever more steeply, it is always a challenge, and you'll often come across someone wearing their shoe cleats out having succumbed to its relentless 20% slopes. But look around you: unique in character and devilish of gradient, Winnats is a true star

of a road which must be enjoyed no matter what pain it dishes out, as you grind past the cattle grid, over the brow, to continue westward.

After a short descent, turn south in Perryfoot into Perry Dale, and follow this road to Peak Forest. Then cross the A623, still heading south, until you turn left onto Wheston Bank to head for Tideswell. Go through this village to Litton, then turn south again on Bottomhill Road to Cresbrook, before dropping down the foot of Monsal Dale. Give yourself a minute to enjoy the calm of the valley road, then get ready to take on the climb at the end.

The venue for the annual Monsal Head hill climb, one of the must-watch and must-ride events on the calendar, this seemingly

insignificant road has seen epic battles since the race was first run back in 1930. From the top, head east through Little Longstone into Great Longstone, where you then turn north to take on Longstone Edge. A long climb, and pretty tough on its lower slopes, it reveals, once you escape the trees on its upper reaches, another of my favourite views in the Peaks. Over the summit, follow Moor Road all the way to the A623; turn right, take the immediate left to pass through Foolow and Grindlow, and then continue north on the B6049. Coming up next is a road that, until I moved north, had remained off my radar, and would have been a worthy entry in any of my climbing guides – and, boy, did I miss a beauty of a climb.

ABOVE *Snake Pass is always the first road in the Peak to be shut if it snows. We were lucky.*

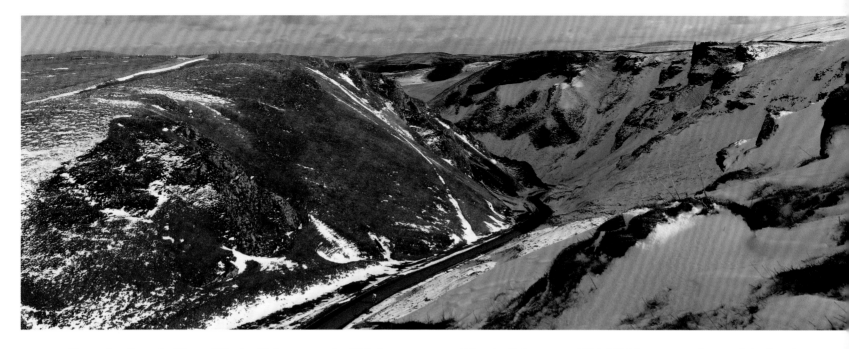

Known locally as the 'Beast of Bradwell', it is a real killer. First, head through the village of Bradwell, and then take the left turn onto Town Lane. Then go left again onto Small Dale, engage your smallest gear and get ready for a fight. A simple straight lane, it takes you in the most direct route back to the top of the ridge, with a wonderful brace of tiny bends at the midway point to spice things up a little more.

Once at the top, carry straight on, then follow the road as it loops back east and down Pindale Road towards Castleton. Don't ride all the way into the village, but instead take the first right to cut the corner to Hope and get back to the now very familiar Hope Valley Road. You'll be glad to be back, because you know it offers you a little

respite. This time you want to follow it all the way into Hathersage, where you could maybe make a second stop before you get stuck into the final flurry of climbs.

Heading south out of town where the B6001 reaches a brow at Leadmill, turn right onto the climb many locals call their favourite: Abney Road. A 6-kilometre ascent, set on an undulating slope which finishes at the open fields that are home to the Derbyshire and Lancashire Gliding Club, Abney is a joy to ride from bottom to top. Once over the summit, turn left towards Bretton, then drop down through Eyam to the A623, and follow this to Calver. Saving a real brute for last, turn off the main road and, passing the Bridge Inn, you find yourself at the base of Curbar Edge.

With 150 kilometres under your belt, there is no question you'll be pushed to the edge by this one, but it's the last serious hill before the finish, if that's any consolation. Hitting 1-in-6 almost straight away, and rarely dropping below it, you ride up to and through the village of Curbar, then turn left to face the rock edge that gives the climb its name, always covered with adrenaline junkies of various persuasions. Aim straight for them, then bend right to search out the summit.

Ouch. You've done it. Well, almost. There's still a slight climb on the run back into Sheffield on the A621 to Owler Bar but, once that is crossed off, it's all downhill to complete my Tour of the Peak.

Wait: did I miss anything out . . .?

ABOVE *If you thought Winnats Pass wasn't already dramatic enough, just add a dusting of snow.*

RIDE 12

THE MIDLANDS
HIGH PEAK

DISTANCE 171KM

CLIMBING +3,296M

DIFFICULTY 9/10

FOOD & WATER | GLOSSOP / HOPE / HATHERSAGE

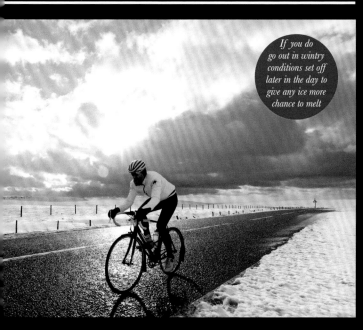

If you do go out in wintry conditions set off later in the day to give any ice more chance to melt

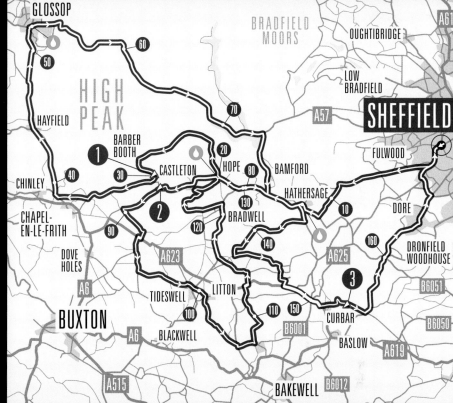

KEY CLIMBS

1 MAM NICK
1,983m +196m

The most beautiful climb in the Peak, this curvaceous beauty is set on an average gradient of 9% as it winds up from Edale in the shadow of Mam Tor. The slope is far from uniform and spikes at close to 20% in a number of places, most notably right at the bottom to give your a proper thumbing

2 WINNATS PASS
1,707m +197m

I make the start of the climb of Winnats Pass as the turn off the A6187 just out of Castleton. From here the gradient creeps up gradually until you reach the entrance to the Blue John Caves and find you have run out of gears just as the final kilometre of 20% starts to bite.

3 CURBAR EDGE
1,780m +187m

With a 10% average Curbar Edge has a fearsome reputation and is the least-used route back to Sheffield from the Peak. With 16% stretches into the village of Curbar then following a slight hiatus some more out the other side it will be a real treat for sore legs at the end of this route.

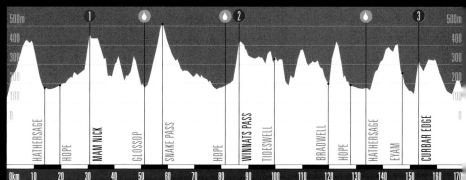

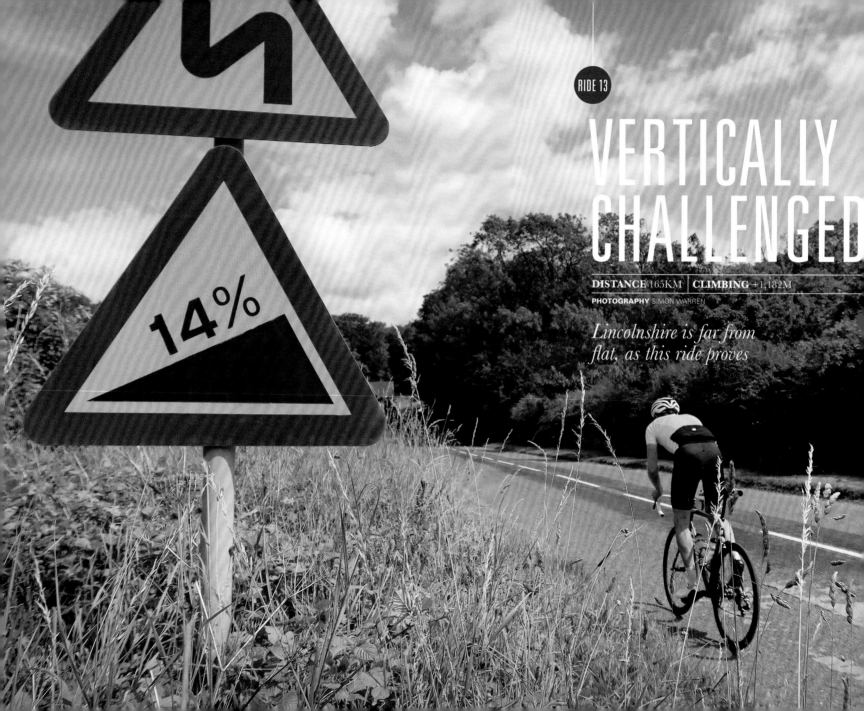

VERTICALLY CHALLENGED

DISTANCE 165KM | **CLIMBING** +1,182M

PHOTOGRAPHY SIMON WARREN

Lincolnshire is far from flat, as this ride proves

In a book of hilly bike rides you may be surprised to see an entry in Lincolnshire, a county with a reputation of being somewhat vertically challenged, but it is far from being so. On a tour which doubles as a spotter's guide to the county's steep-gradient signs, this route takes you through the Wolds and across the Fens, returning via the Lincoln Cliff to deliver you to arguably the most famous cobbled climb this side of Belgium. An AONB, comprising a group of open, steep-sided valleys, the Wolds are criss-crossed by loads of quiet roads just waiting to be ridden.

I spent my formative years as a cyclist tackling these roads, battling the ubiquitous headwinds and searching for scraps of gradient among the vast expanse of barren fields. My early memories of riding are of being dropped off the back of reliability rides, and of having to call home from unknown petrol stations to be picked up, once the owners had explained to my dad where I actually was. I suffered, but more importantly learned to suffer, in Lincolnshire, and, as I will always have a soft spot for the county this ride is my tribute to its varied terrain, and showcases many of the delights it has to offer.

The obvious base for the ride is Lincoln itself, a quaint, sleepy city boasting some of the most beautiful – oh, and steep (more on that later) – streets in the land. As you head out north, what little congestion there is soon fades and, once you're free of the A158, the next 30 kilometres are spent in the peaceful lanes heading north-east towards Market Rasen. Through Scothern, Stainton by Langworth, Snelland, Wickenby and Linwood, the pancake-flat profile won't do anything to trouble your legs, but soon there is the welcome sight of the first hills on the horizon. Once through Market Rasen (a good place for supplies if you need any), you run parallel to the ridge on your right, then turn towards Claxby to face up to your first foe, Normanby Rise.

It's unlikely you'll have heard any horror stories about this lump, and rightly so, as in the grand scheme of things it is hardly exceptional. In the context of its surroundings, however, it presents more than a worthy challenge. Rising steeply, then bending sharp left, before easing right between tall grass banks topped with high hedgerows, it is a stiff climb for Lincolnshire, and one that boasts outstanding views. A perfect example of how even modest elevation gain can rapidly open up the landscape, it takes you to the summit, Wolds Top, which is, for the record, the highest point anywhere in eastern England. Marking the summit is the imposing NATS (National Air Traffic Services) radar installation which, if you've been keeping your eyes peeled, you will have spotted many kilometres away as you approached. Its large white dome is omnipresent on the skyline as you navigate the lanes, spying on you from its perch in the middle of the small clump of rolling hills.

Ignoring the turn to the dominating radar dome, continue north and, following the rapid

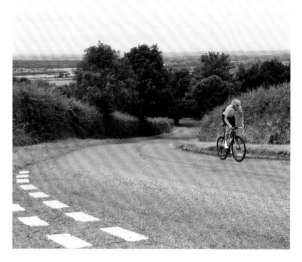

plunge down into Nettleton, it's time for the second ascent of the day, Mansgate Hill. A degree kinder than Normanby Rise, this short, straight ramp takes you immediately back to the high ground, where it joins the B1225 at its summit. Rolling along the exposed tops and now heading south, you'll see the land on both sides of the road drifts away into gullies and clefts, their contours draped with a covering of coarse grass.

To squeeze another climb out of the Wolds (it would be rude not to), the route next drops down Walesby Hill into the village and then, heading further south, reaches the B1203 just below Tealby. Ascending into and through this village, Papermill Lane merges into Bully Hill to climax with a stiff right-hand bend which, at its

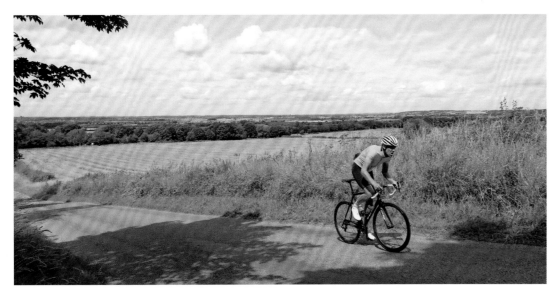

conclusion, boasts a 1-in-7 gradient sign. Such triangular warnings are rare in Lincolnshire, so you know you've tackled (or are about to face) a worthy adversary if you come across one and, as advertised, Bully Hill finishes with a bang.

It's now time to leave the Wolds and commence what is essentially 30 kilometres of gradual descent, passing through East Barkwith (where there is an excellent little shop), Wragby, Kingthorpe and Bardney, before crossing the River Witham to reach the northern tip of the Lincolnshire Fens.

The Fens are what instinctively come to mind when you think of the county, so it would be a shame not to include in this ride a small taster of the spirit-level-flat, featureless landscape. The moment the horizontal, stark and, for us climbers, essentially pointless roads end it's time to thankfully gain some elevation again, as the

route kicks up following the 90-degree right turn in Wasps Nest. For the following 30 kilometres the trajectory of the course continues upwards, albeit slightly, to arrive just above Leadenham on top of the Lincoln Cliff. Running almost 50 miles in length, from the Humber to the boundary of Leicestershire, this sharp edge offers up a plethora of short, sharp hills all boasting magnificent views out over the Vale of Trent.

First up out of the remaining climbs I've worked into this ride is Quarry Lane, a surprisingly nasty beast that kicks up with little deviation from the A607 back to the summit of the ridge, increasing in gradient as it rises. Your legs should now be starting to sting a little as they anticipate the rest of the day's challenges. There are any number of permutations I could have chosen to shoehorn in a handful of the little ramps on this ridge and, from those on offer, I

picked Castle Lane into Boothby Graffoe and, following that, Station Road into Harmston. Both are marked on the OS Landranger map with the infamous black arrow, denoting a 'sharp gradient', and the ascent into Harmston is also bestowed the honour of a 14% warning sign. Neither climb is overly long, at just a few hundred metres, and both can be attacked pretty much full gas from bottom to top but, now you have 140 kilometres in your legs, they will both hurt.

For the finale in Lincoln no trip would be complete without taking in the famous cobbles of Michaelgate, the star in the route of the Lincoln Grand Prix bike race. Hidden, though, in the heart of the ancient city – which is as hard to penetrate as it must have been in medieval times – it isn't easy to find. Once the tangle of roads has been negotiated and you reach Hungate, you'll then see Michaelgate break right ahead, so get ready to rumble. Not to be confused with the even steeper, yet pedestrianised, Steep Hill next door, Michaelgate is all the same a punishing climb, which throws your bike left and right as it hits the rugged stones. At the top of the first ramp you arrive at an opening: be sure to turn left, and not ride straight on into the pedestrian zone. That way you don't run people down, and also follow the same course as the famous Lincoln GP race. Where the tarmac returns, head right back onto the cobbles once more to finish the ride, dwarfed by the shadow of the giant Lincoln Cathedral. See, I told you Lincolnshire wasn't flat.

ABOVE *Quarry Lane, the first of four ascents of the Lincoln Cliff.*

RIDE 13 — THE MIDLANDS

LINCOLNSHIRE

DISTANCE 165KM
CLIMBING +1,182M
DIFFICULTY 3/10

FOOD & WATER | MARKET RASEN / WRAGBY / BARDNEY / LEADENHAM

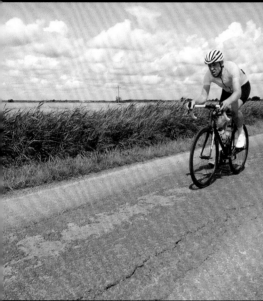

KEY CLIMBS

1 NORMANBY RISE

1,438m +105m

A mere pimple, but arguably the toughest climb in the Lincolnshire Wolds averaging 7% across its length. Climbing gradually steeper up to the 90 degree bend it's here that it hits its maximum gradient of 12%.

2 QUARRY LANE

1,000m +54m

The first of the four climbs up the Lincoln Cliff you start by leaving the A607 from where you will see the whole climb in front of you. Once you begin it ramps up steeper and steeper for 600 metres until it reaches almost 15% before then fading to the T-junction.

3 MICHAELGATE

249m +33m

'Judge me by my size, do you?' It may be only 250 metres long but underestimate Michaelgate at your peril. This famous little cobbled street has dished out more pain than I have had hot dinners and with 100 miles in the legs you need all your power to beat it.

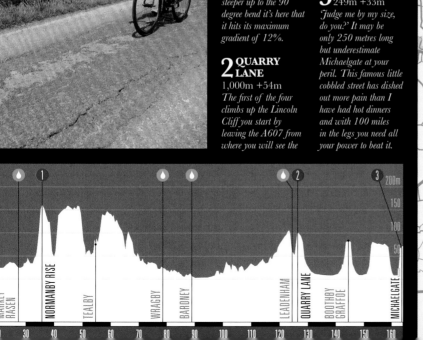

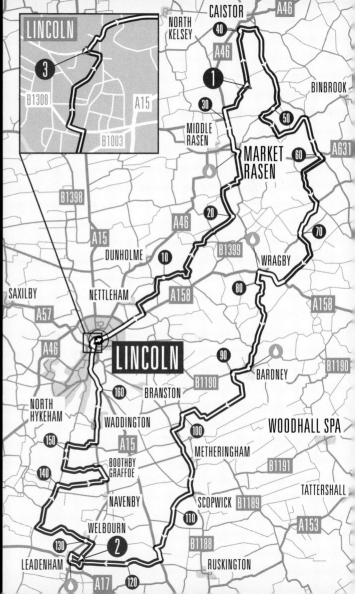

'll always have a great affection for the north Norfolk coast because, long before I rode a bike around its sleepy lanes, this is where my childhood holidays were spent. My dad being an ornithologist meant many a weekend or summer break was spent on the beach, or in the marshes, spying on the local avian life. Ah, the memories of gruelling treks to spend hours of total silence in dusty hides full of twitchers, who would give me the look of death if I so much as breathed loudly. Although as a child I wasn't a fan of life in the hide, I did enjoy the hunt – not to kill, but to catch a glimpse of, birds such as the elusive bittern. To this day I can't walk or ride down to the coast without scanning the marshes, just in case I see its elongated beak poking out between the reeds.

Aside from being a birdwatching Mecca, it's a wonderful place to ride a bike, with a myriad of quiet roads, their verges lightly dusted with fine, white sand. The high hedgerows, ornate town signs, flint-covered buildings and picturesque villages with a penchant for scarecrows make this a simply beautiful place to be.

Whereas pretty much all of Norfolk is flat (bar a few hills in and around Norwich), the north coast has a single raised ridge that runs from Hunstanton to Mundesley which is crossed by a plethora of steep little hills. Starting from the ever-popular market town of Holt, the goal when plotting this route was to accumulate 1,000 metres of climbing over 100 kilometres of distance – yes, in Norfolk. Having tweaked and pulled the course

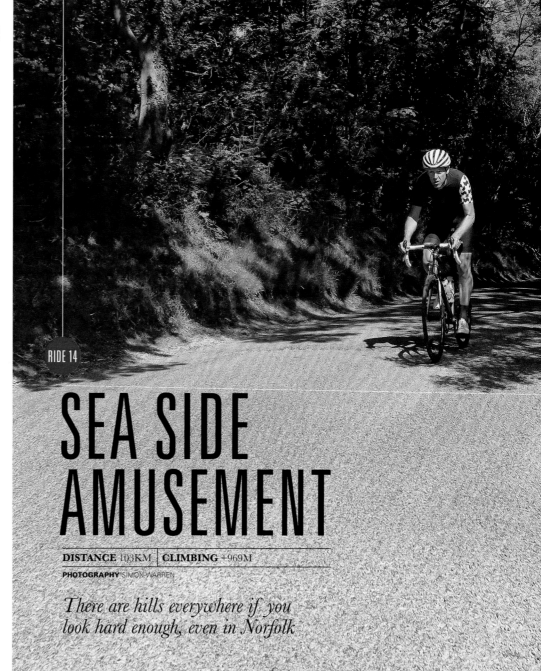

RIDE 14

SEA SIDE AMUSEMENT

DISTANCE 103KM | **CLIMBING** +969M

PHOTOGRAPHY SIMON WARREN

There are hills everywhere if you look hard enough, even in Norfolk

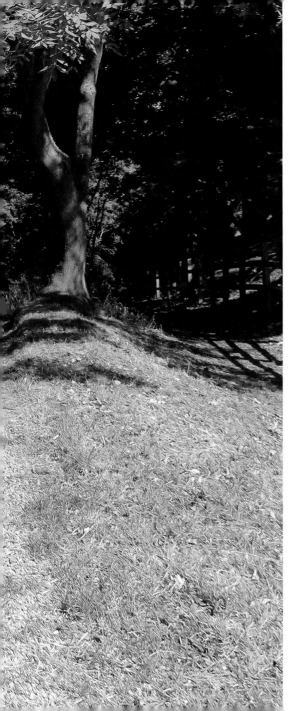

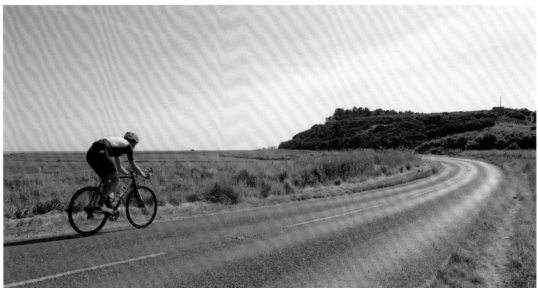

this way and that, and without repetition, I've got as close as I think is possible to the target, with a respectable 969 metres of elevation gain, so not far off. Each of the climbs on the route has its own character, and each is a test for the legs. Think of it as an unstructured interval session with sea views and oh-so-fresh air.

To start, head west on the A148 to Letheringsett, then continue west though Saxlingham, Field Dalling and Binham to arrive in Warham. These first 15 kilometres (apart from the climb out of Letheringsett) are predominantly downhill, a nice relaxing opening to help build anticipation for the hills ahead. Turning right in Warham, head north to join the A149, the coast road, and then turn east to the first of the wonderful villages that adorn it, Stiffkey.

It's in Stiffkey where you'll find the base of

the first of seven climbs over the diminutive geographical feature that you'll soon be exceptionally well acquainted with. This opening ramp is a mere 650 metres of 5% slope, but enough to get the blood pumping if you give it some gas. Arriving in Cockthorpe, at the top press on to Langham, turn left to drop back down to the coast, ride into Morston and onto the A149. Entering Blakeney (an excellent spot for crabbing), turn right to climb up Langham Road. Then, at the crossroads, turn left, then left again to drop back once more into the village. Here, turn right and immediate right again, continuing down to Wiveton Bridge, then turn left on the pan-flat road into Cley next the Sea. With its windmill, deli, cafés and craft shops Cley is a jewel of a village, and after 40 kilometres you may be inclined to stop for refreshment before the climbs

ABOVE *The glorious coast road, sea to the north, hills to the south.*

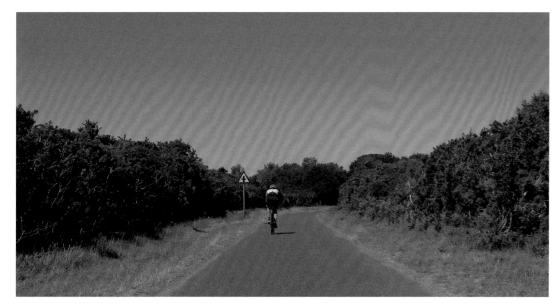

get a little tougher and appear more frequently.

Heading east once more on the coast road, soak up all that sea air, shake the legs a bit and get ready to climb. Up next is my favourite: Bard Hill, a kilometre of testing climbing that averages 6% but is a whole lot steeper in places. Turning south in Salthouse, the road is dead straight, with a lull at half way from where you can give it full beans to the top, before turning left to recover on the descent of Wood Lane into Kelling.

Before you know it, it's time to go again, as you turn right up The Street. Not quite as tough as Bard Hill, this incline delivers you to Bridge Road, where you turn left, then left again down Holgate Hill into Weybourne. Well, almost into Weybourne: you don't quite hit the A149, but take the right just before it, then right again to take on Station Road, which turns into Sandy

Hill Lane. Steady at first, this climb soon rears up into maybe the steepest pitch of any of these tiny but collectively tiring hills.

Turn left to Bodham, then left again via a short rise, before shedding your altitude all the way into the comparatively large town of Sheringham. You'll find supplies here if you need them, but if you don't want to upset the repeated rhythm of up down, up down, head south right away on Holway Road to take on the 'urban' climb up to the A148. After the briefest of excursions on the main road, turn left down Briton's Lane to West Runton to meet the last of this barrage of climbs, Beacon Hill.

The toughest challenge of the day, Beacon Hill was even included on the route of the Tour of Britain one year – not that the professional peloton will have had its feathers ruffled much by its solitary

kilometre of averagely challenging gradient.

Cresting the brow in the woods, keep left, then follow the main road down into the classic seaside town of Cromer. If you can resist the temptation of the arcades and the lure of fish and chips then climb back out of town, past the Royal Cromer Golf Club, along the top of the cliffs to Overstrand. I could tell you a tale of camping on top of these cliffs one summer in a storm, but I don't want to burden you with the nightmares I still have about that night, so we will move on.

Passing through Sidestrand, turn off Cromer Road and head back west on Hungry Hill, and by now you will indeed be hungry if you've not stopped yet; I can guarantee that. More a series of small peaks than a constant climb, this road takes you into Northrepps, from where you continue due east all the way to the B1436. Leave this road to head south to Metton, then back north, this time to climb on the inland side of the ridge up through the woods and return to the top of Beacon Hill.

This somewhat superfluous loop is simply to squeeze that bit more elevation from the area, and it has quite a sharp kick towards the top, where you head left on the main road, then left again to descend through Aylmerton and start the journey home. Passing through Lower Gresham, Lower Bodham and High Kelling, and with all the serious climbing behind you, you can relish these last few undulating kilometres through the impeccable tranquillity of north Norfolk, to finish where you started in the town of Holt.

ABOVE *This network of deathly quiet lanes are simply perfect for cycling.*

THE MIDLANDS

NORTH NORFOLK

DISTANCE 103KM

CLIMBING +969M

DIFFICULTY 2/10

FOOD & WATER | SHERINGHAM / CROMER

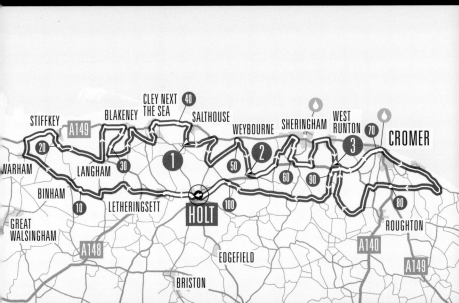

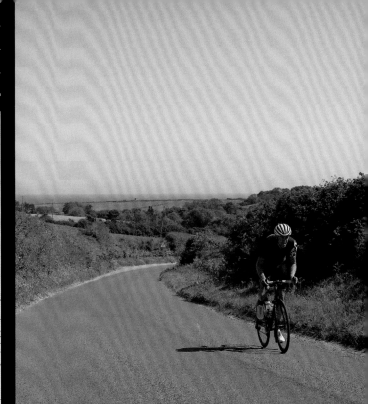

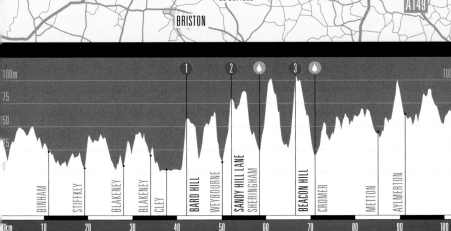

KEY CLIMBS

1 BARD HILL
954m +54m

My favourite of the climbs on this ride Bard Hill is just the perfect little road. The average is 6% but it's much steeper in places. It takes a short while to get going then ramps up close to 10% before easing slightly then resumes on a challenging pitch for another 100 metres before tapering to its summit

2 SANDY HILL LANE
1,594m +66m

The climb starts on Station Road turning south out of Weybourne and the first 1200 metres are very slight. It's when the road turns into Sandy Hill Lane that the gradient kicks in and over the last 400 metres it's proper tasty as the slope ramps up to 15% as it winds towards the top

3 BEACON HILL
1,263m +106m

Climbing a MASSIVE 106 metres this is the toughest climb on the ridge boasting a 5% gradient from bottom to top. The toughest stretch is hidden in the middle of the climb under the cover of the thick canopy of trees where it sits at a maximum of 11% for quite a while

PARADISE FOUND

DISTANCE 105KM | **CLIMBING** +2,601M

PHOTOGRAPHY ANDY JONES

*Heading to the western side of the Peak in
search of beautiful climbs and magical valleys*

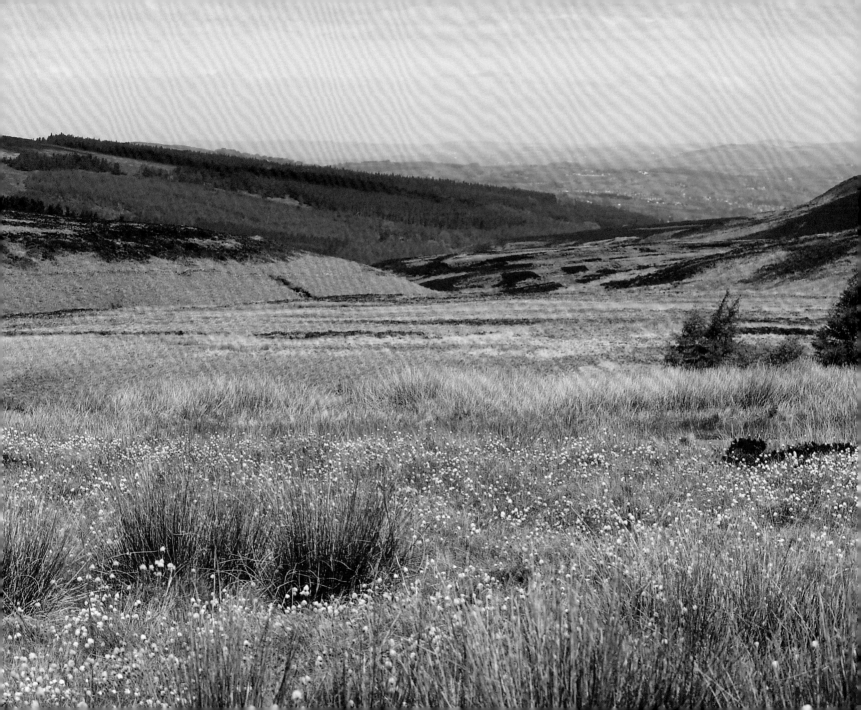

PREVIOUS PAGE
*The magical world that lies at
the top of the Goyt Valley*

Nearly all the riding I've done in the Peak District has been in the northern half around Bakewell, Matlock, Castleton and Hathersage, but there is far more to it than that. Sandwiched between the A515 and A523, the southern Peak is just as full of stunning roads and great climbs as the northern half, as this route proves.

Starting in Leek, the ride wastes no time in its search for altitude, and so immediate is the climb out of town that you may consider bringing your rollers with you to warm up in the car park. Head north-east on the A53, then leave the main road to join Thorncliff Road. Pass through Thorncliff to find yourself on Thorncliff Bank. For 6 kilometres the climb goes up, and it's as steep as 13% in places, so I hope your breakfast is well digested or you may be seeing it again.

After this shock to the system, the ride calms down for a while, as you roll over the top, then take the first right, and then turn right again onto Upper Elkstones. Up high on the exposed hill tops make your way south between the low stone walls, through the village of Upper Elkstone, dropping all the way to the B5053. Turn right here and continue down into the base of the valley, then take the first left turn onto Dog Lane to rise into Butterton. At the top turn left, then first right into the village to join Pothooks Lane. As you Exit Butterton there is a long Ford, so to avoid mishap dismount and walk on the path provided.

Continue on Pothooks Lane to climb across

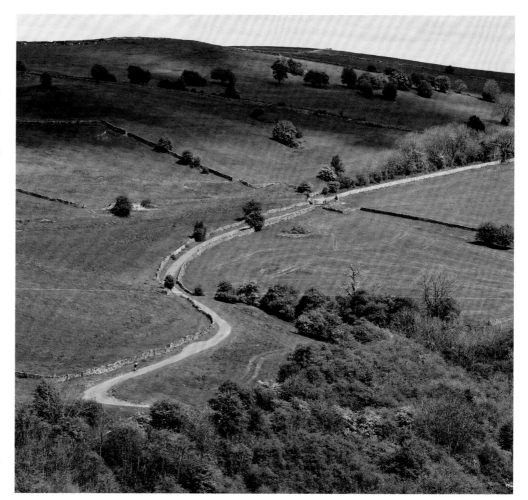

ABOVE *Larkstone Lane
can be seen in all its glory
from across the valley*

Grindon Moor, before turning right, then left, into Grindon village. Continuing east through the village, and dropping down Weag's Bridge Road, it's time to face up to the first signature climb of the day, Larkstone Lane.

From the pit of the Manifold Valley, this wonderful road thrashes its way through two tight bends, over sections of 25% slope, all in its first 500 metres. Trapped between stone walls and intermittent tree coverage the climb heads due east into more long stretches of double-digit gradient, to open up fantastic views out over the rolling hilltops and the snaking passage of the valley below. The summit arrives at the junction with Stable Lane. Turn left here into Wetton, then head right to meet the Alstonefield Road where you head north all the way to the B5054. Turning right, then next left, continue north to climb gradually through Sheen up to Knowsley Cross, then almost into the village of Longnor, before turning right to Crowdicote and, yes, more hairpin bends.

People who live in the Alps may think I'm mad getting over-excited about a couple of sharp corners set on a vicious incline but, as they are as rare as hen's teeth on our small island, you have to shout about them whenever you find them. It's all about the zig and the zag, the climbing back and forth, scaling the mountain side – or in this case the few hundred metres through Crowdicote up the sheer bank, before taking the left-hand turn to Earl Sterndale.

Now, I just love this stretch of road: it's exposed, the skies are huge, and around you the

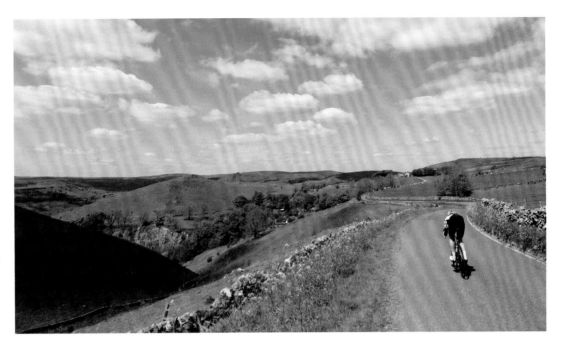

horizon is peppered with tiny grassy hillocks. As you pass first High Wheeldon, then further on Hitter Hill and Parkhouse Hill, the scenery could have you imagining you're riding though Tolkien's Shire rather than Middle England. Above the patchwork of neat fields below, with the odd tree to provide a point of focus, the ever-undulating horizon of smooth grassy lumps is just a joy to behold.

This sublime road continues for some distance, and it's one of those you never want to end, but end it must. Joining the A53, you turn right to race down through Burbage into Buxton. At about bang-on half way this makes a good point to stop if you are in need of refreshment. If not, head directly north out of town on the

A5004 towards Whaley Bridge. First, climbing for 3 kilometres, you are then treated to an 8-kilometre descent down, wait for it, Long Hill.

Long Hill was the venue for the 2011 National Hill Climb Championship but, as it boasts an average gradient of just 3% and competitors that day rode on time-trial bikes with aerobars *in a hill climb*, I have refused to acknowledge it in any of my books, and would never dream of sending a ride up its tame slopes. The descent is a dream, though, all the way into Whaley Bridge, where you turn left on the B5470 towards Kettleshulme.

From the low point of the day's ride, it's time to reclaim some of that lost elevation, and that is achieved by crossing a series of four sharp peaks in a row. The first two, complete with

ABOVE *The Peak District horizon, littered with peaks, naturally.*

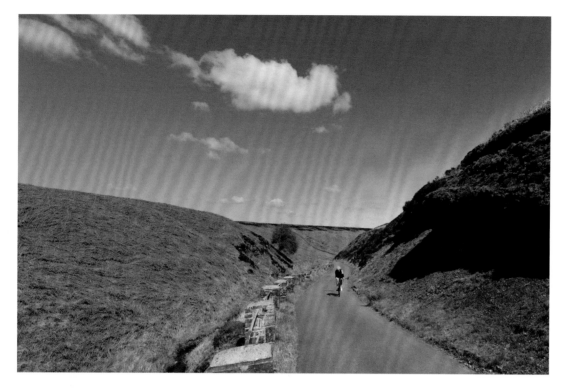

their respective descents on the B-road up and through Kettleshulme, will take you to the top of Blaze Hill, where you turn left onto Pike Road to make your way to the day's toughest challenge: the climb up to Pym Chair. There's one more peak to cross before you arrive, then, dropping down Nab End to Todd Brook, it's time to tighten the toe straps for a beaut of a road.

Also known as Jenkin Chapel, and boasting five severe-gradient arrows on the Ordnance Survey map, this road will make the legs sting as you grind upwards between its high grassy banks in search of the summit. All the effort is worth it,

mind, as, once over the top, you're on your way to a wonderland, and one of the real treasures of the Peak District: the Goyt Valley.

First you descend across the wild moors and into the forest to reach the shoes of the Erwood Reservoir; then, begin the steady climb south, which, and get this, is a one-way road: a 5-kilometre-long one-way road. You may have to contend with traffic from behind but, rest assured, nothing will be coming towards you from here to the top of Goyt's Moss.

At the base of the gently sloping valley sides, butted up against the shore of the lake, the road

begins to rise on an ever-so-shallow pitch, before increasing in difficulty as it enters more wooded surroundings. Twisting through the forest, just wide enough for a single vehicle, this glorious stretch of tarmac keeps progressing upwards. Then, once free of the trees, it will blow your mind. Bisecting the interlocking hills, mimicking every move of the River Goyt a few feet below the exit from the valley, is arguably the most beautiful road in all Derbyshire. Never steep, never hard work, completely dazzling: you'll want to ride it again and again.

At the top turn right, then left, then right to cross the A537, the famous Cat and Fiddle road. Then, heading south-west across the empty moors, take the A54 all the way to Allgreave. After another lengthy downhill, cross Clough Brook, then turn left for a short up-and-over to Wincle. From here, head left to Danebridge and across the River Dane to start the last climb of the day: what is effectively the back route up Gun Hill.

It may have been a stalwart of many a Tour of Britain, but I've never been a fan of Gun Hill from the east. This side is much more interesting, as it winds between farms, through one final hairpin for the day, across 4 kilometres of what is in places serious climbing. Once over the peak there are a couple of tiny blips left to negotiate, but essentially it's downhill now all the way back to Leek. Turning south in Meerbrook, follow Meerbrook Road at the side of the Tittesworth Reservoir, then there's the last of the quiet lanes to meet the A523, where you turn left to end back in town.

ABOVE *Reaching the end of the Goyt Valley, maybe the best one way street in Britain.*

THE MIDLANDS

WHITE PEAK

DISTANCE 105KM

CLIMBING +2,601M

DIFFICULTY 6/10

FOOD & WATER | BUXTON

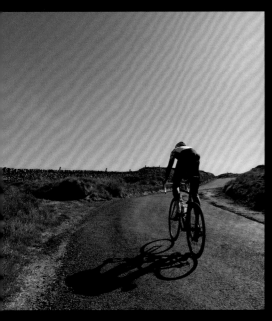

KEY CLIMBS

1 LARKSTONE LANE

1,914m +126m

Rising out of the Manifold Valley this climbs begins with a brace of tight hairpins and slopes that approach 25%. After this violent start the gradient eases a little as you climb between the high stone walls to the summit at Ashbourne Lane.

2 PYM CHAIR

1,477m +160m

Starting the climb as you cross Todd Brook the first ramp takes you up to Jenkin Chapel where there

is a slight rest. From here the profile ramps up gradually until it reaches 20% towards the end as you weave between the high grassy banks to Pym Chair.

3 GOYT VALLEY

4,592m +184m

A long steady climb running north to south with no serious gradient but spectacular scenery. It starts to climb as you reach the end of the Erwood Reservoir meandering through the woods then across open ground all set on a sublime 4% average.

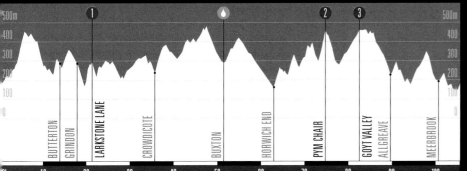

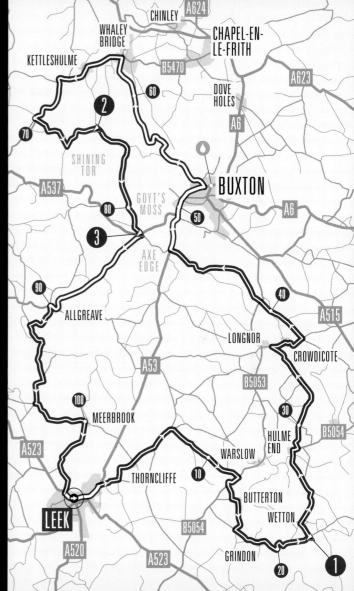

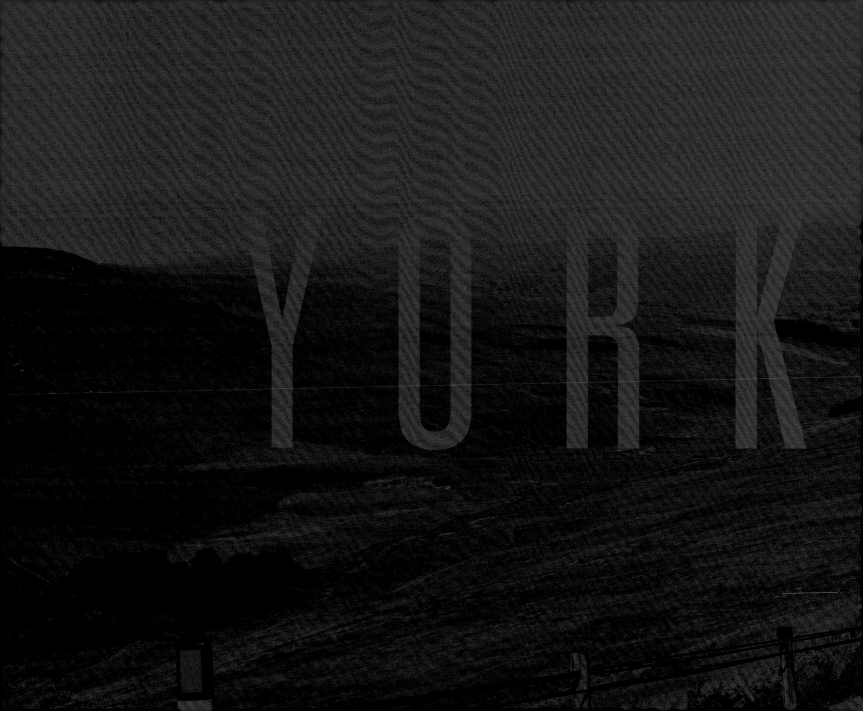

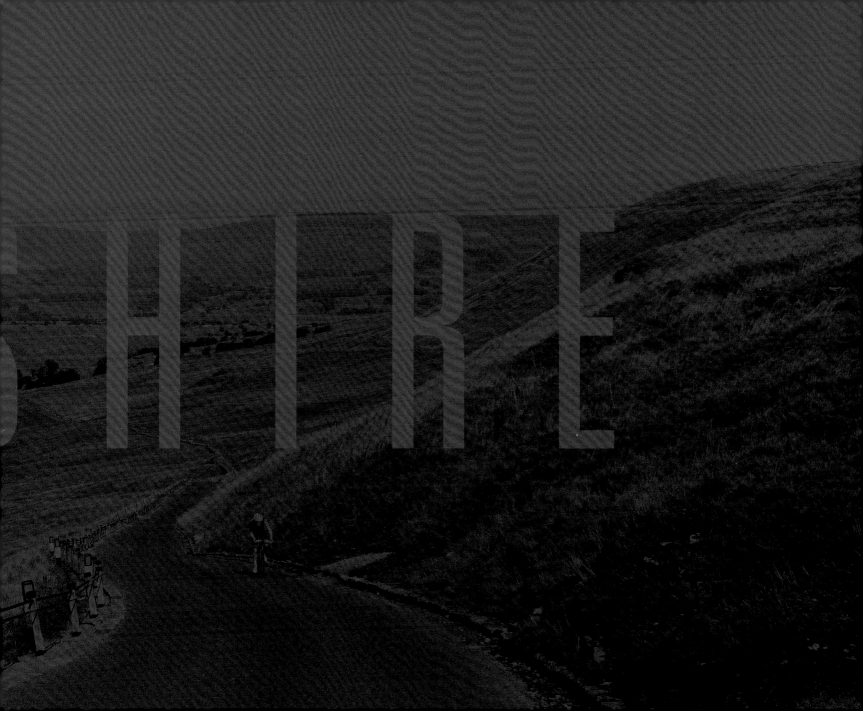

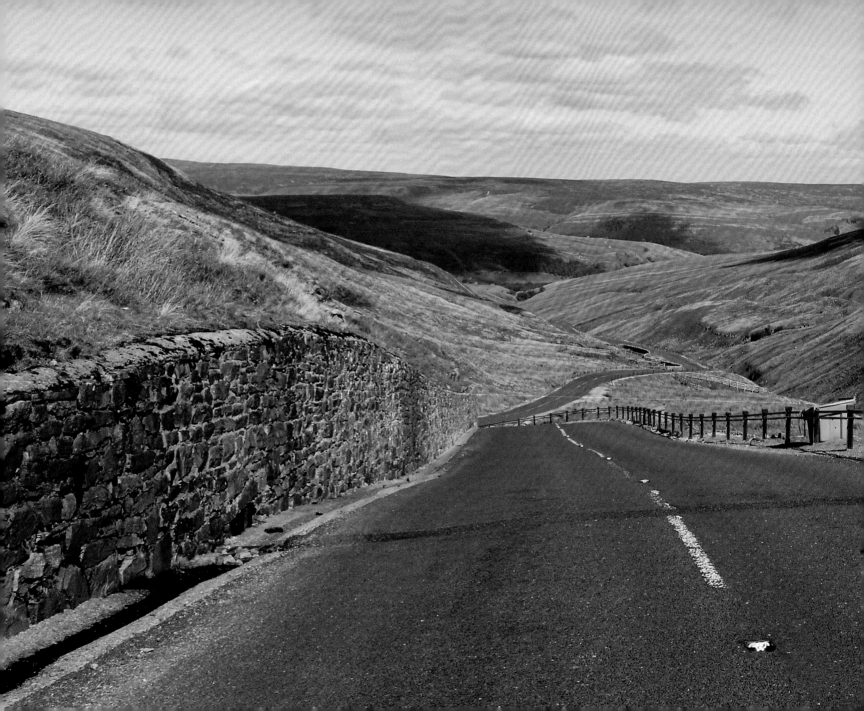

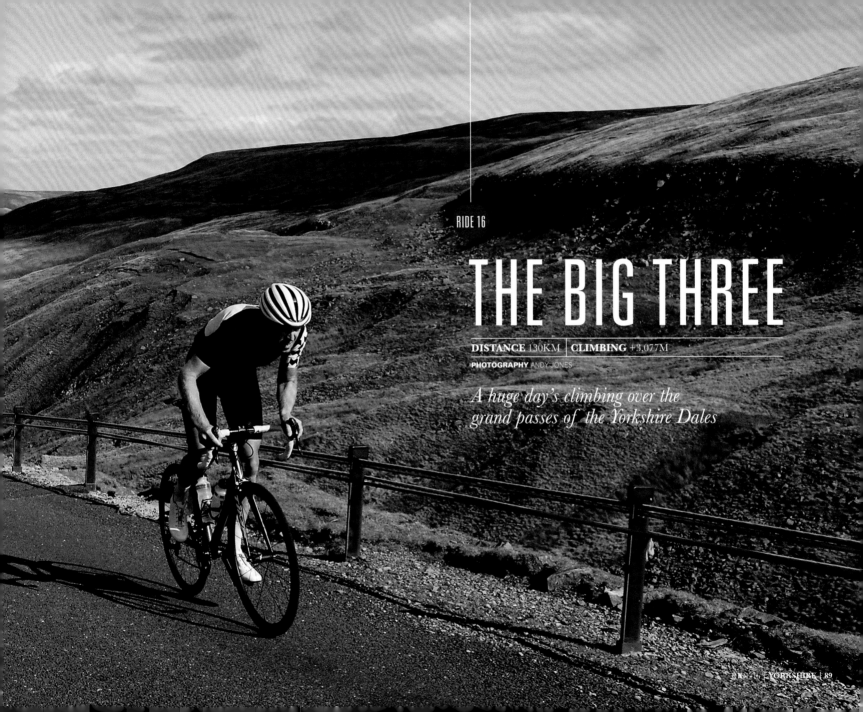

THE BIG THREE

DISTANCE 130KM | **CLIMBING** +3,077M

PHOTOGRAPHY ANDY JONES

A huge day's climbing over the
grand passes of the Yorkshire Dales

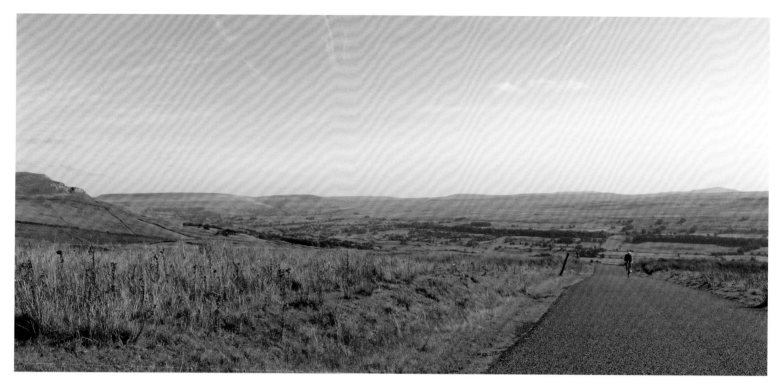

Of all the giant climbs in the Yorkshire Dales three, in my opinion, stand above all others, with an X-factor that, for one reason or another, the rest lack. They are, in no particular order, Buttertubs Pass, Fleet Moss and Park Rash. These fearsome arteries that have linked the Dales for the transport of livestock, produce and people for centuries are naturally the perfect playground for some serious type-two fun of the cycling kind.

Initially I was going to use Hawes as the base for the ride, but the thought of the hate mail I'd receive for sending riders' cold legs straight up Fleet Moss changed my mind, so I picked Leyburn as the start–finish point. It's still uphill right from the off, but on a more sedate gradient, as the route makes its way onto Leyburn Moor and through the Bellerby shooting ranges. As you cross the moors, the first peak of the day is passed as you enter the Yorkshire Dales National Park. Then begins the long descent to Grinton, via the small bridge that was replaced following floods in 2019. In the village, just shy of the junction with the B6270, turn west and take Swale Hall Lane to run south of the river into the depths of the valley. Rising up, then dropping down, your passage delivers you to the foot of the first giant pass of the day (not one of the Big Three), a climb that had slipped under my radar for many years: Fleak Moss.

Neither as abrupt and arduous as Fleet Moss nor as famous as Buttertubs, nor as steep as Park Rash, this climb is arguably more beautiful. The road is quiet, deathly quiet, as it starts its journey, with just a couple of nasty patches of harsh gradient, and also a few small dips to allow you to recover as you traverse Whitaside Moor. The upper slopes are spectacular as the road begins to squirm through the contours of the

PREVIOUS PAGE
*The last ramp of Buttertubs Pass
following the short fast mid-climb descent.*

ABOVE *Giant climbs
and immense views are
everywhere in the Dales.*

hills, revealing vast views out over Swaledale and beyond. Topping out at 541 metres, this is the second-highest point of the day, and it feels like it as you reach the exposed summit, before the twisting descent down the other side.

I should point out at this juncture that all the descents on this ride must be treated with caution: some are more hazardous than others, but all are capable of catching an inattentive rider off guard, so just remember it's work tomorrow and keep your fingers close to the brake levers. Once safely back in Wensleydale, turn immediately right and head north up onto Askrigg Common and the stunning formation of Oxnop Scar. Framing your descent, this large outcrop of rocks dominates the skyline as you plunge down the undulating road once more into Swaledale to start 8 welcome kilometres on the level.

Once you're through Gunnerside and Low Row, this fleeting period of calm comes to a shocking end as ahead – and you'll see it from a mile off – the road breaks left and hits the 20% slopes of Feetham Bank. I know few more abrupt transitions from horizontal to vertical, and this ramp knocks the wind out of your sails as you panic to find a comfortable gear. As you ascend through the woods, the vicious beginning eases once the cattle grid is crossed; then you can continue your quest for the summit at the top of Turf Moor. It's not a straightforward climb, this one, as, following the initial kick up, the profile drops to cross Surrender Bridge, then climbs again, only to fall again soon afterwards, this

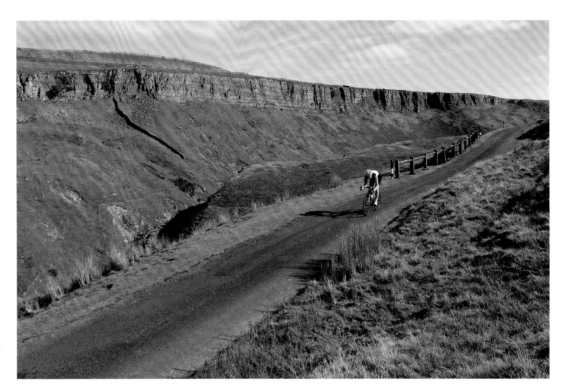

time to cross a notoriously slippery ford.

I'd usually take the bridge here rather than ride through, as it's just wide enough and just unpredictable enough to take your wheels away, but sometimes this isn't an option. Once, during the Etape du Dales, I'd formed an alliance with two very strong riders, both ex-pros, and I just knew they were going to take this obstacle at full gas. I had two choices: wimp out, and lose the quality wheels I was sharing the pace with, or blindly follow them and just hope I made it. On that occasion I went for it and survived, but many don't, and either way, immediately after

this hazard you have the twin hairpins of Fore Gill Gate to contend with, the last hurdle on this tough and eventful climb.

Over the top and into your third dale of the day, Arkengarthdale, and the next climb could not be more different from the last. Turning west, you begin the 10 steady kilometres of the dazzling Tan Hill, across the giant expanse of the moors, to the solitary inn at the summit. In a headwind this climb is hell; in a tailwind – and be warned: they are few and far between – it is pure joy. Famed for its extended 'lock-ins', due to the unpredictability of the weather, the Tan Hill Inn at the summit

ABOVE *Oxnop Scar provides a stunning backdrop for the descent into Swaledale.*

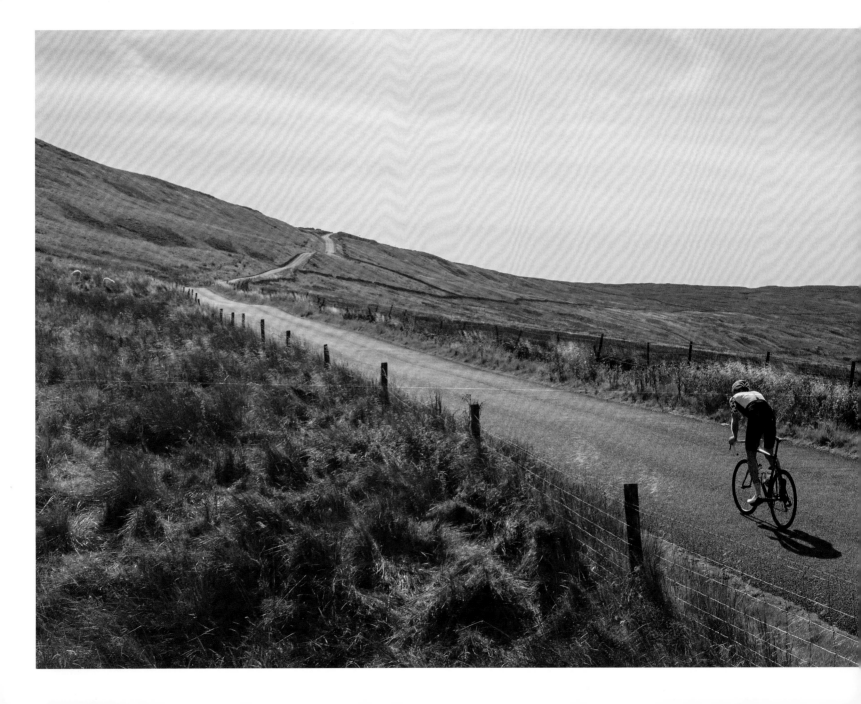

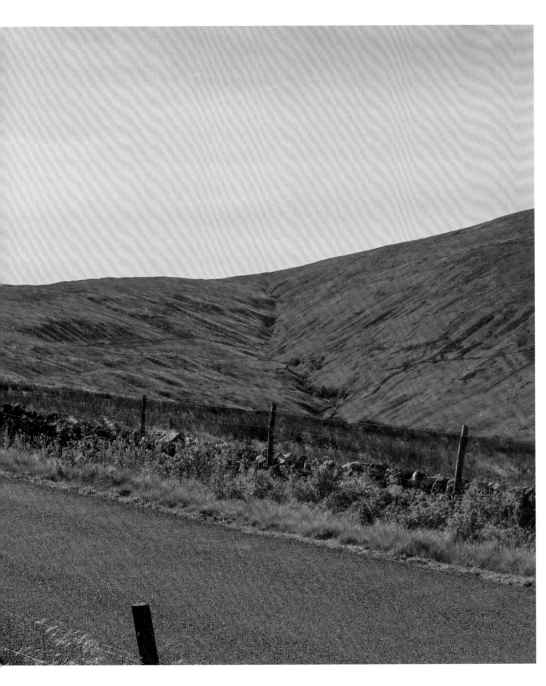

LEFT *The formidable sight of Fleet Moss strikes fear into the hearts of all that approach.*

will welcome your patronage if you need to stop before heading south down to Keld.

Once back again in Swaledale, make your way further south on the B6270 to the base of the first of the 'big three'. Up to this point you will have already climbed 1,790 metres but, and here is the good news, the biggest climbs are still to come! First up it's Buttertubs Pass, which you may have seen during footage of the 2014 Tour de France when it came to visit the dales of Yorkshire. Well, that day the race climbed the easy side out of Hawes; this route, though, takes the tough side, the true Buttertubs Pass.

Lurching up and out of the valley, it packs a killer start, then settles down for a while as it creeps dead straight towards the twin giant bends ahead, carved out of the rock and set on a double-digit gradient. You head right, then left, then right, to a distinct crest that marks a hiatus in the climbing but not the top of the pass. Following a short yet rapid descent, any momentum you gained soon vanishes as you start to pound the final slope to the top. Passing the Buttertubs themselves – 20-metre-deep limestone potholes once allegedly used by travelling farmers to keep their butter cool on the way to market – the road arrives at the summit, set amid the vast splendour of the Yorkshire Dales.

Crossing the expansive moorland and the subsequent descent into Hawes are magical experiences and, once in the valley floor of Wensleydale, the popular village makes a perfect place for a pit stop. Don't get too settled, though,

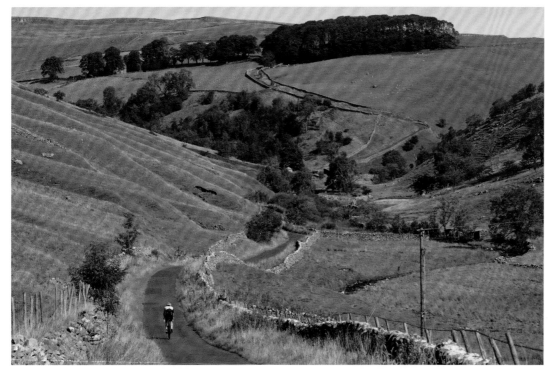

B6160 to Kettlewell. What comes next will have you, with 100 hard kilometres in the legs, screaming for mercy. Before you reach the lowest point there's the harsh climb out of the village to contend with. Then, tracking the path of Can Gill Beck, you make your way to the foot of what in profile looks like a ski jump. Get ready to take on Park Rash.

Turning hard right at the bottom, fight your way to the first 30% corner and pull yourself round – but don't under any circumstances go full gas here, or very soon you'll be in all sorts of trouble. Many times I have made the mistake of going too deep on these initial bends, most notably in the 1991 National Hill Climb, only to spend the rest of the race in utter agony. There is a nice break after two-thirds distance where, if you haven't heeded my warning and have pushed too hard, you can recover somewhat, and then you can let rip to the summit.

At the summit you'll find my favourite spot in the Dales: the simplicity of the uninterrupted 360-degree views and the sheer amount of nothing on view are the perfect tonic to the relentlessness of modern life, and ideal for releasing the pressure of a cluttered brain. You'll also be able to rejoice at having ticked off all the climbs.

Now you have 26 wonderful kilometres of downhill, bar a couple of short ramps, all the way back to Leyburn, and the reward of a huge meal to replace the massive amount of calories you will have burnt to climb over the best the Dales have to offer.

because, the longer you stop, the more your 'café legs' will hurt when you climb straight away out of town to take on the high point and highlight of the day, the second of the 'big three': Fleet Moss.

Following the initial skirmish of bends that ascend out of Gayle, and after negotiating the perpetually dirty road between the farms on the lower slopes, you crest a small brow, where the prospect of the remainder of the climb smacks you in the face like a wet fish. What a road! Cutting a single straight line right across the huge hillside in front of you, this, the highest pass in Yorkshire, is simply a monster, and one

that gets angrier and angrier until it touches close to 20%. The horizon is greeted with blessed relief, as is the subsequent plateau, but the sight of another 20% sign brings you right back down to earth: Fleet Moss is not finished with you yet. This beast has one more surprise in its locker, one more wicked ramp, until you can finally cross the summit and take in the epic views in all directions.

You'll be thankful of the long break before the final instalment of the 'big three' as you drop down into Langstrothdale, follow the River Wharfe all the way to Buckden, then take the

ABOVE *No turning back now. Approaching the fearsome opening slopes of Park Rash.*

RIDE 16 YORKSHIRE

YORKSHIRE DALES

DISTANCE 130KM

CLIMBING +3,077M

DIFFICULTY 8/10

FOOD & WATER | TAN HILL / HAWES / KETTLEWELL

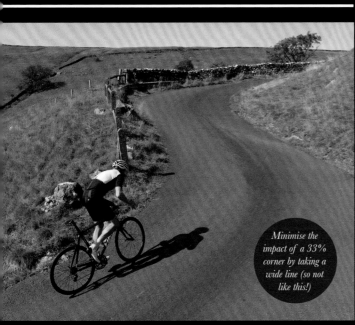

Minimise the impact of a 33% corner by taking a wide line (so not like this!)

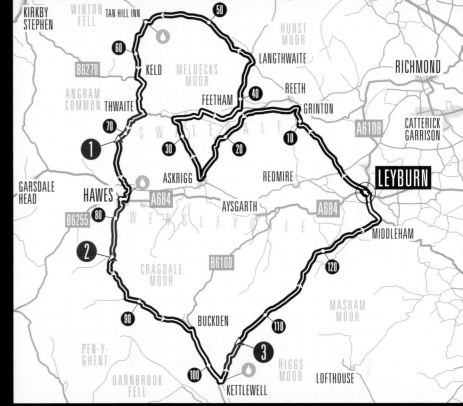

KEY CLIMBS

1 BUTTERTUBS PASS
3,857m +215m

The north face of Buttertubs averages 9% from bottom to top but that statistic is heavily skewed by the brief descent towards the end. Either side of this momentary relief you have some extremely tough climbing which at its steepest touches 20% in places.

2 FLEET MOSS
5,387m +320m

The highest pass in Yorkshire is a monster. It starts with a 16% climb out of Gayle then relaxes for some time before the giant ramp to the summit comes into view. Climbing incrementally steeper and steeper until it reaches 25% before a brow it then levels before kicking up to 25% once more.

3 PARK RASH
2,089m +211m

The secret to mastering Park Rash is not to go too hard and blow up round its first 30% corner, which is easier said than done. If you can survive the early slopes unscathed there is a nice break to refresh the legs at about two-thirds distance before the final ramp to the empty summit.

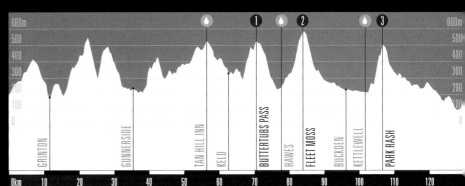

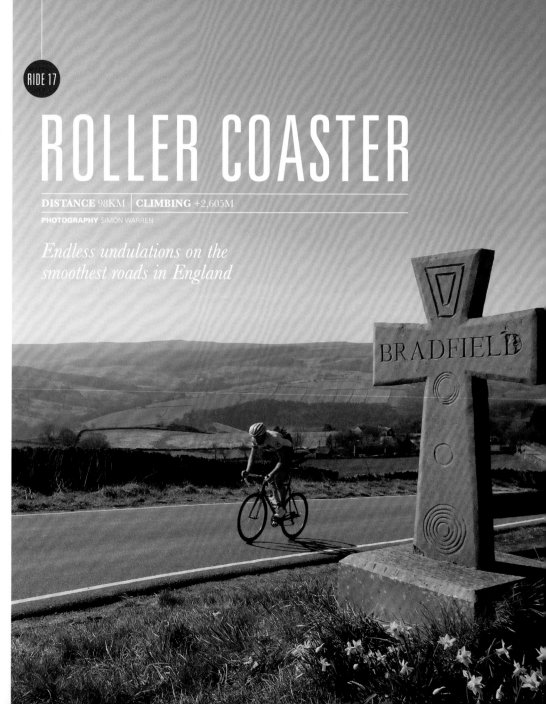

RIGHT *Passing the cross at the top of Kirk Edge Road on asphalt as smooth as a baby's . . .*

RIDE 17

ROLLER COASTER

DISTANCE 98KM | **CLIMBING** +2,605M

PHOTOGRAPHY SIMON WARREN

Endless undulations on the smoothest roads in England

T he first time I heard of the Strines was reading about ex-pro Russell Downing's epic training rides when he was at the peak of his power. He didn't bother with modern training aids like heart rate monitors and power meters. He wasn't concerned with watts per kilogram or functional thresholds: he was like Rocky in *Rocky IV* – he just headed for the hills and smashed his legs to bits on them 'old school'.

Sitting just above Sheffield, bordered to the north and east by the A616 and A6102, in the south by the A57, and to the west by the High Peak, the tangle of exquisitely surfaced lanes that surround the area's nine small reservoirs is the perfect cyclist's playground. It was 2014 when I first visited these amazing roads, in the run-up to the arrival of the Tour de France, but it wasn't until I moved to Sheffield that I really got to grips with this wonderland of peaks and troughs, all set on the best asphalt you will have ever seen.

At first glance the route appears almost impossibly complicated, and, well, it is, but pay attention and hopefully I can talk you through it. Starting from Low Bradfield, climb out of the village heading east on Lamb Hill to cross the first peak of the day, then gently drop down Loxley Road to enjoy the briefest period on level ground, before buckling up as the roller-coaster ride really begins. Turning left, head up Long Lane, which is a lane and long, and rises dead-straight on a stiff gradient to deliver you into the small village of Worrall, from where you fall right away down into Oughtibridge.

This next climb is my favourite on the whole route – I should have saved it for later but, then again, you'll enjoy it more with fresh legs. The base of Coldwell Hill is hidden: it's a bit like Platform 9¾ in *Harry Potter*, so keep your eyes peeled. As you turn to drop down Church Street into Oughtibridge you need to turn left first onto Wheel Lane but – here is the trick – you have to mount and cross the pavement, as there is no direct junction onto the road.

Rising as steep as 20%, and thrashing through a succession of tight bends, this wonderful climb cuts between the houses and their gardens that line either side. There is some respite at the T-junction, where you head left, but you are a long way from the top, which lies where Lumb Lane meets Onesmoor Road.

Turn right at the junction, then right again, to descend through Brightholmlee to momentarily join the A6102, before leaving it at the first opportunity to start the next climb. At the junction you are faced with two paths, and you need to take the right. More Hall Lane turns into Sunny Bank Road and grinds all the way up into Bolsterstone, a village you'll pass through three times in all. This time you want to leave on Cockshot Lane, to ride into the heart of Stocksbridge, home to the dreaded Pea Royd Lane: venue for the National Hill Climb Championship three times in the space of ten years. 'When in Rome . . .' – so that's of course where the route heads next.

You'll not find many people with a nice word to

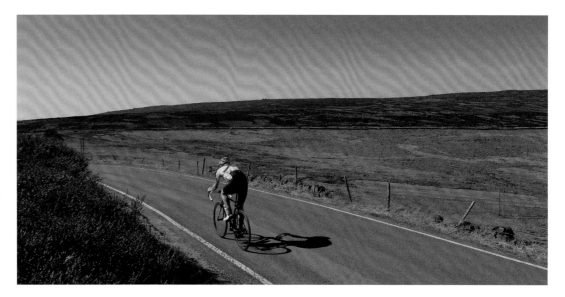

say about this road: it's dished out too much pain to too many legs. Kicking up from the Fox Valley retail park, with two tight bends and multiple 20% ramps, it was also once used at the start of the Tour de Yorkshire sportive, and had half the entrants walking within a kilometre of the start. Oh, and, to make matters worse, the event car park was at the top, so they had to walk up it again when they had finished (no sniggering).

Once you've crossed it, you're allowed a slight period of calm along the top of the ridge, before dropping down to join the A616 to Langsett. Take real care as you turn onto the main road, then leave it to head south across the dam wall, through Upper Midhope. Then it's onto Shaw Lane, to meet up with Mortimer Road again. Turn left, then right onto Oaks Lane, and begin the long, steady climb up to the second passage through Bolsterstone. Turn right once in the

village, drop rapidly down Yew Trees Lane, then take the first left onto New Mill Bank. Continuing to plummet downwards, you'll reach Ewden Village; pass the end of More Hall Reservoir, then start my second favourite climb of the day, Fairhurst Lane.

Even though I love its sharp corner and vicious inclines, it does hold bad memories as, during the aforementioned Tour de Yorkshire sportive, I somehow managed, while shifting onto my largest sprocket, to push my rear derailleur into the spokes of the back wheel, resulting in it being torn from the frame. Stranded with a bike that couldn't be ridden, I had no choice but to take the walk of shame back to HQ. Thankfully, I wasn't too far away, but as I trudged up the final hill, in my socks, the sizeable crowd of people near the top saw me and broke into applause. 'Come on – you can

ABOVE *Looking out over Strines Moor and wondering where the next climb will be.*

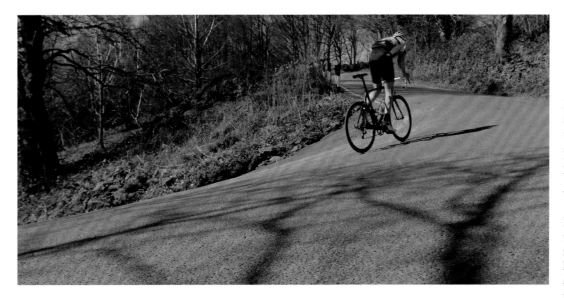

do it!' 'Almost there – great effort!' Head hung down, I shuffled past them, trying to smile. I just wanted the world to swallow me up.

At the top of Fairhurst Lane, turn right onto Bank Side, then left onto Onesmoor Road, then right to the high point of the day below West Nab. Dropping down via High Bradfield into Low Bradfield, you reach almost the halfway point, so this is all the excuse you need to stop at the Flask End tea room at the base of the descent. After refreshments, head east on New Road past the Damflask Reservoir, to turn right and climb up the hairpins into Dungworth, then right again on Sliding Hollow to Ughill, then on Ughill Wood Lane and Hoar Stones Road to return to Low Bradfield.

The next section of the ride radiates around the village, reaching out and back in a series of loops rather like the petals of a flower. The first petal starts with the climb of Blindside Lane. A long, steady incline with stunning views at the top, it takes you all the way, via Sugworth Road, back to Mortimer Road, where you can enjoy the passage along the base of Strines Moor. To the left the High Peak; to the right, drop-dead views out over the Strines reservoirs: this is indeed a very special piece of road. Heading north, you cross Strines Dike, climb out the other side, then take the first right back again towards Low Bradfield. Just before hitting the village, however, turn left up Windy Bank, then at the top turn right onto Mortimer Road. Then take the next right back once more to Low Bradfield, to begin the final phase of climbing.

Instead of saving the best hills for last, I've saved the hardest, and the first of the remaining challenges is Woodall Lane (well, three-quarters of it). Home to the annual Bradfield Summer Hill Climb race, it's a nasty little ramp and, although said event may end in High Bradfield, the climb doesn't: continue left out of the village, and then take the right back up to West Nab. From here turn left, and left again, all the way to Wigtwizzle, climb Moor Lane back to the final visit to Mortimer Road – and take a deep breath.

Next is the climb the locals like to call Deliverance, (after the terrifying 1972 movie of the same name). Ewden Bank rises ferociously from the gully across Ewden Beck up to its first left-hand bend, which is easily 30% at the apex, and just the start of things to come. Although never as steep again, this punishing ascent, with two more distinct bends, didn't get its fearful name because it's a walk in the park: it got its name for chewing up riders' legs and delivering them into Hell.

Turning immediate right after the summit, return to Bolsterstone for the third and final time. Then, after falling all the way down to the Broomhead Reservoir, it's time for one last climb – and another brute. Turning right off New Road, begin the climb of Dwarriden Lane, at first through the woods, then, turning left and right at the junction, continuing across the moors to peak at Penistone Road.

Feel free to slump over your bars here, or collapse at the side of the road, as that's the climbing done, in the bank, finished. All you need do now is plunge back into Low Bradfield for second and third helpings of cake.

Now, shall I go over it all once more?

ABOVE *The first left-hand bend on 'Deliverance' makes the eyes water and legs scream!*

RIDE 17

YORKSHIRE
THE STRINES

DISTANCE 98KM	
CLIMBING +2,605M	
DIFFICULTY 8/10	

FOOD & WATER | STOCKSBRIDGE / LOW BRADFIELD

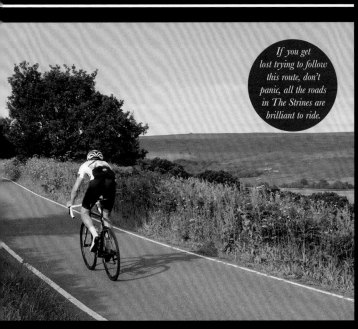

If you get lost trying to follow this route, don't panic, all the roads in The Strines are brilliant to ride.

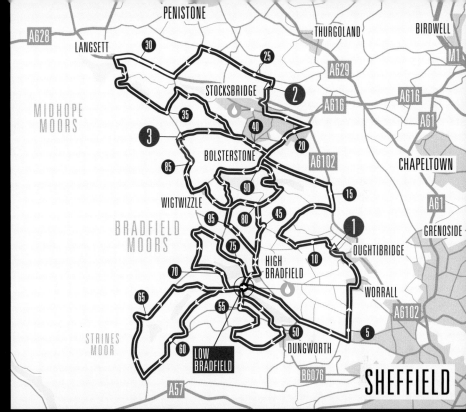

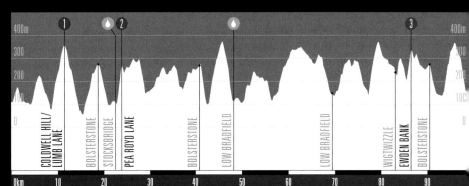

KEY CLIMBS

1 COLDWELL HILL /LUMB LANE
2,630m +235m

A climb in two parts: the first twists up the steep slopes of Coldwell Hill through its 20% bends to the T-junction. Catch your breath here then turn left to follow the significantly steadier gradient to the eventual finish at the junction with Onesmoor Road

2 PEA ROYD LANE
1,130m +135m

Packing a 12% average this climb is a beast from base to summit. The gradient is just about comfortable at first but then at the right turn the 20% slopes arrive. Following these there is the mother of all false flats across the bridge before the lung-busting and leg-breaking journey to the summit.

3 DELIVERANCE
1,012m +139m

Also known as Ewden Bank this road kicks up from the gully into its wicked 25% left-hand bend which puts you in trouble right away. Following this it's very steep for a short while longer, eases midway then hits you hard though the pair of bends that finish off this killer ascent.

THE LAWS OF PHYSICS

DISTANCE 100KM | **CLIMBING** +2,667M

PHOTOGRAPHY ANDY JONES

Searching for the toughest climb
on the North York Moors

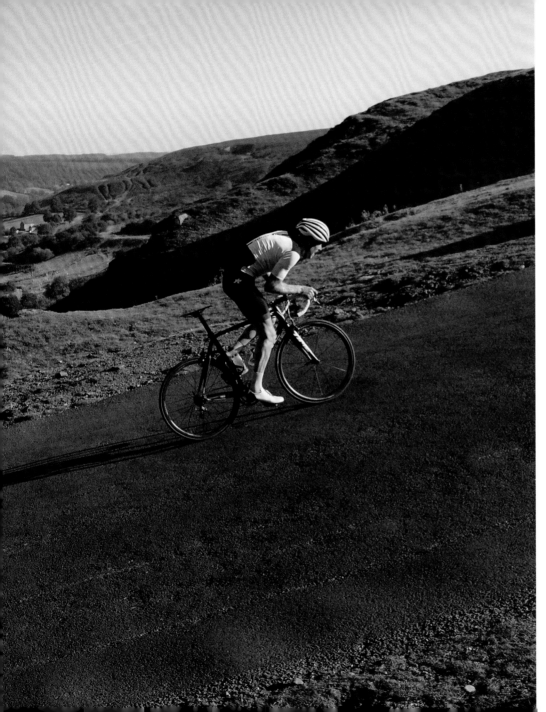

LEFT *The 33% gradient of Rosedale Chimney, and no – I haven't tilted the picture.*

Of all the climbs in Britain, the one I'd heard the most about, and seen more photos of before I got to ride it, was Rosedale Chimney. Also going by the name Chimney Bank, this beast of a road has attained mythical status after being incorporated in the old Milk Race and Kellogg's Tours, not to mention playing host to the 1987 National Hill Climb Championship. Back in a time before compact chain sets, when bike frames and riders' legs were made of pure steel, this road was a battleground feared around the globe. One could draw the conclusion, though, that, owing to its notoriety, and the column inches and now YouTube minutes dedicated to it, Rosedale is a solitary peak in the North York Moors: a single savage climb surrounded by lesser lumps.

You could not be further from the truth. The Moors are littered with such inclines – in fact, any journey you make between any two points within the National Park has a profile resembling the cardiograph of a hyperactive hamster.

So why does Rosedale get all the plaudits? Is it really that much harder than the rest? Well, that question is the cause of much debate, and I'd say there are two other climbs that could, in my opinion, lay claim to being a tougher challenge – Blakey Bank and Caper Hill – and, handily, all three feature on this route.

Starting in Hutton-le-Hole, head north on Blakey Road, then take the second left to drop down through Low Hill into Church Houses, to the base of the first contender to Rosedale's

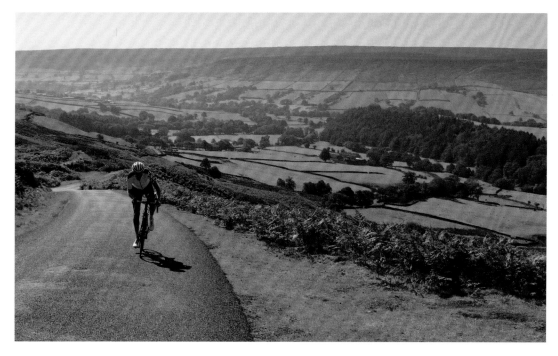

crown: Blakey Bank. Once at the bottom, where you pass the first of the day's ubiquitous severe gradient warnings, you'll see the road head straight up from the bottom of the dale to the top of the moor. With only the faintest alteration in direction to neutralise the pitch of the slope, it's obvious right away why this and all its peers are so bloody steep. The climbs of the North York Moors must have been constructed by Romans following a crow. Adorned with multiple stretches of 20%, the narrow road, kinking ever so slightly left and right, crosses a number of fake brows as it crawls up to the summit. At the top, and with that as your starting reference, it's time to head on to the next challenge, once

you've spent a blissful few kilometres in the emptiness of the moor and raced down into Rosedale – Abbey, that is.

The first of two visits to the village isn't to tackle the Chimney, though – that comes later. This time, the route heads east to take on the often overlooked Heygate Bank. Lying literally in the shadow of Chimney Bank, this perennial bridesmaid may not pack quite as savage a punch as its illustrious neighbour, but it's a serious ramp all the same. With a couple of corners thrown in to take a modicum of sting out of the ascent, it still ramps up over 20% on its way to the vast open spaces of Hamer Moor.

High on the plateau, the North York Moors

are a magical, peaceful place. However, I am forever reminded of the classic scene in *An American Werewolf in London* when the two hitchhikers are dropped off by their ride and given the fateful warning, 'Boys, keep off the moors, stick to the roads, and best of luck.' Which always makes me click up a gear and press on, especially in inclement weather.

It's nigh-on impossible to include all the killer climbs in the Moors in one ride (trust me, I've tried), so I've had to incorporate some as descents in order to join the dots, and one such climb is Egton High Moor. With its 33% corners it is a real beauty, but today all they will do is test the power of your brakes as you drop through them, not the power of your legs as you attempt to drag yourself up.

Arriving in Egton Bridge, take the first right over to Grosmont via Lease Rigg Lane, then cross the ford that lies at its far end. Fords come in many guises, from the short and narrow to some that resemble what Moses faced as he looked across the Red Sea. This one, when the river is in full flow, falls into the latter category, but thankfully there is a very good foot-bridge you can use to avoid being swept away.

Once in Grosmont it's time to climb again, up and out of town on Fair Head Lane towards Sleights Moor. Taking the right fork as the main carriageway bends left, you pass one of the famous 33% gradient signs. This should, and likely will, put the fear into you, but in this case whoever erected the warning oversold what lay

ABOVE *Blakey Bank may LOOK pretty!*

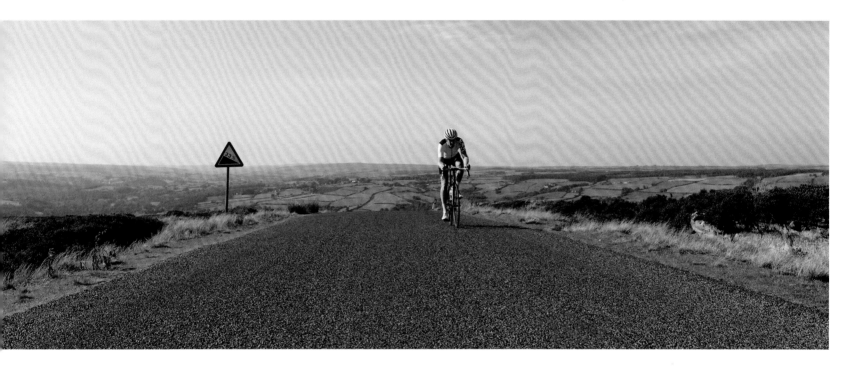

ahead. In my opinion it only just makes it to 20% – maybe the council got a buy-two-get-one-free deal, and just stuck it there to scare people off. A bit like primitive tribes would do with severed heads on spikes in days gone by. Although the 1-in-3 never arrives, that detracts nothing from this stunning road, which finishes on a nice shallow gradient, once again surrounded by the beauty of the empty, windswept moors.

The route continues north and drops down the A169, before turning right into the tangle of lanes and sharp gradients that surround Littlebeck. The target amongst this mêlée of roads is Lousy Hill Lane, a wonderful climb that twists away from the village to reach the

junction with the B1416, where the route turns north, then heads west into Ugglebarnby, then Iburndale and Sleights, before arriving for a second time in Grosmont. To squeeze in another climb the route rises to Egton, then falls back down into Egton Bridge, before making its way via yet one more, further into the valley of Glaisdale, home to the one and only Caper Hill.

The ascent of Blakey Bank stored in your legs' memory will confirm this as the second challenger for hardest climb in the Moors. Caper Hill is the textbook Yorkshire Moors road, and can roughly be split into three parts: the viciously steep straight part at the start; the two slight bends in the middle; and the viciously

steep straight part at the end. With zero regard to the angle of the bank, and crossing exactly perpendicular to its contours, Caper Hill goes from bottom to top using as little asphalt as possible. One can only assume this was a precious commodity at time of construction – either that or the company charged with laying it was local and living up to the famous Yorkshire stereotype of just being tight. Your legs will be a little more jaded than when they climbed Blakey Bank, but, even so, you should be able to ascertain which of the two you believe toughest before making your way to number three.

Yes, next it's the big one, but not until you've thrown away the hard-earned gradient you've

ABOVE *You wait all day for a 33% sign to come along then five turn up at once.*

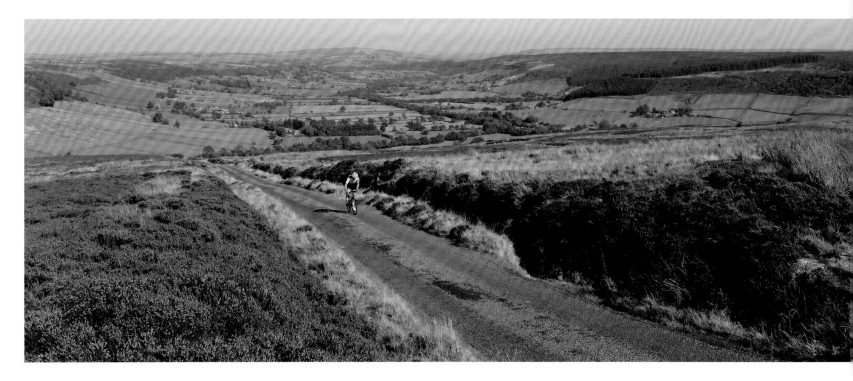

just accumulated by descending into Street, through the wonderfully named Great Fryup Dale, and then climbed out the other side all the way up to Danby High Moor. Joining Knott Road, you retrace a part of the route you rode earlier and arrive in Rosedale Abbey again, this time to take on the hallowed slopes of its most famous attraction, which are guarded by prominent signs warning anyone using any mode of transport that, essentially, what lies ahead will cause them distress.

What I like to call 'base camp one' is reached after you cross the cattle grid to arrive at the small car park on the first bend. Here you

can have a breather, gulping in as much air as possible before carrying on. Next comes the bit that makes Rosedale so famous. By means of a snaking S-bend, the road climbs rapidly into one of most formidable lengths of asphalt in Britain: 50 metres of pure, unadulterated 30% gradient. You don't dare put a foot down here because, once you unclip, the walk of shame is long and slow. You must keep fighting with all your might to get to where 30% turns to 20% and, even though it's still pretty damn hard, some semblance of normality is regained. No matter how your legs feel, once you beat this pure 10/10 climb, you'll be grinning from ear to ear,

I guarantee. Grab a selfie with the famous sign that adorns the summit, then, with all the hard work behind you, tick off the last few kilometres across Spaunton Moor back to Hutton-le-Hole.

So which was the hardest? As it came at the end and is still fresh in your legs, your instinct may be to say Rosedale – but was it Blakey, or Caper? Or any of the multitude of others you have crossed? For me it's always Rosedale: the others may have longer, steeper sections, but in my opinion nothing is quite as hard as that formidable stretch of 1-in-3. Oh, and if throughout all this you've been screaming, *'What about Boltby Bank?'* then just turn the page.

ABOVE *Caper Hill, taking the DIRECT route out of Glaisdale.*

RIDE 18

YORKSHIRE

NORTH YORK MOORS

DISTANCE 100KM

CLIMBING +2,667M

DIFFICULTY 9/10

FOOD & WATER | GROSMONT / ROSEDLAE ABBEY

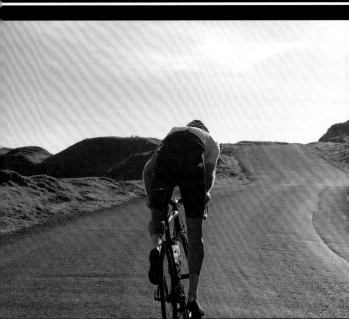

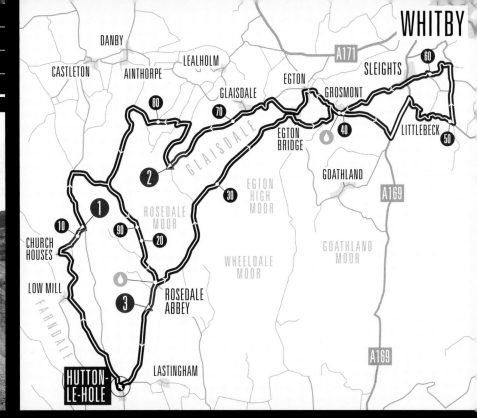

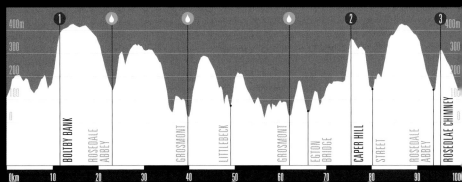

KEY CLIMBS

1 BLAKEY BANK
1,822m +210m

Leaving the village of Church Houses this climb wastes no time getting started and then turns really tasty once you pass the 20% sign. With an average of 11% it lets you take a breather here and there in between the extensive sections of 20% gradient which make such a formidable foe

2 CAPER HILL
1,342m +182m

A straight line of savage gradient with statistics to match. With a 14% average and maximum slopes of 25% Caper Hill requires some real brute force to master. With the harshest slopes either side of the minuscule rest midway make sure you use this to both recover and gather your strength

3 ROSEDALE CHIMNEY
1,340m +168m

What sets Rosedale apart from the other North York Moors climbs is the stretch that comes after the excruciatingly steep left-hand bend. This wall of 33% tarmac has appeared in more than one of my nightmares and it never ends well for me or the bike

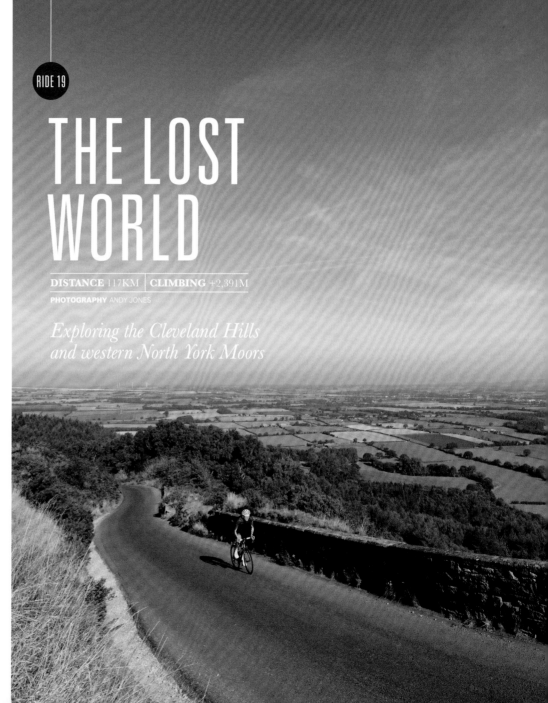

THE LOST WORLD

DISTANCE 117KM | **CLIMBING** +2,391M

PHOTOGRAPHY ANDY JONES

*Exploring the Cleveland Hills
and western North York Moors*

In the previous ride I weighed up the merits of what I considered the three hardest climbs in the North York Moors: Rosedale Chimney, Caper Hill and Blakey Bank. All the while I was writing, however, I could hear in my head the screams of 'What about Boltby Bank?'

When I was compiling *100 Greatest Cycling Climbs*, Boltby Bank was the last climb I rode, and my appraisal split opinion more than I managed on any other (apart, maybe, from Rowsley Bar). When I say 'split', though, it's me on one side and everyone else on the other. I awarded the climb an 8/10 as that, given the legs I had that day, and after applying the algorithm I keep in the dark recesses of my brain, I believed to be a fair assessment. It seems, however, that I was the only person on two wheels to agree with me. Everyone else gives it a 10. So now, placing it first in line on this route, I offer you the opportunity to tell me again I was wrong.

Based on Thirsk, this loop takes in the western half of the North York Moors, criss-crossing the Cleveland Hills while ticking off some very familiar and other less-travelled roads. To start with, though, it's time to head to Boltby Bank, and you've close to 11 kilometres to loosen the legs up for their impending torment. Leave the town heading first east on the A170, then taking the left turn following the signs to Felixkirk and Boltby. Ahead you will see the Moors, an elevated landmass rising abruptly from the Vale of York, spanning the full width of the horizon, and resembling Arthur Conan

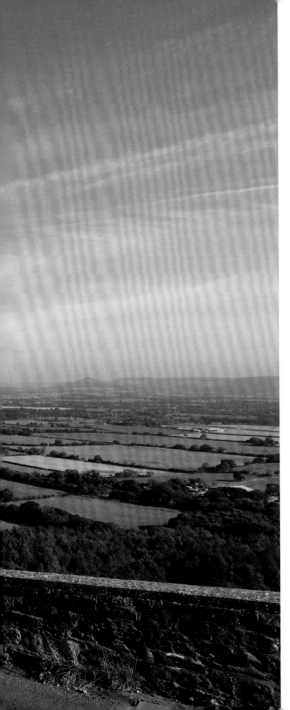

LEFT *It's impossible not to stop and take in the view from Carlton Bank.*

Doyle's Lost World.

The plateau is hidden, and there is no easy way onto it: all routes are arduous, and all have their pitfalls. From the west, the obvious route is on the A170 up Sutton Bank but, and I will say this only once, avoid it at all costs. This is the terrible main road, and I can guarantee you'll find yourself stuck in a jam on its 25% slopes as either a truck or, God forbid, a caravan crawls up with a row of cars behind filling the air with the stench from their burning clutches.

So it's best to take either White Horse Bank (we'll come to that later) or, of course, this climb, Boltby Bank. Climb up through Felixkirk, then into Boltby, before hitting the base just outside the village. It's not a pretty climb: there are no spectacular views or dramatic corners – it's just a wall of unforgiving tarmac which, once across Lunshaw Beck, kicks up for close to a kilometre and a half on an average gradient of 13%. Peaking at between 20 and 25% in a couple of places, this is, there is no question, a bloody tough road to take on – but harder than Rosedale? Really?

Once it's in the bag, it's time to search out more delights, by first heading down into Hawnby, then following the route across the moor in and out of the small patches of woodland that break up the otherwise sparse hillsides. With only one road to follow it's impossible to get lost, as you ride in the shadow of the imposing peaks of Black Hamilton across Thimbleby Moor into Osmotherley. Punctuated by a slew of little ramps, this section

of the ride is all about getting you into the right place to take on the star of today's show, and one of my all-time favourites: Carlton Bank. Heading up to the A172 briefly, you then drop down to Faceby, skirt underneath Carlton in Cleveland, and then hit its slopes.

Venue for the 1996 National Hill Climb, where Stuart Dangerfield won the fourth of his five titles, Carlton Bank is a brute, but rewards you with easily the best views in the North-East. Once on its winding upper slopes, trapped between the high bank on your right and the stone wall on your left, you can cast your eyes out as far as you can see across the pan-flat plains of Teesside. Although I'd never normally condone stopping and putting a foot down on a climb, for this one I'll make an exception, because the views, even though predominantly industrial, are just magnificent.

With a tactical breather taken, press on to the top, and then get stuck into 10 glorious kilometres of descent through Chop Gate for a slight detour up a climb that lies well off the beaten track. As you head south down the B1257 crossing the top of the Moors, on your right, towering high above anything else, and some would say sticking out like a sore thumb, is the Bilsdale transmitter. Whenever I see such a structure I immediately think, well, if they built that up there and they need to service it, then there must be a road – and in this case there is, and it's a beauty.

Ignoring the 'Private road' signs at the entrance where you turn off the main road – it

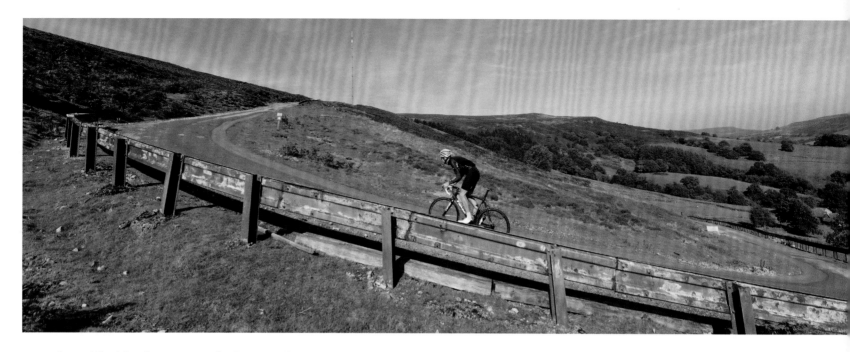

is a public right of way – pass a few houses and a farm to then start the ascent. The surface is rough, seemingly always covered in effluent, and there is a gate to open near the bottom before it kicks up viciously to a glorious hairpin, arcing right and opening up exceptional vistas out over the moors. Once round its 25% apex you are lined up to head directly for the transmitter. Deathly quiet, rugged and, yes, tough, this road delivers you to the highest point in the Moors, so make sure you stop for a while, weather permitting, to take it all in. Take real care on the sketchy descent, back through the gate, then up to the main road to head right, and resume your southward progress through Laskill all the way to Helmsley, for a foray into the Hamilton Hills.

An annex to the North York Moors, these hills lie to the south and are home to a handful of great climbs, two of which are fast approaching. After another brief excursion on the A170, leave it to ride into Oswaldkirk, then on to Ampleforth, where you turn right up High Bank. Kicking off with a nasty kilometre of over 10% slope, you wind up through the trees to the edge of the 'Lost World' once more, before looping almost immediately back down again. Dropping down Wass Bank (which is a great climb if you fancy going rogue and heading back up and down), you carry on to Coxwold and Kilburn for the final challenge of the ride, and my favourite way up onto the Moors: White Horse Bank.

Climbing out of Kilburn, this hill does indeed feature a giant white chalk horse, although from the road views are limited to a few glimpses on the way out of the village before you get lost in the tangle of the woods. The climbing starts from the junction where you head left, and on a slope that touches 20% in places you snake upwards through no fewer than eight distinct bends to summit alongside the Yorkshire Gliding Club airfield.

And that's the climbing done and dusted, all in the bag. All that's left to do is ride across the pan-flat tops and, again avoiding Sutton Bank, cross the A170 to make your way to the top of Boltby Bank and then retrace your way back to Thirsk. Of course, you could give Boltby one more try, just to be doubly sure of your own appraisal.

ABOVE *Traversing the grand Alpine hairpin up to the Billsdale transmitter.*

RIDE 19

YORKSHIRE

CLEVELAND HILLS

DISTANCE 117KM

CLIMBING +2,391M

DIFFICULTY 7/10

FOOD & WATER | OSMOTHERLEY / HELMSLEY

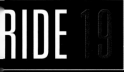

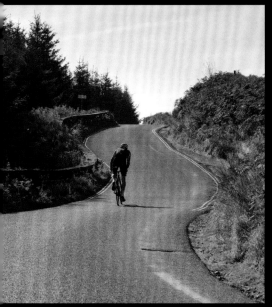

KEY CLIMBS

1 BOLTBY BANK

1,230m +150m

This road never goes much above 20% but it does hang around that gradient for an awful long time. After a brief lull at around half distance the last 500 metres are relentlessly steep into the brace of bends that deliver you to the summit.

2 CARLTON BANK

2,013m +198m

Boasting just about the best view from any climb in the UK Carlton Bank has a 10% average gradient and peaks at around the 25% mark in places. The first half climbs gently then after bending left the gradient ramps up and barely relents until you cross the top.

3 BILSDALE TRANSMITTER

2,247m +236m

A dead-end that passes through a farm yard, is blocked by a gate at the bottom and covered in animal sh*te is enough to put most people off but this beast of a road reveals one of the best views of the North York Moors there is.

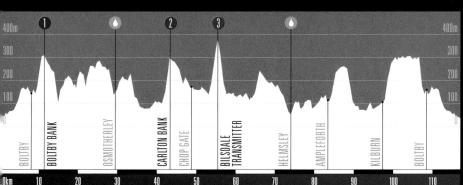

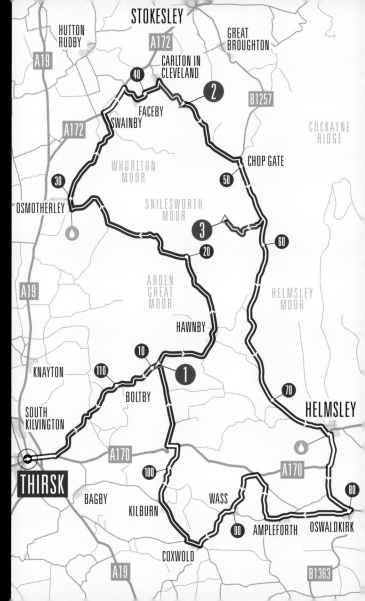

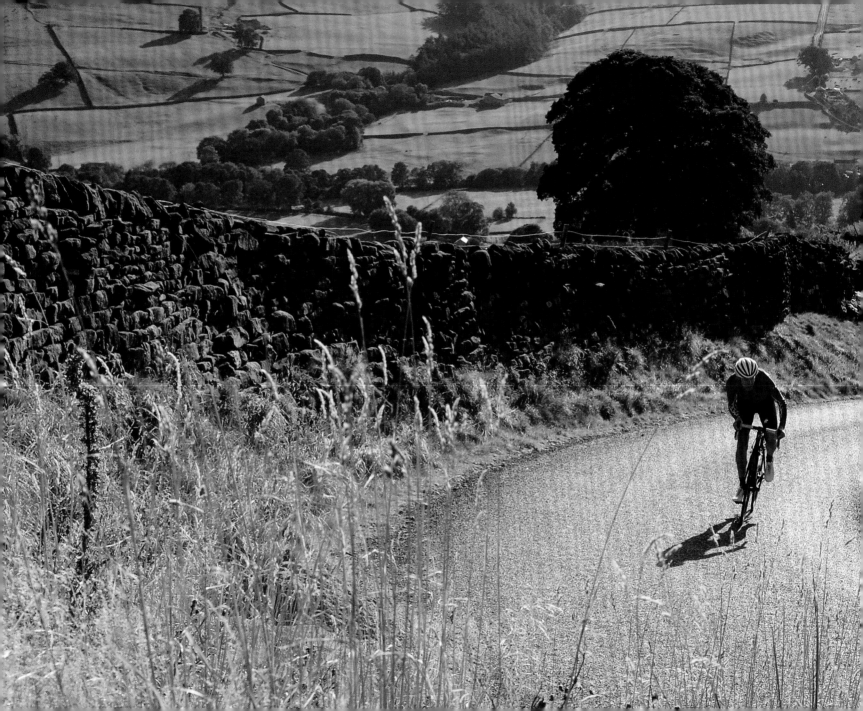

BEAUTY AND THE BEASTS

DISTANCE 154KM | **CLIMBING** +3,000M

PHOTOGRAPHY ANDY JONES

Crossing the hills of the southern Yorkshire Dales and Nidderdale

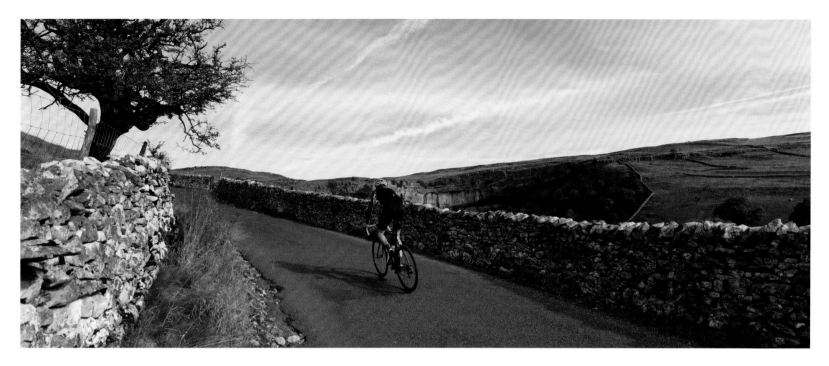

The joint barrier of the A59 and A65 running from Harrogate in the east to Kirby Lonsdale in the west forms a man-made boundary holding back the ever-expanding Leeds/Bradford conurbation. I see this line as the true border with the North, and this, the second ride in the Yorkshire Dales, kicks off right from its imaginary edge in Ilkley to guide you around the southern reaches of the National Park and into Nidderdale.

Ilkley has cycling running through its veins, and you'll always bump into other riders here, especially on the route out of town on Denton Road. Following the line of the A65, it allows relatively safe passage away from the heavy traffic on the main road, and is the default way into the hills. Crossing the River Wharfe, take the first left, then follow the road as it becomes Common Holme Lane and all the way through Nesfield and Beamsley, along its undulating path, to meet the A59. Take a left on the main road, drop down to the roundabout, then take the third exit to Bolton Bridge and Bolton Abbey. The further north you travel, the quieter the roads become, but you're not inside the National Park – not yet.

Climbing past Halton Gill Wood, passing through the gate that splits the climb in two, head on to Halton East and Embsay, with slightly more gain in elevation but nothing to ruffle any feathers, all the way to join the B6265.

The beginning of this ride does lack a certain amount of drama, but is a necessary process to deliver you into the Dales and escape the gravitational pull of the South.

The drama is just around the corner, though, and comes in the shape of the first giant climb of the day, Malham Cove. After you've navigated through the villages of Rylstone, Hetton, Winterburn and Airton, you turn north through Kirkby Malham to face one of the most beautiful climbs in the country. On any day Malham will be teeming with walkers, all kitted out with 50-litre backpacks stuffed with God knows what, poles and compasses as though heading for Everest base camp. In the centre of the village

PREVIOUS PAGE
The star of this ride, the bends of Trapping Hill in Nidderdale.

ABOVE *Climbing past Malham Cove, it doesn't get much more Yorkshire Dales than this.*

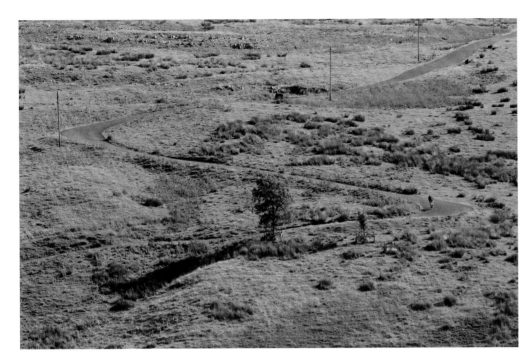

the road forks: both directions take you up fantastic climbs, but you want to head left, the classic way up what is the most quintessential Yorkshire Dales road of all.

Rising above the cove on your right, hitting gradients close to 20%, bending back and forth between the high dry-stone walls, this road is just perfect and, better still, delivers you to even more delights at the top. Once you're through the dramatic steep bends the pitch of the slope fades, but it's a long slog to the eventual summit, on the open, sheep-covered plains beneath Malham Ings. Up ahead, carry straight over the crossroads, past the tarn and, as you begin to lose some altitude, your next challenge comes into view.

You'll spy this climb from afar, and in direct profile it looks simply vicious. In fact, it's one of the most dramatic sights in the Dales: a simple ramp lying perpendicular to your direction of travel, scaling the wall that blocks your progress. As you plunge into the gully, try and take some speed back up the other side, but do be careful over the tight bridge. Then try and stay on top of your gear through the twin hairpins to summit at Nab End. Continuing east, it's impossible not to stop and take a photograph of the views ahead: they are outrageous, and sometimes, indeed, too much of a distraction as you dodge sheep, cross cattle grids and deal with sharp corners and adverse camber on the

fast descent to Arncliffe. Arriving in the bottom of Littondale, head south, following the River Skirfare into Wharfedale, then, after a brief stint on the B6160, turn to Conistone to take the quiet back way into Grassington. At the 63-kilometre point, this makes a handy place for a stop, and you'll find everything you need in this wonderful little village with its period shop fronts and cobbled streets.

Moving on, the route heads for Greenhow, because no route in the southern Dales would be complete without visiting Greenhow, but before you scream, relax: we're not climbing the tough side, thankfully. Apart from, say, Chapel Fell up in County Durham, there's no climb I hate more than Greenhow Hill: it's a total bitch and, when tackling it from Pateley Bridge, you always have a headwind. Since we are travelling in the opposite direction, logically you should have the wind on your back, as you spend almost the entire next 12 kilometres gaining altitude. Not without interruption, and surrounded by the rolling moors, your climbing ends as you leave the confines of the Yorkshire Dales National Park, and enter the Nidderdale AONB.

Running north to south, bisecting the area in two, lies Nidderdale itself and, turning left in Pateley Bridge, you begin to ride through it. Following the shores of Gouthwaite Reservoir, there is only one way into the valley and, unless you double back, only one way out, up Trapping Hill.

My favourite climb on the ride and, naturally, the toughest, longest and highest, Trapping Hill is

ABOVE *The hairpins on Nab End look worse from a distance than they actually are.*

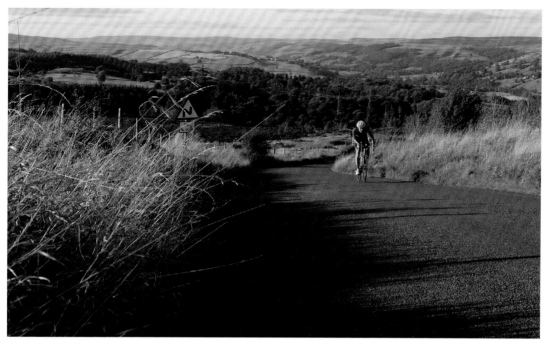

a spectacular road in every way. The lower slopes are savage, hitting 20%. The road twists beneath the omnipresent towering stone walls at the base of a giant grassy trench which, when pro races have visited, forms the perfect amphitheatre from where to watch the riders' legs burn. Once you're through the lower slopes, the struggle may ease, but it's far from over, as the protracted journey to the final peak lasts an eternity across the empty moor. You'll love every minute of it, though, as the scenery just gets better the further you climb. Plunging down to Leighton Reservoir the other side, with 100 kilometres now in the bank, you are two-thirds round, but there is still a multitude of climbs left to cross.

The first handful are small. Passing through Ilton, you make your way to Kirkby Malzeard, where you begin the long climb up and over Dallow Moor and back once more into Pateley Bridge. You may be in need of some more sugar now to help you tackle the final part, so grab a Coke (other sugar-delivery devices are available), then leave town up the last true brute of the day, Nought Bank Road. A regular hill-climb course, gaining the same elevation as its neighbour Greenhow Hill but on a much quieter road, at this late stage it will take some proper grunt to get over. Its fluctuating gradient, which kicks up from the T-junction after crossing Fosse Gill, will have you and your tired legs wishing for a

smaller gear, no matter what you're packing. Twisting through the woods and between a small canyon of tall rocks either side, you reach a false summit at the look-out on the left-hand bend. Before continuing to climb right, cast your eyes out for one last look over Nidderdale, then revert them to that metre of asphalt in front of your handlebars as you grind it out to the top.

Heading across the last of the day's open moors, the slope fades gradually to the peak and, as you pass the large stones either side of the road, it's time to descend, briefly. You have 250 metres of altitude to lose before arriving back in Ilkley, but you don't dump it all in one go – in fact, there are still a couple more peaks left to cross before the finish.

The first of this final flurry of climbs comes as you rise up into Padside, then drop down to Blubberhouses to cross the A59, and hit the next horrible little ramp. This one always knocks the stuffing out of me, so make sure you drop your chain down to the small ring, as from the main road the start is instantaneous. After this rude little kicker there are two more: the remainder of Rues Lane, and finally Snowdon Bank, and then that is it – done. All your elevation has been gained for the day, and all that is left is the fast descent, via Askwith, back into Ilkley, where you enter town on Denton Road, then turn left across the River Wharfe. When you roll to a halt, check the altitude gain on your computer: it should read 3,000 metres – a typical day on two wheels in the Yorkshire Dales!

ABOVE *With the toughest part of Nought Bank Road completed you are almost home.*

YORKSHIRE

YORKSHIRE DALES

DISTANCE 154KM

CLIMBING +3000M

DIFFICULTY 8/10

FOOD & WATER | MALHAM / GRASSINGTON / PATELEY BRIDGE

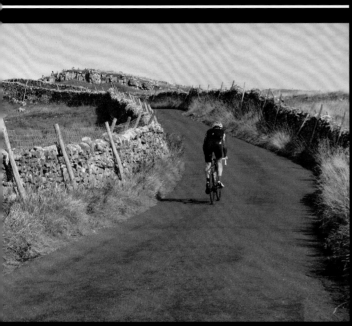

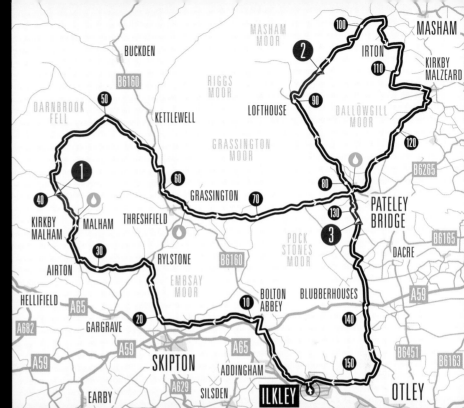

KEY CLIMBS

1 MALHAM COVE
3,307m +205m

The perfect Yorkshire Dales climb set in stunning scenery between immaculate dry stone walls. With a 6% average it is no real killer but along its length on its multiple kinks and turns there are a couple of stiff 20% sections before the very shallow last kilometre to the eventual summit.

2 TRAPPING HILL
3,163m +259m

Hidden away at the end of Nidderdale lie the delights of Trapping Hill which ramps up immediately through the village of Lofthouse. All the really hard climbing is crammed into the first half with twisting slopes as steep as 19%, then the second half is much easier.

3 NOUGHT BANK ROAD
2,293m +206m

Of the three ways that climb west out of Pateley Bridge this is my favourite. The start is pretty tough, the middle section the toughest where the 18% slopes can be found, then rounding the sweeping left-hand bend the final part is much easier to the summit.

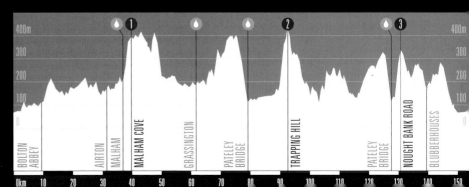

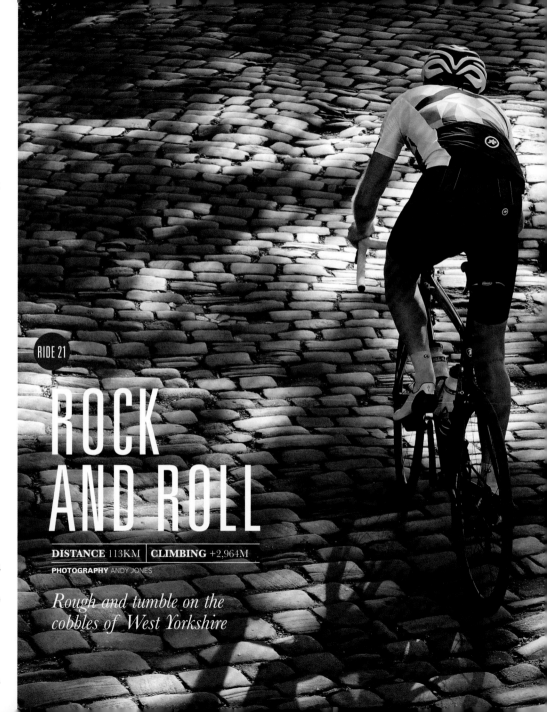

Think cobbles, think Belgium, think Flanders. Think the Oude Kwaremont, the Paterberg and the Koppenberg: the famous roads that have wreaked havoc beneath cyclists' tyres for generations. Yes? No. Think Yorkshire. Don't tell the Belgians, but in and around Halifax and the Calder Valley there are beasts that make those legendary Belgian hills look like new-born puppies. Stones the size of asteroids, gaps big enough to lose an army in, not to mention 30% gradients and cambers you can ski down – it's these roads that should be legends, not the little Belgian efforts. I'm not the first to plot a route linking these monstrous roads together: far from it – events such as the Ronde van Calderdale have been entertaining riders with the local delights for many years. To pay my respects to them I have cherry-picked my favourite cobbles, left out a few of those that need mountain-bike gears to tackle, and for good measure thrown in a few tasty tarmac climbs to build this route.

Halifax is the hub for the ride, and also where the largest concentration of cobbled hell lies and, starting from the magnificent Piece Hall, the route makes a beeline for the bumps right away. Halifax is a complicated place to navigate through, a carbuncle of roads that all seem to have been built on top of one another like layers of sediment over the years, but once you find the A58 and head east you'll be on your way out of town. After turning left onto Keith Lane, then immediately right onto a road simply named Hough, within a few hundred metres the cobbles start, a nice, gentle introduction,

RIDE 21

ROCK AND ROLL

DISTANCE 113KM | **CLIMBING** +2,964M

PHOTOGRAPHY ANDY JONES

Rough and tumble on the cobbles of West Yorkshire

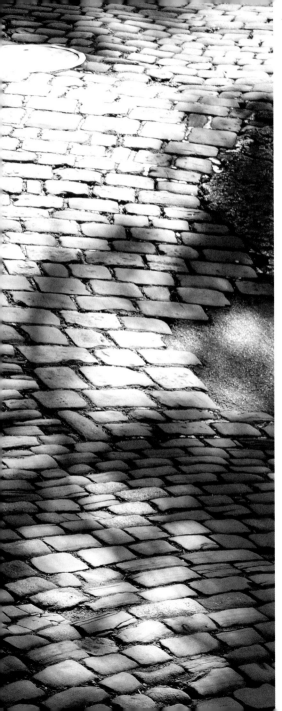

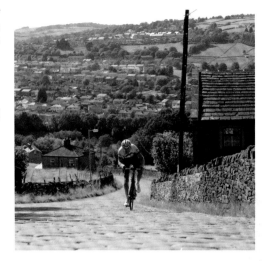

neatly laid on a shallow slope but a long stretch, bending around the corner until they are enveloped by tarmac and disappear. Keep climbing, break left onto Upper Lane, then take the next left onto Howes Lane to drop down Blake Hill, all the way to Shibden Brook and the bottom of a true beast, the Shibden Wall.

While the majority of the climbs on this route have largely passed under the radar, the Shibden Wall has had its share of time in the limelight. Having paid host to the Tour of Britain and Tour de Yorkshire, this famous stretch of stones has been treating the world's best riders to a taste of true Yorkshire cobbles for decades. Set with huge stones, featuring two tight corners and gradients approaching 20%, the Shibden Wall deserves every ounce of its fearsome reputation. However, your fresh legs will make mincemeat of it, I promise. At the top the route turns right, and that's it for rough-and-tumble for a while, as we head north in search of the next challenge in the town of Keighley.

Passing Queensbury, Bottomley Holes and Harden, the route descends all the way into Bingley, then follows the River Aire west into Keighley to what are, in my opinion, the best cobbles this side of the Arenberg Forest: those of Thwaites Brow. Starting from the mundane settings of a small industrial park, then rising like a phoenix, comes a twisting road set with utterly random stones that cover its multiple kinks and turns. With 25% corners and total chaos beneath the wheels it is madness to climb but, oh, so much fun.

Turning right at the top (which is a significant

distance after the end of the cobbles), drop back into Keighley before turning left, and then left again, for the next helping of hell, Hainworth Lane. Far more ordered than Thwaites Brow, these cobbles are large and well set and the gradient is a degree kinder, allowing you to sail up them, just like the pros do on TV. (Warning, this may not actually happen.) From here take Bingley Road down into Haworth, to ride the quaint, photogenic cobbles of Main Street, before making your way to Oxenhope for the first of three big asphalt climbs. The crossing of Oxenhope Moor takes you high above the congested valleys for a brief period of calm and big open skies, before you plunge down the other side into Hebden Bridge.

Once in the town take the left past Eiffel Buildings, then left at the top onto Birchcliffe Road to follow this out of town, to climb almost all the way to Midgley. With the legs now well and truly softened up, drop to cross the River Calder in

LEFT *Negotiating the absolute chaos of Thwaites Brow.*

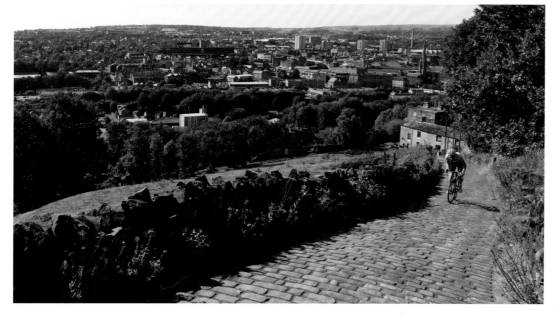

Mytholmroyd, then ready yourself for Cragg Vale, the longest single ascent anywhere in England (it even has a sign to prove it). Over the next 9 kilometres, on an average gradient of just 3%, you'll gain 288 metres, so it's never too steep – but when the wind is in your face, which it frequently is, this road can really dish out some punishment.

After a brief foray on the A58, turn south across Baitings Reservoir, skirt round the edge of Rishworth Moor, cross the M62 and travel a little further south to loop underneath Scammonden Water. What may seem like an elaborate detour has a very specific purpose, and that is to deliver you, in the correct orientation, to the base of Steele Lane. A hidden wonder in the jumble of tiny roads that rise and fall from this small valley, the cobbles of Steele Lane hit your front

wheel shortly after you begin to head upwards. Although this fantastic road has provision for riders to avoid the jarring stones by riding the metre or so of smooth surface either side, I can categorically state that this is NOT ALLOWED under any circumstances.

It's now time to head for the killer finale, but first you must negotiate the fall and rise in and out of Sowerby Bridge, before arriving back in Halifax for a triple bill of pulsating cobbles: Gibb Lane, Ploughcroft Lane and the one and only Trooper Lane. Once you've got out of Sowerby Bridge and found your way to Fountain Head, the pleasures of Gibb Lane start as you pass Riding Lane. Wide like a giant boulevard, what starts out as Overdub Wood Road rises round a sweeping right-hand bend, then breaks

left onto the narrower Gibb Lane. On the whole the cobbles are large, even and well set at first, then, as Gibb Lane starts and the gradient ramps up towards the unpleasant, they become a little more chaotic and random.

With this one tamed, make your way to Moor End, then double back into town and through Ovenden to the A647 and the base of Ploughcroft Lane. Short, straight and with smaller, neatly set stones, this penultimate climb should be a breeze. By now your legs will be stinging but your technique, your ability to tame the anarchy of the cobbles, down to a T, which is good, because you'll need all your experience to get you up the last one, Trooper Lane.

Until I saw this climb I thought I'd seen it all, but I'd seen nothing. *Nothing.* Trooper Lane is the Muur van Geraardsbergen on steroids. Just the right side of ridiculous, the cobbles start about halfway up the climb, where the already narrow road is compressed even further, and on a pronounced camber the stones begin to hammer your wheels. If it's not hard enough already to ride on cobbles and a sloping camber, just wait until the gradient tips up to 30% – yes, 30%! If you keep clipped in on this road then you will have passed one of the greatest challenges the British roads can throw up, so good luck. Once at the top, with either slightly worn cleats or an intact sense of pride, all that is left is to drop back to the Piece Hall to finish what could one day become a classic route to match anything the Belgians can muster.

ABOVE *Trooper Lane rewrites the rule book for crazy roads. 30% gradient and cobbles!*

YORKSHIRE

WEST YORKSHIRE COBBLES

DISTANCE	113KM
CLIMBING	+2,964M
DIFFICULTY	9/10

FOOD & WATER | BINGLEY / OXENHOPE / HEBDEN BRIDGE / SOWERBY BRIDGE

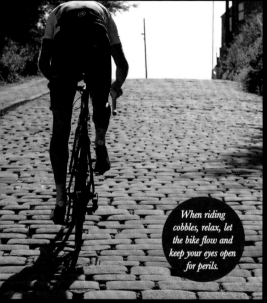

When riding cobbles, relax, let the bike flow and keep your eyes open for perils.

KEY CLIMBS

1 SHIBDEN WALL
878m +119m

A true classic. The Shibden Wall has it all, 25% gradient, tight bends and in places huge irregular cobbles. Take as much speed from the tarmac start then try to preserve your momentum for as long as you can.

2 THWAITES BROW
1,215m +126m

Weaving through multiple 25% corners, finding a clean line on Thwaites Brow is a constant challenge. It jars and jolts, twists and turns like no other road in Britain.

3 TROOPER LANE
769m +123m

A brutal finale, Trooper Lane will push you right to the limit. As soon as you hit the stones the slope rises to 20% and it goes on and on. The really steep stuff, the 30% section, arrives as you approach the houses at the top so just cross your fingers you have a small enough gear to preserve forward motion. You'll love it!

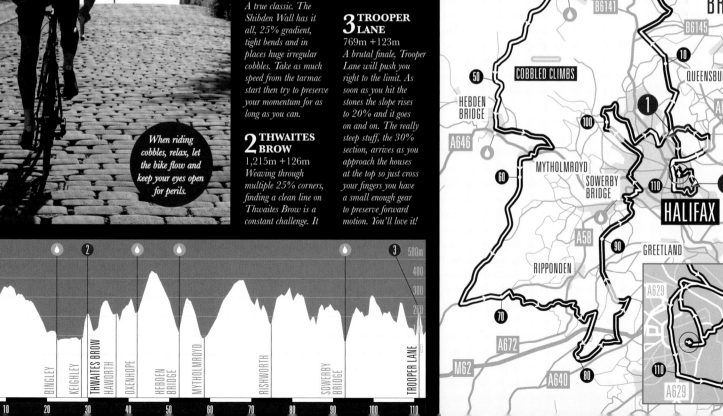

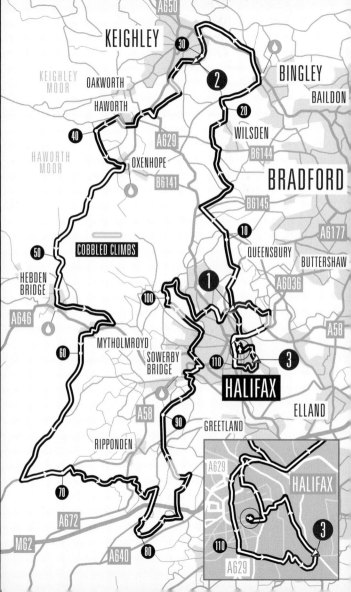

NORTH

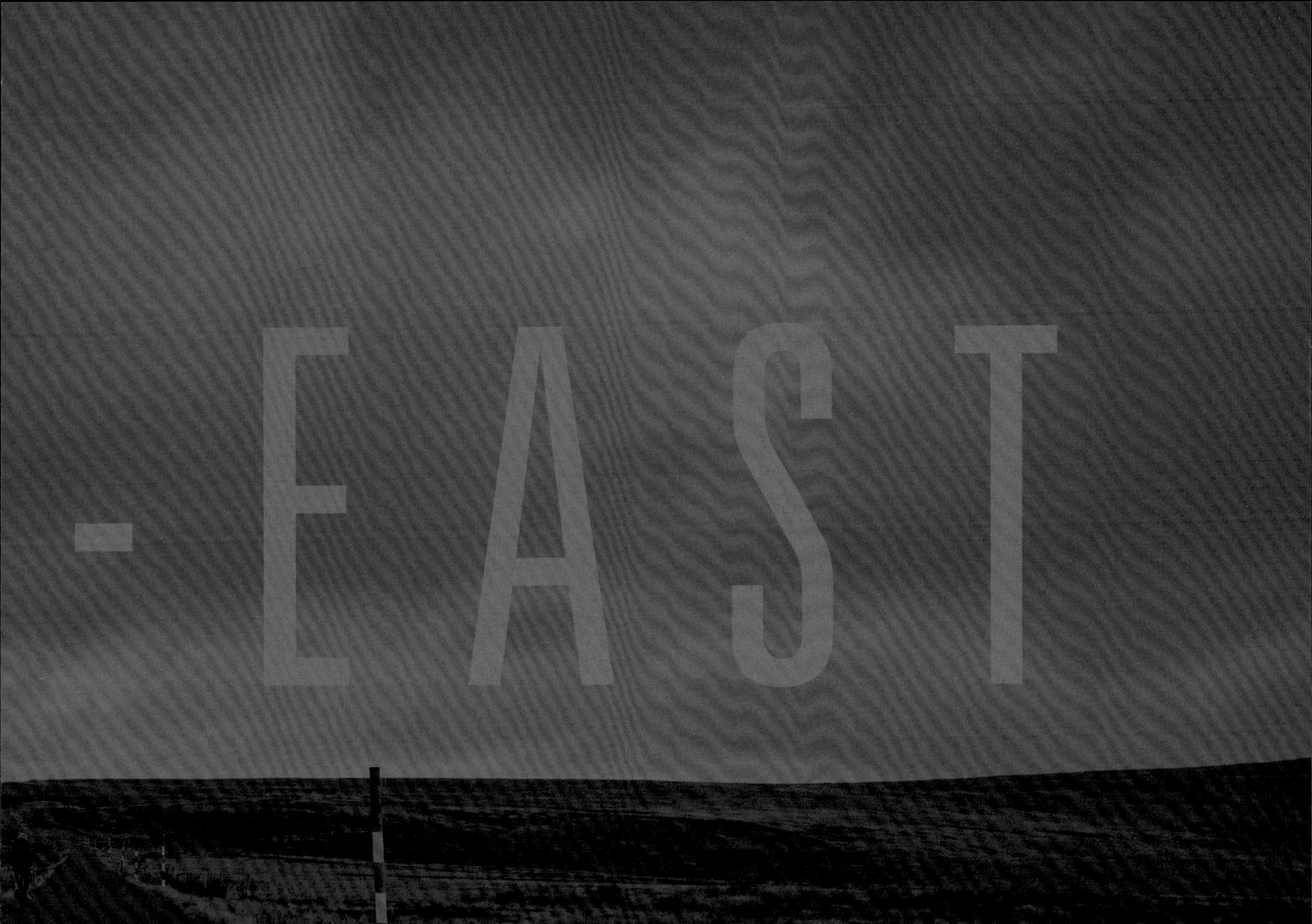
-EAST

KNOW YOUR ENEMY

DISTANCE 121KM | **CLIMBING** +2,514M

PHOTOGRAPHY PHIL HALL

*A journey across the highest
and wildest passes in England*

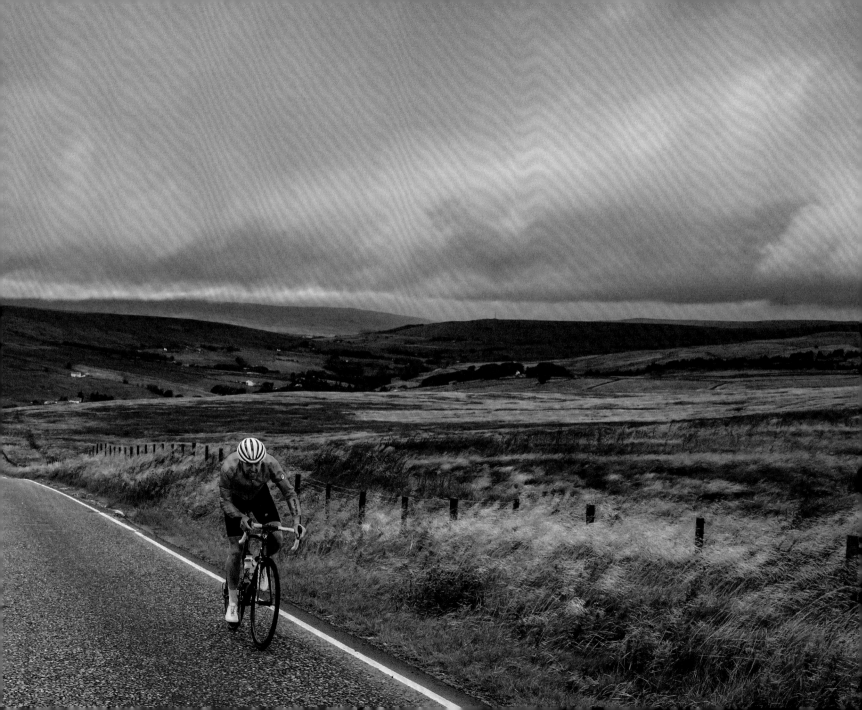

PREVIOUS PAGE
*Reaching the top of Killhope
Cross, the highest pass in Cumbria.*

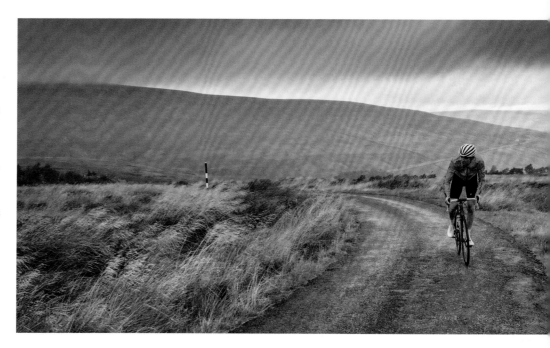

On the morning of 25 October 1992, I awoke in a B&B just outside St John's Chapel in Weardale to draw back the curtains and see the land covered with a foot of snow. Out of nowhere, and seemingly without warning, the valley had been paralysed by nature, and from the looks of things I was well and truly stuck.

Now, on any standard day this wouldn't be such a problem, but that day the National Hill Climb Championship was due to be held in a couple of hours' time on the highest pass in England, the infamous Chapel Fell. I was in great shape, and my mate Nick and I had driven to what seemed at the time the most northern extremities of the realm and the absolute middle of nowhere. It was pretty obvious the race was not going to be happening – in fact, once we had slid my old VW Golf down to the HQ, the talk was focused not on racing but rather on evacuating the valley before we all became trapped.

After I'd somehow escaped back to the Midlands, it would be almost seventeen years before I would return, to at last tackle Chapel Fell. That first ride marked the start of a tortured relationship that would have me hating this road more than any other in Britain.

The focus of this loop has to be Chapel Fell, as it is both the toughest obstacle and the high point of the day, but of course there's far more to get your teeth into round here, as the roads cross back and forth between Weardale and Teesdale. Immersed in some of the most striking landscape in England, and traversing arguably its most inhospitable passes, this ride is as beautiful as it is challenging, and one I would recommend if at all possible be ridden in favourable conditions.

We start and finish in the town of Stanhope, and the initial 10 kilometres are nice and steady, rolling west towards Daddry Shield on the minor road that shadows the A689. After this relatively placid introduction, you reach the base of the first of the giant climbs and turn south, to take on the road up to Swinhope Head. Broken into two sectors of climbing separated by a lengthy hiatus, this glorious road will take you to an altitude of 607 metres as it bisects Swinhope Moor and Westernhope Moor. As we enter the final stage of the climb, past the last buildings the road breaks left, and rises up to a gate that blocks your progress. Once that's negotiated, the scenery opens up dramatically, as you face Black Hill dead ahead, and the huge views out over Weardale on your left. Up and through the sweeping right-hand bend, cutting though the sparse grassland, the pitch of the slope hits its maximum just before the summit, which ushers in your next stupendous landscape, this time looking out across Teesdale.

With the first huge climb in your legs, it's time to plunge down the long descent across Newbiggin Common and into the heart of the neighbouring valley. The next stretch of the ride follows exactly the same path as a substantial part of Ride 32, as you climb the long ascent through Teesdale up Yad Moss to Burnhope

ABOVE *Leaden skies and howling winds hinder progress on Swinhope Head.*

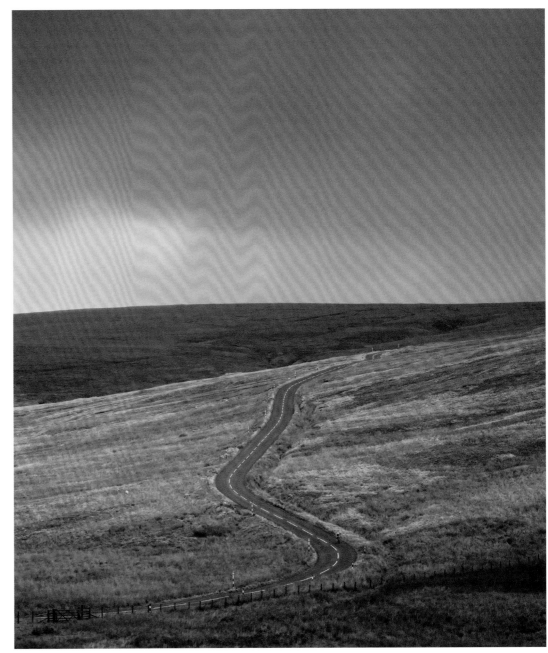

Seat. These 18 kilometres of almost consistent altitude gain get wilder and wilder as they rise to peak at the border with Cumbria and the Yad Moss Ski Tow. Dropping down the other side, the route heads into Alston which, after 50 tough kilometres, is perfectly placed for a pit stop should you desire, but don't take on too much fuel, as I've worked in a nasty little climb right out of town which could see you dumping it if it's not settled in your stomach. The short, sharp ramp of Coatly Hill will sting the legs, of that you can be sure, but, once over the top, they will be allowed some respite before they take on the giant Killhope Cross.

The highest road in Cumbria, this wild climb hits you with multiple waves of punishing gradient, one after another until you snap. Heading east from Nenthall, the giant tarmac staircase ramps up in five distinct stages, each set on a gruelling double-digit gradient. The peak stands at a lofty 623 metres, and in challenging conditions it is not a place for spending time dithering, so, stunning though the views are, quickly grab some photos then, before you get exposure, head back into the shelter of Weardale, where you can prepare to face the monster that is Chapel Fell.

Since 1992, the National Hill Climb Championship has only ventured to the high passes on a couple of occasions, instead favouring climbs that will likely have more benign conditions because, let me tell you, and tell you once only, it is always wild on Chapel

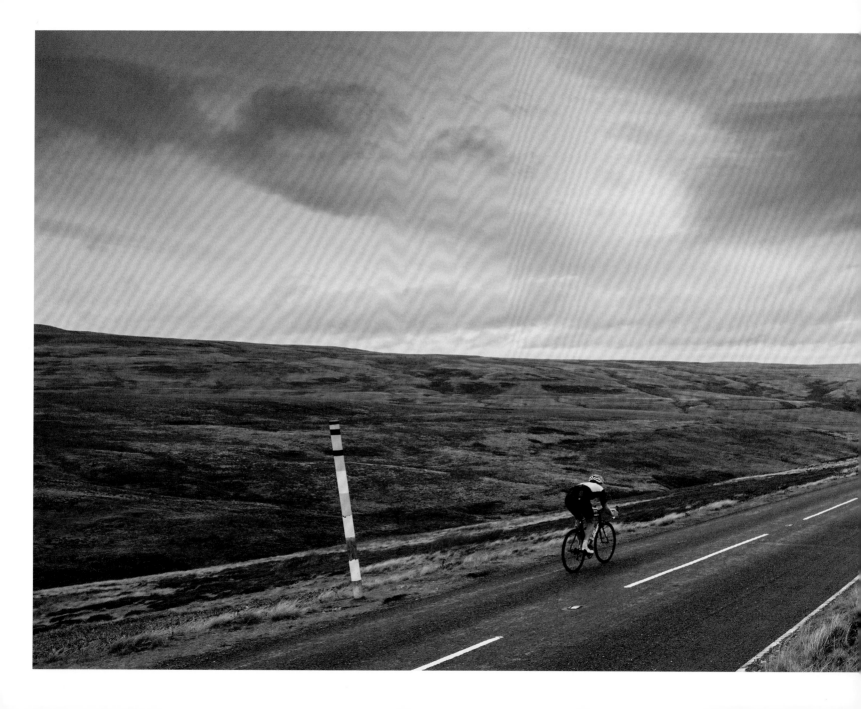

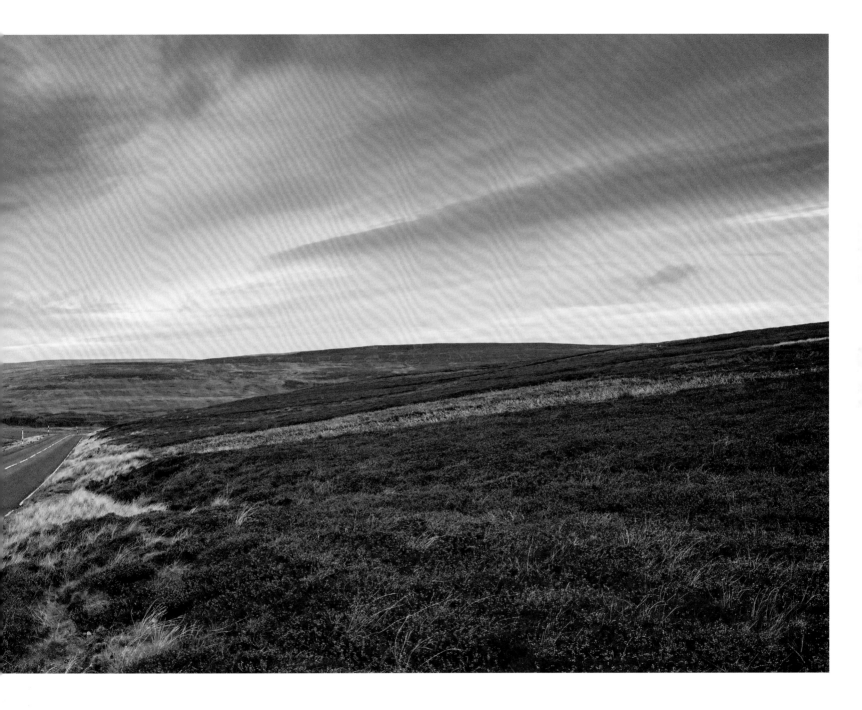

PREVIOUS PAGE
*Descending across Bollihope
Common whilst eyeing up the
last climb before home.*

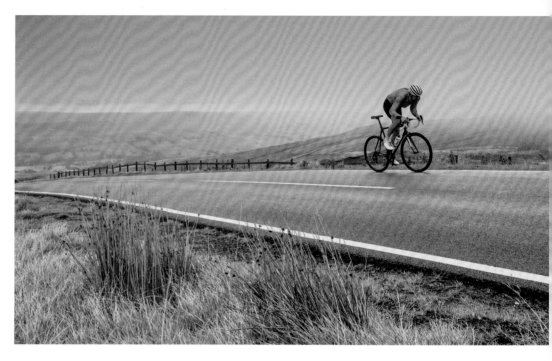

Fell. To date I've ridden this beast just the five times, and every one of them has been into the teeth of a monumental headwind, every time I've been lashed by rain, and every time I have said, never again.

Of all the hills in England I have crossed, this is the one that has hurt me the most. A glutton for punishment, of course, I continue to return, if only in the vain hope that one day it will be kind to me. But that day is yet to arrive, so until then I'll just have to take the beating, as I slog away on the unforgiving gradient. Climbing 323 metres in 4.1 kilometres, laced with multiple stretches over 15%, it would be hard enough without adverse weather but, with the constant force of nature pushing against you, it simply breaks you down. From the time you crest the first stiff rise out of town, you see the climb in its entirety and the enormity of the task before you, laid out in a single line up the hillside. With no deviation to lessen the slope until you close in on the summit, it's a straight line of remorseless attrition that messes with the mind like few other climbs can.

The views from high up are, needless to say, exemplary and, once the summit is conquered – in this case the word is not an exaggeration – it's back to Teesdale once more, to take on a series of short and very sharp spikes on the way east. First there's a foray on the B6277 and then I've – and you can thank me later – diverted the road through Newbiggin to treat you to the joy of Miry Lane. Although only 800 metres long, this nasty ramp boasts an average of 13%, and peaks at 20% to further roughen up your tired legs.

Continue east and, instead of cutting through Middleton, I've shoe-horned in two more harsh lumps on the exquisite loop round Hudeshope Beck. Diverting north into the cul-de-sac, then back south, this allows you to discover yet more rugged scenery, before turning east to cut the corner over Raven Hills to join the B6278. If you are in need of supplies, though, you could miss this out and instead divert into Middleton, before joining up with the main road north to begin what is arguably the most beautiful part of the day's ride.

This long climb takes you up above 500 metres altitude again, before throwing you down the other side for the dazzling passage across Bollihope Common. It's fast, straight and lined with the ubiquitous snow poles, and you will cascade down to cross Bollihope Burn, then abruptly hit one last hurdle. On your way you'll have spied this final ascent in the distance, as it appears like a wall rising from the valley floor, but, fear not, it isn't quite as tough as it appears. It's also, as I said, the last climb of the day, so you're safe in the knowledge that if your legs fall apart here you'll still get home, fingers crossed. The ride is then completed by snaking down through the tight hairpins of Unthank Bank to return to Stanhope exhausted, yet hopefully exhilarated, after a day spent in immaculate scenery of epic proportions.

ABOVE *Battling the infernal
wind to the top of Chapel Fell.*

RIDE 22 — NORTH-EAST

WEARDALE & TEESDALE

DISTANCE 121KM

CLIMBING +2,514M

DIFFICULTY 8/10

FOOD & WATER | ALSTON / ST JOHN'S CHAPEL / MIDDLETON

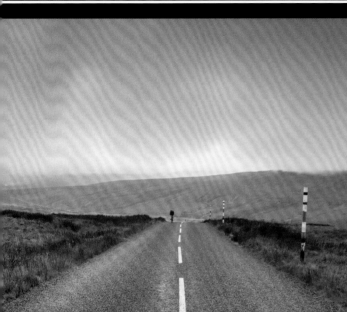

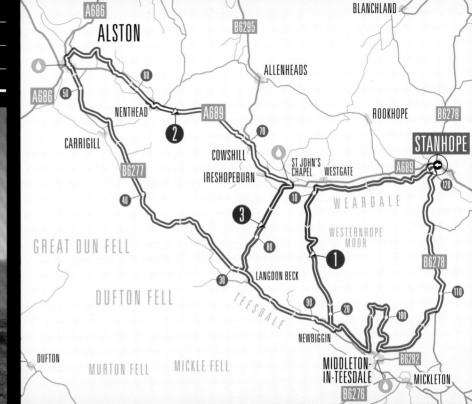

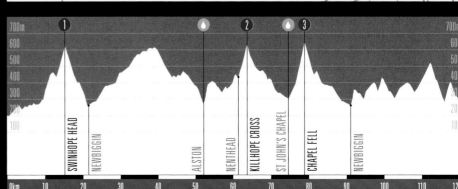

KEY CLIMBS

1 SWINHOPE HEAD
5,497m +318m

The climbing comes in two parts, the short gentle first part then tougher, longer and more exposed second part. With a gate to negotiate at midway if you are going for the KOM get a mate to hold it open for you; h and save some gas for the p 15% ramp to the finish

2 KILLHOPE CROSS
5,204m +249m

Linking Cumbria to County Durham, this pass seems to have its own micro-climate at the top, one a fair few degrees cooler than down the bottom. With an average gradient of 5% but slopes approaching 17% its climbing comes in waves separated by periods of rest

3 CHAPEL FELL
3,940m +320m

My Nemesis. This road seems to have it in for me and as a result I just hate it! Once out of St John's Chapel and with the full enormity of the climb in plain sight it's best not to look up. Just grind away on the unforgiving slopes that reach 16% for what seems like an eternity

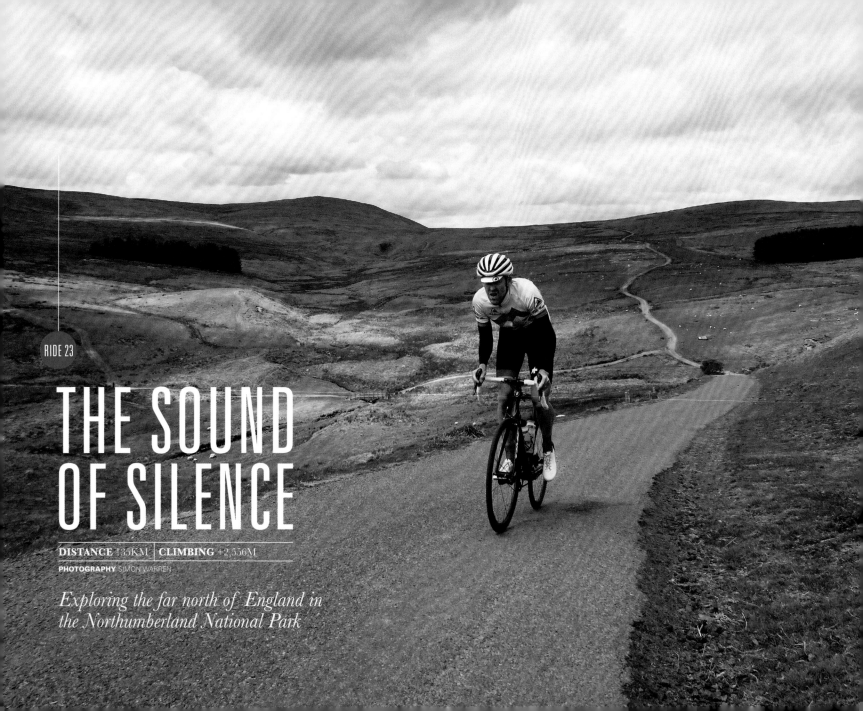

RIDE 23

THE SOUND
OF SILENCE

DISTANCE 135KM | **CLIMBING** +2,556M

PHOTOGRAPHY SIMON WARREN

*Exploring the far north of England in
the Northumberland National Park*

When I first cast my eyes to the far north of England in search of hills to conquer, I was somewhat disappointed. The further towards Scotland, I naïvely imagined, the more inhospitable the scenery – but actually, after all the razzmatazz of County Durham, the topography calms down somewhat on the way to the border. There are hills out there, though, and this ride picks off the best of them. However, it's not the hills that draw people up here, but the deathly quiet roads that Northumberland has in abundance. Formed of two loops with an interconnecting passage, and set almost entirely within the Northumberland National Park, this ride uses the village of Bellingham as its base, which, although small, has all the facilities for pre- and post-ride nutrition.

To start, head out west on the B6320, then take the first right turn, still going west just above the River North Tyne, through Charlton to Lanehead. Here, turn right to Greenhaugh and, once through the village, take the right-hand turn to start the first climb of the day. Rising in two distinct sections, the climb of High Green takes you onto the wild, windswept fells where there's nothing between you and the sky. Passing Highgreen Manor, then bisecting Blackburn Common and Troughend Common, keep climbing until you can climb no more, then press on over the summit to soak up the colossal views out over the Cheviot Hills. Proceeding in a dead-straight line, with nothing more substantial than a blade of grass for protection from any weather, descend into

Redesdale to meet the A68, then turn right, then first left, on the B6320 to Otterburn.

Turning right here on the A696, then left onto the B6341 to Elsdon, the route wastes no time before reaching climb two of the day, the sinister Winter's Gibbet. Standing at the summit is said gibbet: a macabre monument erected in 1792 to display the corpse of William Winter after he was convicted of murdering Margaret Crozier (although it has been destroyed and replaced many times since). The climb to the top is close to 3.5 kilometres and, although only averaging 4%, it does ramp up to 10% in places, and was the venue for the 2004 National Hill Climb Championship – indeed, the most northerly climb ever to host the event. Keep your eyes on the horizon to spot the gibbet which, if you're lucky, might have a fibreglass head swinging

from it. Once over the summit, get stuck into the long straight descent to join the B6342, then, at the Rothley Cross Roads, turn north, still on the B6342, all the way into Rothbury.

With four spikes in gradient, this 15-kilometre trek north over sleepy roads, between the rolling farmland and clumps of forest, will really begin to sap your energy. The last of these series of lumps crossing Garleigh Moor takes you back briefly onto exposed ground, before the plunge down into Rothbury, where at 55 kilometres refreshments could be taken before the killer climb of Cragpit Hill.

This is a beast of a road: a real slog, which starts in the forest around the Cragside Estate, then, following a few undulations and false starts, hits you with a triple whammy of tough ramps on its way to its empty summit. With that

LEFT *Returning from the isolation of the High Knowes summit, a remarkable road.*

ABOVE *The huge empty landscapes of Northumberland are heaven to ride though.*

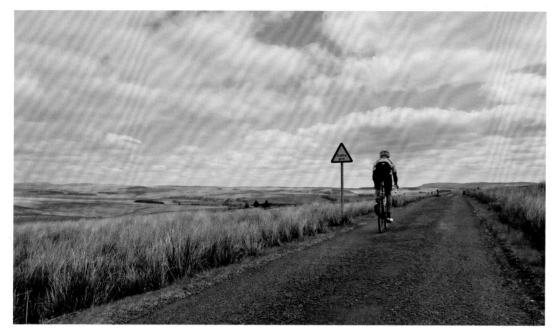

across the bare hillside to the horizon. Breaking up the climb is a small yet sharp descent (which will bite you on the way back), then it kicks up into another couple of kilometres to the top.

Once you reach the summit, have a look around, then turn to retrace the route back to Alnham, where you turn right to head south to Netherton, Burradon and Warton to reach the B6341. Turning right at the T-junction, follow the B6341 to Hepple, in Coquetdale, ride through the village and cross the river to approach the wicked climb up to Bilsmore. At 2 kilometres long, with an average gradient of 7%, it gets wilder the higher it climbs, to open up grand views before falling over the other side for the second visit of the day to Elsdon. Through the village to Otterburn you go and, continuing to trace your tracks from earlier, head south to the A68, where this time you pass straight across to continue on to the last climb of the day.

Heading directly up this final ramp, this final punishment for your legs is close to 6 kilometres from bottom to top: never steep – just a consistent grind onto yet more splendidly barren moors. Can you ever have too many hills crossing empty scenery? No, of course not, and I'd go as far to say this is the best part of the entire route. Under huge skies, with perpetual views in all directions, this is just perfect Northumberland. As you cross Troughend Common, breathe in the clean air and empty the clutter of your mind, before rolling over the top for the rapid drop back to base in Bellingham.

significant obstacle out of the way, you're almost at the most easterly point of the route. Crossing the A697, there's one more climb to get there, up past Corby's Crags. With gradients as steep as 13% on its lower slopes, this is another stiff examination for the legs. Once over the brow, turn left down Lemmington Bank, back across the A697, and ride through the villages of Whittingham and Little Ryle.

The route now travels due west on a largely benign profile, passing from farm to farm on the narrow, agricultural (dirty) roads, and the next target is the climb up to High Knowes. A one-way road, this is a diversion off the loop, which takes you as far as you can ride on tarmac into this part of the Cheviot Hills. The

border between Scotland and England has few crossings and even fewer roads, so when one presents itself you must take the opportunity to ride it. At the junction that leads you to the base beside a farm, there is a sign for the Northumberland National Park, and another noting that it is indeed a dead end. From here you head north into nowhere.

The tiny road starts between low stone walls, then, as these end, you approach a cluster of grass-covered mounds. Squirming its way between them, the road climbs around the contours among the decidedly rugged scenery, deeper into the unknown. Around the fourth – yes, fourth – hairpin the road begins to straighten, and heads out on its isolated path

ABOVE *Far from the madding crown Northumberland is a joy to ride through.*

NORTH-EAST

NORTHUMBERLAND

DISTANCE 135KM

CLIMBING +2,556M

DIFFICULTY 5/10

FOOD & WATER | ROTHBURY / OTTERBURN

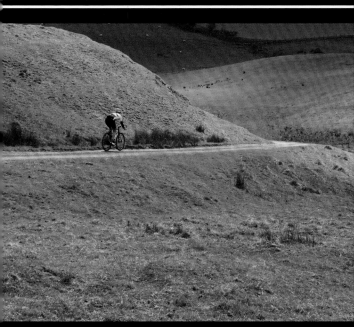

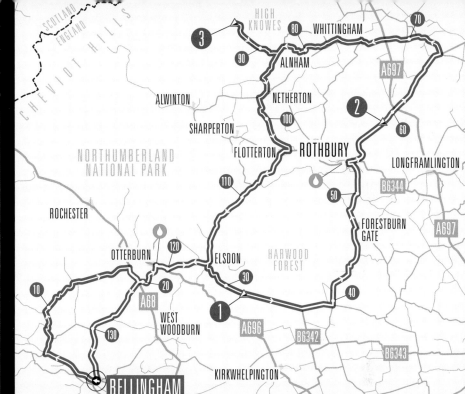

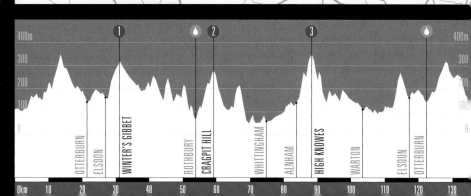

KEY CLIMBS

1 WINTER'S GIBBET
3,354m +139m

With a 4% average it doesn't look much on paper but hidden in there are a couple of tough stretches of 10% slope. Hardest is the first part and with a nice, almost level sector in the middle you can click up a couple of sprockets for the final 1,500 metres to pass the famous gibbet at the top.

2 CRAGPIT HILL
5,072m +206m

Once out of Rothbury the climbing comes in three distinct bursts, the first of which ramps up to 16% on the wide road that cuts through the forest. The average is only 3% because each hard ramp is followed by a gentle stretch where you can recover a little before tackling the next.

3 HIGH KNOWES
3,799m +200m

A road to nowhere this climb has a bit of everything from twisting bends to a small mid-climb descent. Most of the changes in direction come through the hairpins at the bottom then the slope increases in severity, up to 18% before the tiny drop which leads you into the lonely slog to find the summit.

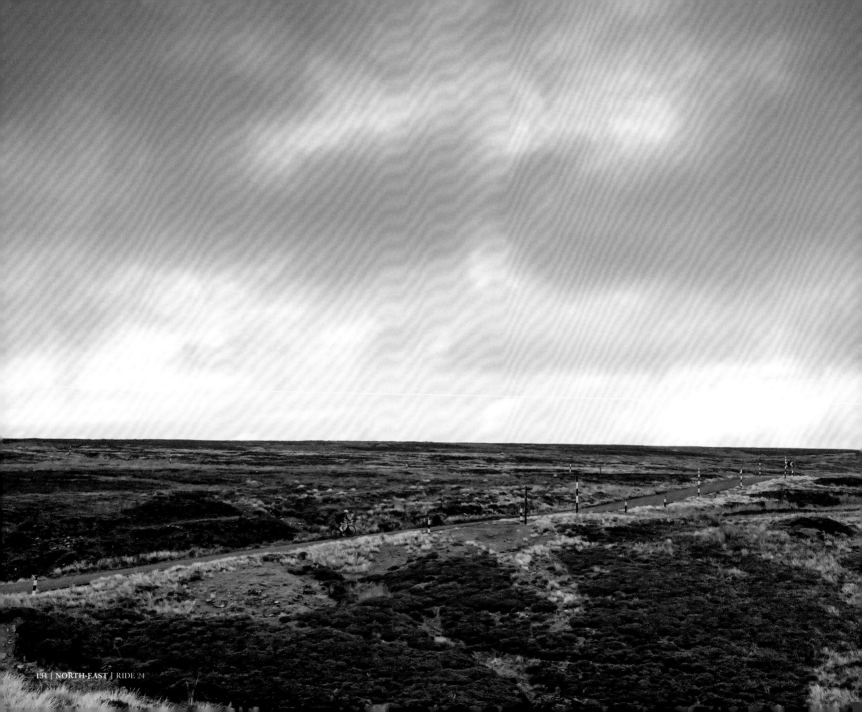

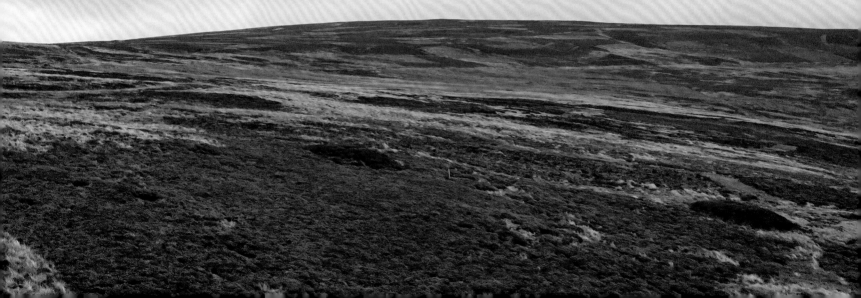

INTO THE VOID

DISTANCE 136KM | **CLIMBING** +2,892M

PHOTOGRAPHY PHIL HALL

*Travelling from Northumberland to County Durham
in search of adventure in the North Pennines*

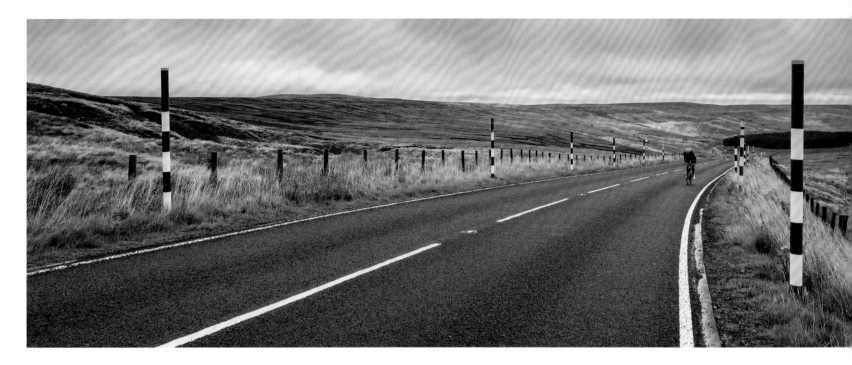

The further north you travel in the Pennines, the bleaker the scenery becomes, but don't for one minute think bleak is a negative adjective. In this context bleak is 100% positive. Bleak means less development, quieter roads and fewer people. Bleak is solitude, unspoilt nature, huge vistas and huge climbs. Although the weather may be harsh at times, bleak is to be embraced and soaked up, for it is something the densely populated parts of the country would give their eye teeth for.

The first time I ventured into Weardale, into what was at the time a mystical far-away kingdom, I really did feel like an intrepid explorer. It was mid-March and, while the North was trying to free itself from the grips of winter, some late snow had fallen to throw a spanner in the works. I was working on my second climbing guide, though, and had a deadline to meet: there were hills I had to ride and, as time was running out and my trip could not be postponed, I had to head north and cross my fingers the roads would be rideable.

As it turned out, although the moors were white and the temperature was just a couple of degrees above freezing, the roads were miraculously and immaculately clear. The harsh contrast of black asphalt against the surrounding white-out, all trapped under a claustrophobically heavy sky, helped frame one of the best days on a bike I've ever had.

To show off the best of Weardale and its surroundings, and to chuck into the mix what is in my opinion the best hill in the North-East, I have picked Hexham for the start–finish point and, to kick things off, the ride heads due east towards Newcastle. To warm the legs up, there are a few kilometres of flat on the A695, but this gentle opening is only brief as, before you know it, you arrive at the first test, Prospect Hill.

I kick myself every time I think of this hill, because it should have been in my original *100 Greatest Cycling Climbs* book. I'll never forget the moment I first spotted it on the map: I couldn't believe it was real. What I saw was – is – a geometrically perfect zigzag, composed of seven

PREVIOUS PAGE

This is why you head to the North Pennines.

ABOVE *Fighting gravity and the wind up to Killhope Cross.*

straights and six corners, which from above resembles a road being crushed in a vice. The fun begins when you leave the A695: heading south, you go from bend to bend to bend on the unforgiving gradient until you arrive at the top, dizzy from the constant switching of direction, not to mention the effort needed.

With this early excitement out the way, it's time to leave the relative 'hustle and bustle' of Northumberland and head for the barren lanes of County Durham. Heading to Slaley, and then to the banks of the Derwent Reservoir, the route climbs a little, but there's nothing too much to trouble the legs – yet. When you reach Blanchland, though, the first big climb of the day starts, Bale Hill, which will take you all the way up onto Edmundbyers Common. Peaking at 499 metres, and with more than one stretch of high double-figure gradient, this is a serious ascent set in remarkable surroundings.

Once this is crossed, you drop rapidly down into Stanhope in the bottom of Weardale, where there are shops if you need them, before pressing on west, following the valley upwards. To avoid the busier road, the route sticks to the back lanes that lie below it, and heads through Brotherlee to Daddry Shield past the multitude of farms that punctuate the journey. Once in this village, and to continue avoiding the A689, cross over the River Wear and keep heading westwards, this time north of the main road, all the way to Cowshill.

In Cowshill you now have no choice but to join the A689, to extract yourself from the valley

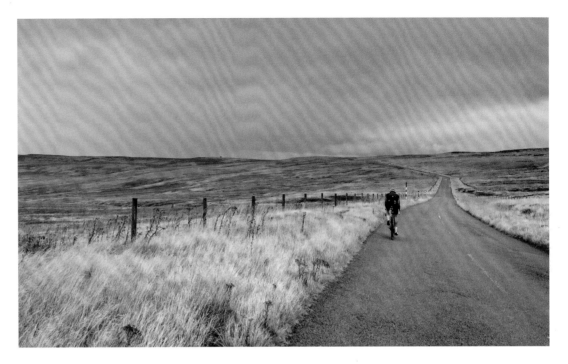

heading all the way up to Killhope Cross and the border with Cumbria. It's an easier ascent than its Cumbrian flank, but one more likely to be ridden into a prevailing westerly, which always makes the higher slopes of this climb a serious challenge. Once the small stone cross that marks the summit has been reached, it's time for the thunderous drop over the other side that leads to the right turn into Coalcleugh Moor. Heading north towards Allendale Town and back into Northumberland, you'll see on your right the beautiful, yet fearsome sight of Coalcleugh Hill cutting its way over the hillside.

Now, I'd love to say the ride heads over this climb, but unfortunately not: its fate lies in the

blissful solitude of the path across Dryburn Moor, so you can breathe a sigh of relief if you are already tired. Instead of heading into Allendale, I plotted a bypass to pick up a brace of wonderful little hills, cutting the corner to reach the B6295 and cross the East Allen river. Following the road south as it then follows the path of the East Allen river, you arrive in Allenheads for the next big climb, the crossing of Burtree Fell. Dividing the small interlocking hills via a handful of slight direction changes, this charming climb finds its way to the summit and delivers you back once more into County Durham.

This time, as it's predominantly downhill, the route utilises the main road to make the

ABOVE *Heading north across the beautifully barren Dryburn Moor.*

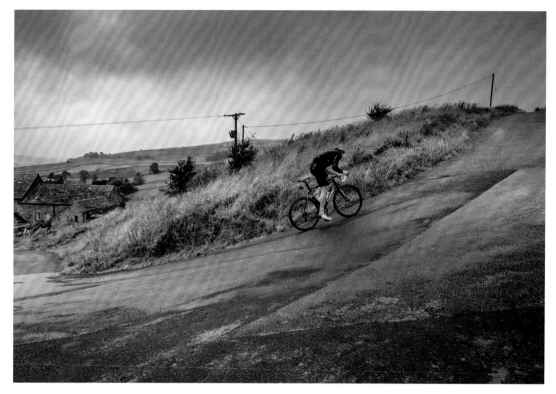

transition to the first of two killer climbs that usher in the final part of the adventure. Descending through Wearhead and St John's Chapel (which makes for the perfect pit stop after 100 kilometres), you arrive in Westgate, where it's time to take a few deep breaths. Hidden between the houses in the centre of the village there is a small road heading north; it may look inconspicuous, but this is the base of the fearsome Peat Hill.

From the moment your wheels turn left, you'll see the tarmac ahead vanish upwards, dividing the houses as it climbs. A faded 20% gradient sign sees it rear up into its initial vicious pitch before, free of the buildings, twisting first right, then left, then right again into the real meat of the climb. Beyond the farm on the left, you crawl up to an abrupt hairpin, which must be ridden wide to minimise its impact, and then, and only then, does the slope relax. At the abandoned mine of West Rigg Opencut it is still a way to the eventual finish, which you'll find at the junction in the shadow of Windy Hill. Turning right here and careering down across Lintzgarth Common,

in the blink of an eye you'll arrive at Rookhope Burn to take on the second big monster, Cuthbert's Hill.

It was on this climb all those years ago that I truly fell for these roads. This perfect stretch of asphalt that links Rookhope with Blanchland across the desolate Hunstanworth Moor is simply exquisite. Your experience begins with a bit of 20% slope to further weaken your now surely tired limbs, throws in a couple of nice bends, then, once the climbing is done with, it's time to cross the lonely moorland and enjoy the bleakness. Under leaden skies, and with nothing for company but the chatter of grouse and the whistle of the wind, this is a truly special place to be. Once you have drunk in every last drop of your surroundings and become 'at one' with nature, you must unfortunately leave it all behind and plunge back down into Blanchland to begin the trip back up to Hexham.

Immediately out of town comes the climb of Park Bank, which packs a double punch of sharp gradient. Then, crossing Blanchland Moor, you reach the Slaley Forest, which ushers in 10 sublime kilometres of downhill. All rides, in my opinion, should end with a good long downhill: it helps the production of endorphins, ensures you finish at speed and on a high. However, and I am sorry, you've got one more hill (anyone who has ever ridden with me will know there's always one more hill): the small climb up Linnels Bank from Devil's Water – and then it's done. Your adventure is over, I promise.

ABOVE *The last of the steep bends on Peat Hill is a real beauty.*

RIDE 24

NORTH-EAST

NORTH PENNINES

DISTANCE 136KM

CLIMBING +2,892M

DIFFICULTY 8/10

FOOD & WATER | BLANCHLAND / STANHOPE / ST JOHN'S CHAPEL

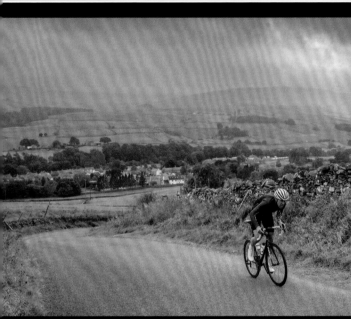

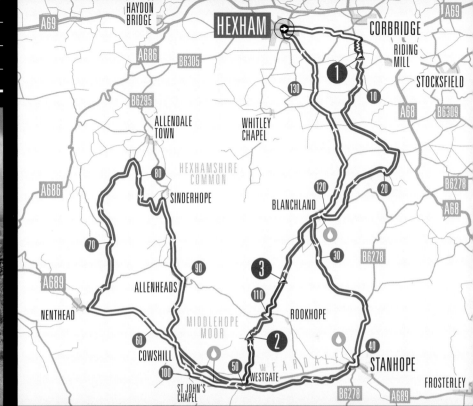

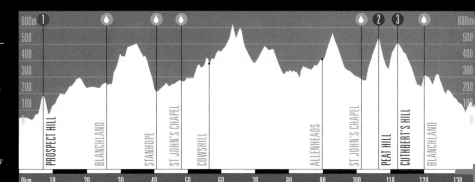

KEY CLIMBS

1 PROSPECT HILL

1,673m +124m

The glorious Prospect Hill boasts an amazing six hairpins in the space of just 1.7 kilometres of climbing. With an average gradient of 7% and a maximum of 15% there is nothing to be afraid of when you arrive at the base but everything to be excited about as you start to climb.

2 PEAT HILL

3,547m +262m

The first 700 metres of Peat Hill are an all-out battle as the rugged narrow road squirms up violently from Weardale. With a maximum gradient of 25% these early slopes are brutal but the rest of the climb is nowhere near as hard and the overall average works out at 7% from bottom to top.

3 CUTHBERT'S HILL

2,759m +150m

Much like Peat Hill, the tough slopes of this climb come right away as it tears itself out of the valley up onto the moor. Hitting 20% through the corners the tough gradient is with you until almost half way then the last 1,500 metres are a breeze to the final summit.

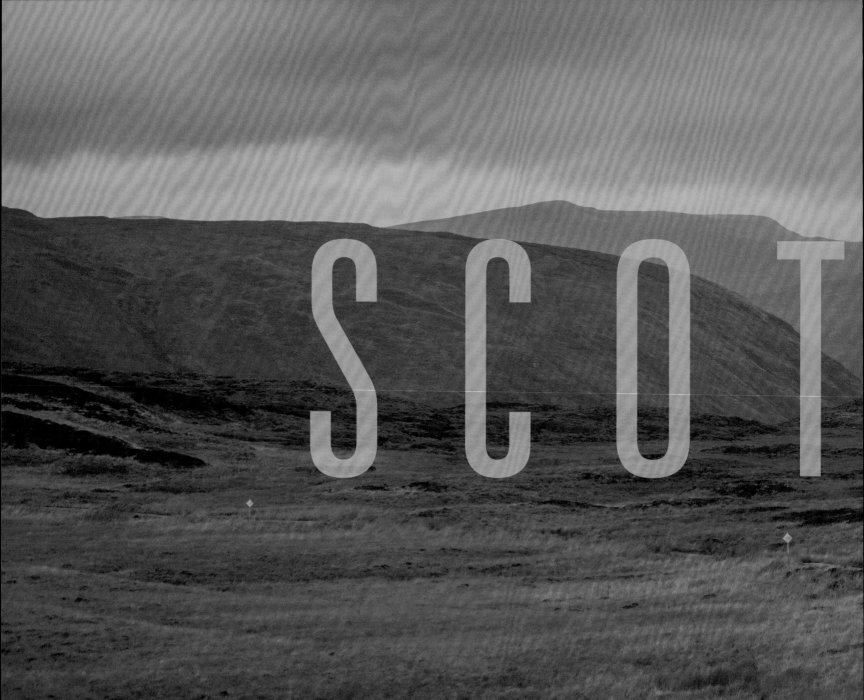

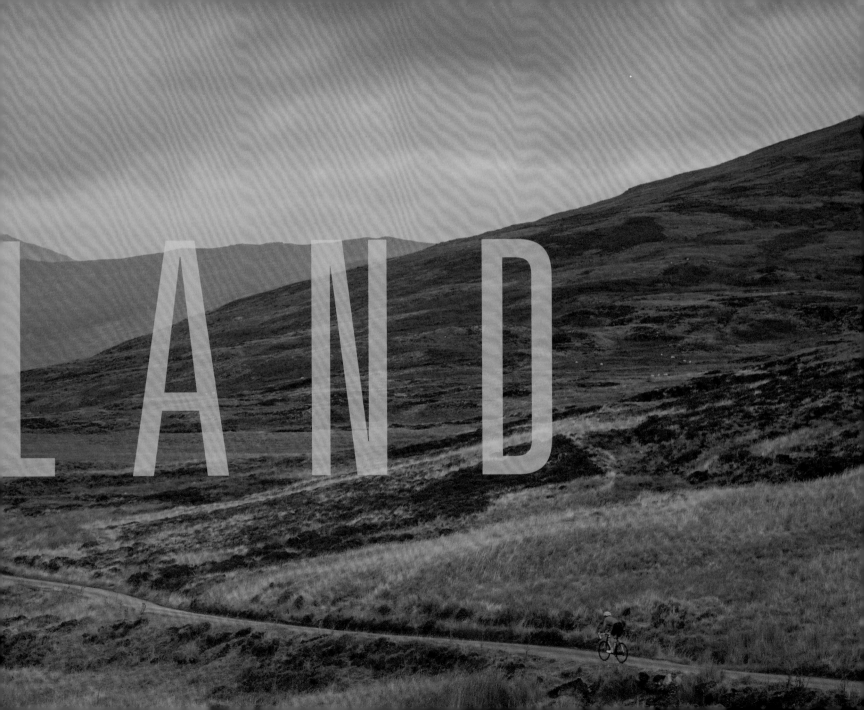

IT'S A LONG WAY TO THE TOP

DISTANCE 204KM | **CLIMBING** +3,827M

PHOTOGRAPHY PHIL HALL

Wonders of the Scottish west coast,
and the biggest climb of them all

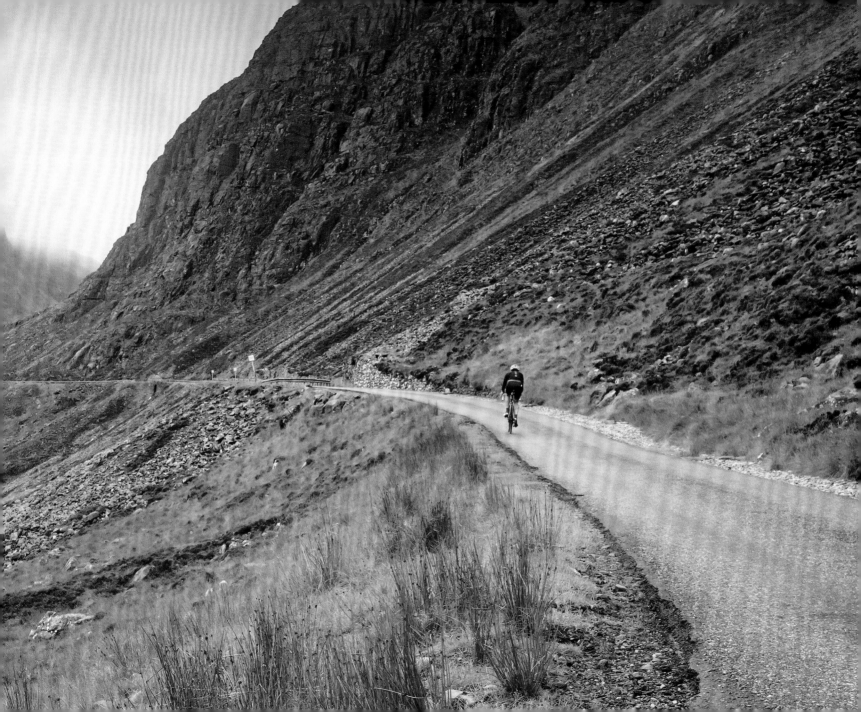

PREVIOUS PAGE
*Riding into the clouds on the
higher slopes of Bealach na Ba.*

The most northerly of the routes in the book, and likely to be the wildest, the central loop of this ride has often been labelled 'The best in Britain' and, to be honest, I can't argue with that. It has absolutely everything any lover of life on two wheels craves in spades, including the only climb, and one of the toughest, Bealach na Ba. Although this mighty road is enough of a challenge on its own, as is the loop around the Applecross peninsula, there are so many great roads in the vicinity that I have ended up creating a giant 204-kilometre course that takes them all in. Be warned: this ride is for high summer, when the days are long, and will also require some logistical planning when you get towards the end (I'll come to that later).

Starting and finishing in Kyle of Lochalsh, the day begins by heading north, following the rugged coastline, via the villages of Badicaul, Erbusaig and Achmore, to meet the A890 at the mouth of Loch Carron. We join the larger road for a while, tracing the edge of the loch all the way north to Strathcarron, where you join the A896 to double back down the other side to the village of Lochcarron. As I have mentioned, at 204 kilometres this loop is a *huge* challenge, so if you think you may not be equipped for that distance, but still want to see the imperious Applecross peninsula, then I'd suggest starting and finishing here (as marked on the map).

Whether you are riding the short or the long route, after leaving the small fishing village it's time for the first significant climb of the day: just

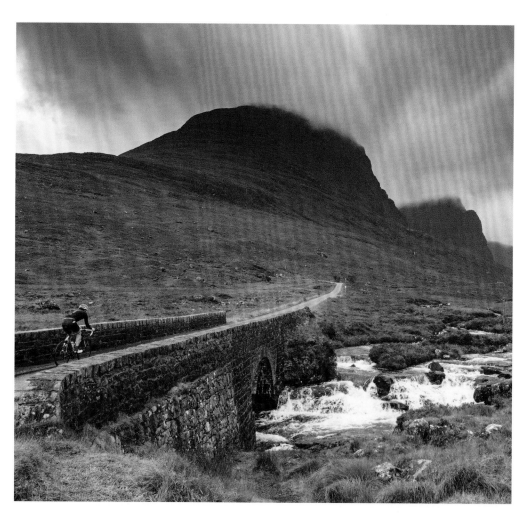

ABOVE *Dark skies are
standard all year round on
the Scottish west coast.*

over two kilometres through the narrowing of the glen, on the way to the *big* one. The nerves will be jangling now as you drop down the other side, pass Ardarroch and roll north to the head of Loch Kishorn and the Tornapress café. Stopping at the T-junction, you'll see the giant road sign warning of the dangers ahead: almost obliterated with stickers, it marks the base of the biggest, baddest road in Britain.

Some are steeper, some longer, but nothing, *nothing* trumps the one and only Bealach na Ba. *NOTHING*. It's epic, it's wild, the weather is *always* bad, it's 9 kilometres of total hill-climbing heaven. Riding at full gas, the best riders can get to the top in just under 30 minutes, but I'd leave an hour to be comfortable (to take loads of photos, of course). If you've not ventured to ride in mainland Europe, chances are you will never have tackled anything of this magnitude before, so make sure you pace yourself at the start as you wind across the rolling foothills beneath the giant peaks above you.

For the first 5 kilometres the slope is set on an agreeable 6–7%, a classic Alpine-style gradient, but then, rounding the right-hand hairpin teetering on the edge of the cliff, you turn north and there, laid out in front of you, is the true magnitude of this climb. Cut from the raw beauty of the hillside, visibly increasing in pitch as it rises, it appears all but overwhelming. We are now way above the valley below, and what was 7% soon turns to 10%, then, approaching the dramatic switchbacks, closes in on 20% to

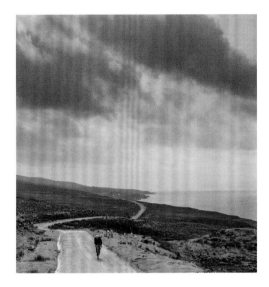

rip your legs to pieces. The sight of the hairpins fills you with dread but, fear not, once you reach them, 'most' of the hard work is over and this section, although steep in the corners, does ease off on the straights, as a proper mountain road should. Beneath cascading waterfalls and jagged rocks, you can cast your eyes out over the grand valley down to Loch Kishorn, to drink in the size of your achievement, before inching through the final bends, then heading inland to eventually reach the summit.

Like I said, this giant climb on its own is enough to satisfy most cyclists for the day, but the wonders this ride contains have only just begun.

ABOVE *Tracing the rugged coastline up towards Fearnbeg.*

The descent over the other side is long and rapid, falling into two distinct sections separated by a vast plateau. Down through the pristine scenery you fall, to the shore at Applecross (which, if you are doing the full distance, makes for the perfect place to refuel), dumping in minutes the entire 608 metres altitude you spent so long accumulating.

It's now time to take the more sedate route back, to trace the circumference of this magical peninsula by heading north along the weather-beaten coastline. The horizon punctuated with rugged islands, the road undulating, with the odd spike in gradient to allow you a fleeting foray out of the saddle, this road is utter perfection. As you reach the northern point of the peninsula and turn south-east, the character of the landscape changes, as the smooth, grass-covered hillsides now become progressively more uneven and dotted with patches of exposed rock. Twisting and turning alongside Loch Torridon, rising and falling past Fearnbeg, Kenmore and Ardheslaig, you navigate this prehistoric landscape interspersed with tiny lochs and craggy bluffs.

Thirty-five kilometres have passed since you crested Bealach na Ba, and it's only now you have to face the next meaningful climbs, as the profile begins to spike and trough once more. On the journey back inland the scenery morphs again, as trees appear on the harsh barren hillsides. As you make your way south towards Tornapress, the Highland peaks over to your left begin to dominate the skyline. This is Scotland at

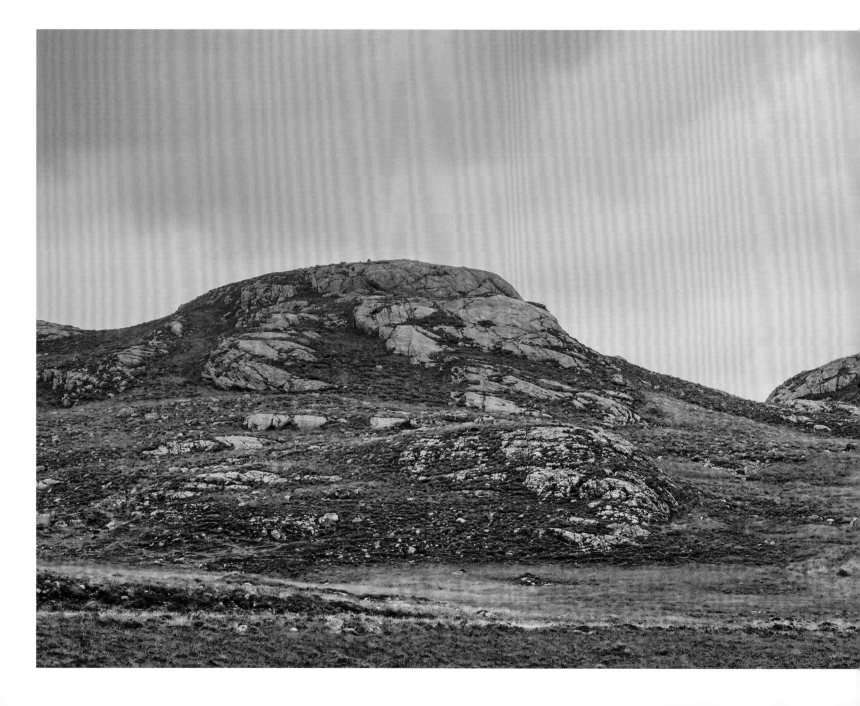

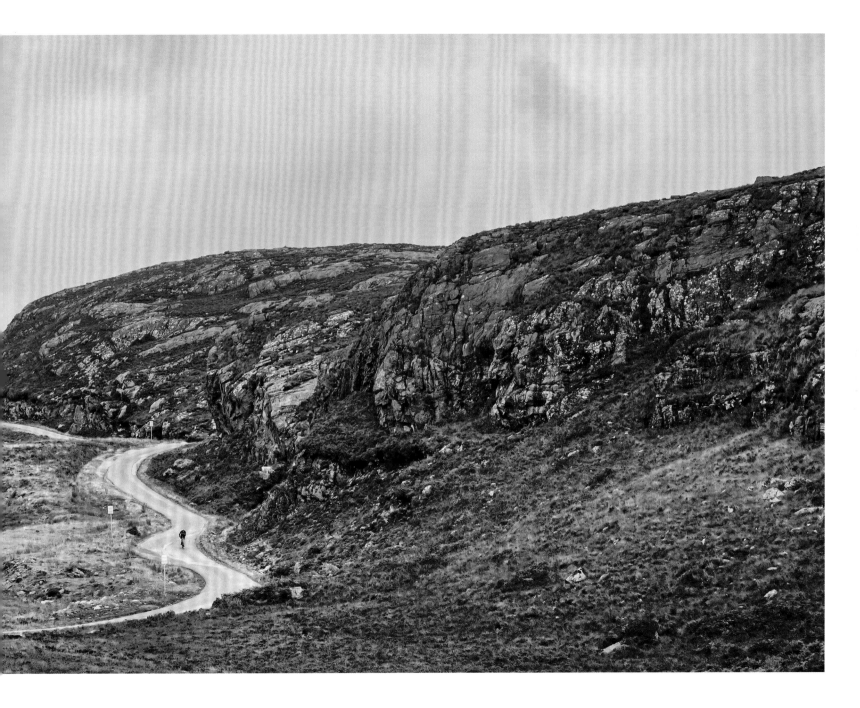

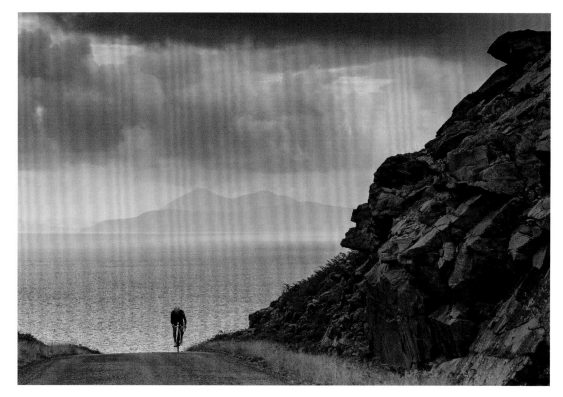

First, though, ride south-east past the world-famous Eilean Donan Castle, and keep heading east all the way to Shiel Bridge, to leave the A87 and head into the forest. Here lies the base of the Bealach Ràtagain, a climb plucked straight from the high mountains of the continent and plonked down in Scotland.

Packed with bends, lined with tall conifers and boasting giant views out to sea, it has everything you can dream of within its 4.5-kilometre journey to the summit. Once over the top, plummet down to the banks of the Glenmore River, and follow this to the shore, where you'll need to catch the ferry to progress. Providing it is running, the *Glenachulish* ferry is the last manually operated turntable ferry in Scotland, and will transport you the very short distance across the Kyle Rhea strait, but, again, you *must* get there during the hours it operates, or you'll have to double back, or swim!

Once across the other side, and without warning or warm-up, you start the last climb of the day and, you'll thank me for this, the second toughest on the ride! Right from the banks of the loch, through a small collection of houses, it's up and away on this fierce ramp out of Kylerhea Glen. Crossing Bealach Udal amidst the dark stone and harsh spikes of heather, you are almost at the finish, and all that is left is to drop through Glen Arroch, then turn right to take the Skye Bridge back to Kyle of Lochalsh, to complete one of the most amazing rides you may ever do. That I can guarantee.

its absolute finest in every way.

Beneath your wheels a succession of nasty little ramps do their best to weaken you on the journey to meet up with the A896 again. At Loch Dughaill comes a glorious climb up through Glen Shieldaig, 3 kilometres of sublime gradient between the sloping banks either side that, with a tailwind, you will be able to rattle off as though your bike is fitted with a motor. Over the top you cascade down to Tornapress and back to the aforementioned road sign, where you can now take a selfie as you've conquered the

beast, before continuing south.

Back around to Lochcarron, then Strathcarron, then Attadale, and follow the A890, via a brace of challenging lumps, all the way south to the A87. If your legs have gone then there is an option here to take the escape route west back to Kyle of Lochalsh. If you are feeling brave, head east to complete the final 50-kilometre loop, which contains two glorious climbs and a ferry. Yes, a ferry, and, to determine whether you can complete your ride, you must check the sailing times in advance (see contact details opposite).

ABOVE *The insignificance
of man and machine.*

RIDE 25

SCOTLAND

APPLECROSS AND SKYE

DISTANCE 204KM

CLIMBING +3.827M

DIFFICULTY 10/10

FOOD & WATER | LOCHCARRON / APPLECROSS / SHIEL BRIDGE

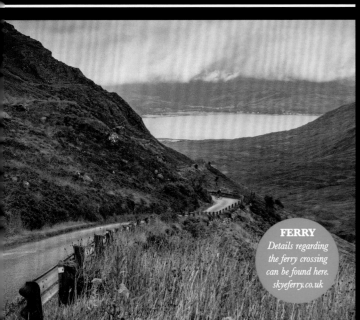

FERRY
Details regarding the ferry crossing can be found here.
skyeferry.co.uk

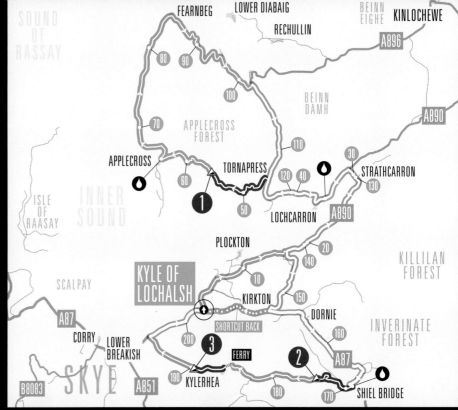

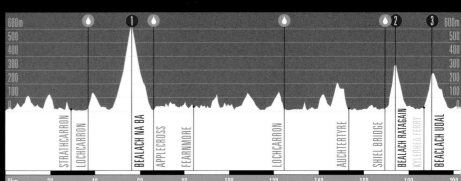

KEY CLIMBS

1 BEALACH NA BA
9,204m +608m

You can split this climb into four sections. 1: The gentle lower slopes to the first 90-degree left-hand bend. 2: The tougher 7-8% gradient as it climbs around the mountain to head north. 3: The increasingly punishing stretch of 20% that will put you to the sword. 4: To finish the hairpins that

deliver you to the summit of the ultimate British climb.

2 BEALACH RÀTAGAIN
4,452m +319m

Set in thick forest on snaking bends this climb hits a maximum of 15% in places before breaking free of the trees to reveal grand views out over Loch Aleh and the surrounding peaks.

3 BEALACH UDAL
3,909m +277m

With no chance to get a run up this climb begins its journey upwards on a stiff gradient then eases before gradually ramping up to the brutal finale. The last kilometre gets steeper and steeper until it hits 20% to have you crawling to the summit.

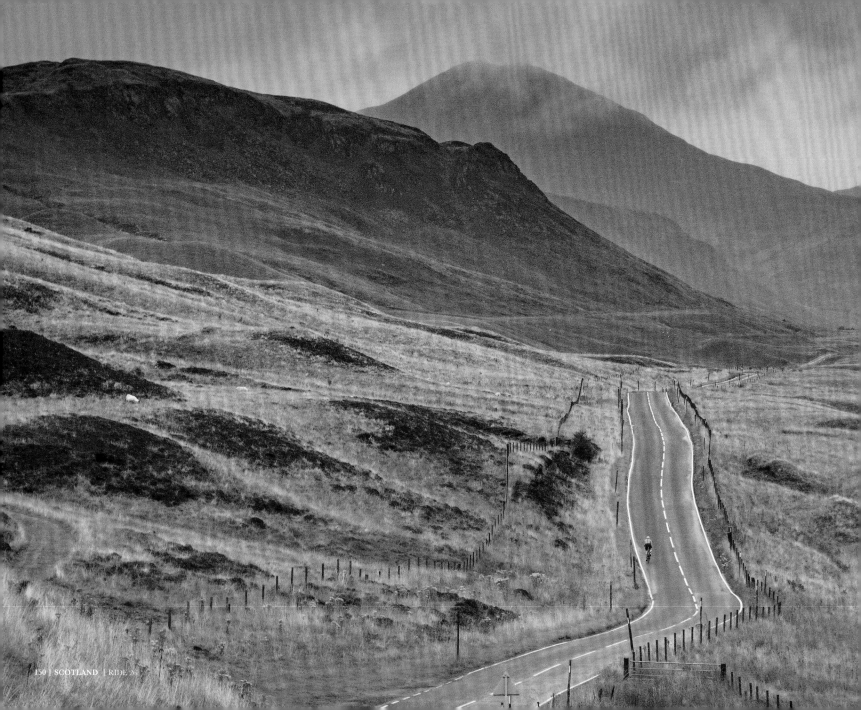

FULL CIRCLE

DISTANCE 274KM | **CLIMBING** +3,497M

PHOTOGRAPHY PHIL HALL

*A colossal circumnavigation of
the mighty Cairngorm mountains*

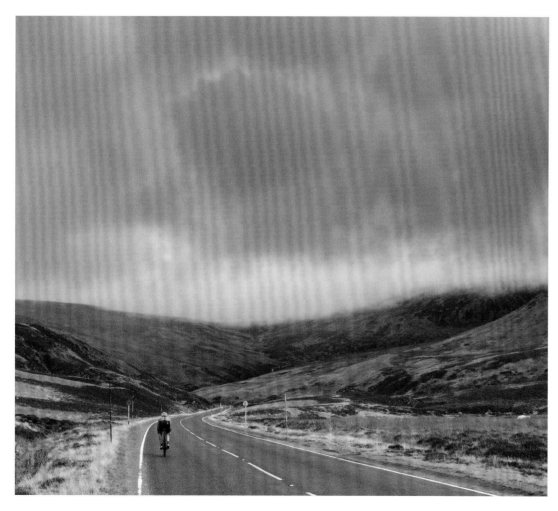

Hearing about the camping trips my dad
and his birdwatching mates made to the
Cairngorms in the Sixties, I've always
imagined them a far-away land, unspoilt
and hostile. Equipped with canvas tents and little
more than layers of jumpers, they journeyed
into the wilderness searching for such exotic
species as ptarmigan, capercaillie and, of course,
the golden eagle. One of the very few places in
Britain to experience year-round snow fall, and
officially classed as an arctic, alpine environment,
they are home to not only fabulous wildlife
but also five of the six highest mountains in
Scotland. This route, by far the longest in the
book, circumnavigates the giant land mass and in
places dives deep inside it.

Although all 40 routes in the guide are
designed to be tackled in a single ride, it would
be perfectly reasonable to split this one in two
if you wished, with a stop-over in Aviemore to
recharge the batteries at half way. The challenge,
though, is to do it all in one go.

Starting in Pitlochry, the giant loop heads
east, immediately climbing into the mountains
by taking the A924 over to Glen Brerachan,
then following the River Ardle to Kirkmichael.
Heading further east, you take the B950 to
meet the A93, then, after diverting through
Blacklunans and Cray, rejoin it to continue
northwards to the Spittal of Glenshee. The
junction of Shee Water and Black Water, where
there has been a settlement of some sort for
centuries, marks the start of the colossal climb

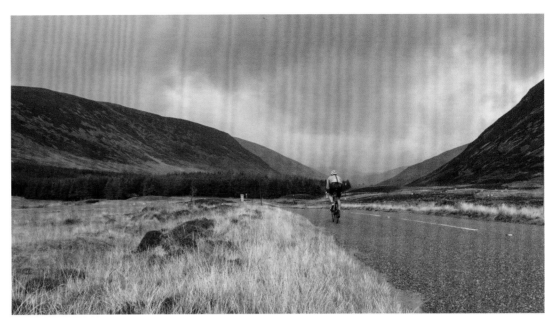

of the Cairnwell. Rising all the way up the giant glen to the Glenshee Ski Centre, the Cairnwell road ascends through the magnificence of the mountains to a lofty altitude of 665 metres, before falling suddenly away into Glen Clunie the other side.

Surrounded by the splendour of the tall peaks, you descend almost effortlessly all the way to Braemar, which is a perfect place for a break after 65 kilometres, as there will be little else on offer for a while once you delve back into the wild. Carrying on down into the valley, you pass the Queen's pad at Balmoral, then leave the A93 at Crathie to ride north over the first of three huge peaks, each one bigger than the last. Up first is Crathie Hill, which rises out of the valley to open up yet more views over the mountains. Then, after meeting up with the A939, you climb again into the shadow of Carn Fiaclach before falling down to the River Don.

With two of the three of climbs done and dusted, you must now line up for the third, which, I won't lie, is practically the entire point of this ride. The initial inspiration for the route was simply a route in the Cairngorms that included this climb but, to create a loop that had the same start and finish point, it turned out at 274 kilometres! Yes, up next is the one and only, the benchmark for a 10/10 climb, the hill all other Scottish hills must be judged against: the infamous *Lecht*.

Arriving at Cock Bridge to cross the River Don again, and passing the novel sight of the ice-white Corgarff Castle, you see the road disappear up into the woods. Faced with this formidable-looking foe, you immediately search out your smallest gear, then begin your quest for the summit by passing the huge gates that close the road when it's snowed over. Bending right, then left, this swine of a road, which at close to 20% in places will test the resolve of any rider, emerges from the trees, turns to a crest, then – just when you think it's over – reveals the remainder of what you still have to climb.

This sight hits you in the face like a frying pan and, with legs already screaming and lungs already burning, what can best be described as a giant tarmac staircase lying across the mountainside is enough to make you want to turn back. There is no way to sugar-coat this one: it is tough, really tough, and in bad weather you'll be left questioning your choice of hobby on more than one occasion as you fight its monstrous slopes. The Lecht is and will always be in my top five British climbs, though, because, no matter how much effort it takes, as you pass your second ski station of the day, the sense of achievement in cresting the summit is palpable and always well earned.

Nothing else on the route will test you as much as that, but you are still a long, *long* way from home, so it's not time to pop the champagne just yet. Next stop is Tomintoul in the Glenlivet Estate (a key stop on the Whisky Trail), a small town entirely laid out on a geometrically perfect grid pattern, reminiscent of a settlement in the old Wild West. Supplies can be taken on board here, then it's on to the northern point of the

NEXT PAGE
The Lecht, NUFF SAID.

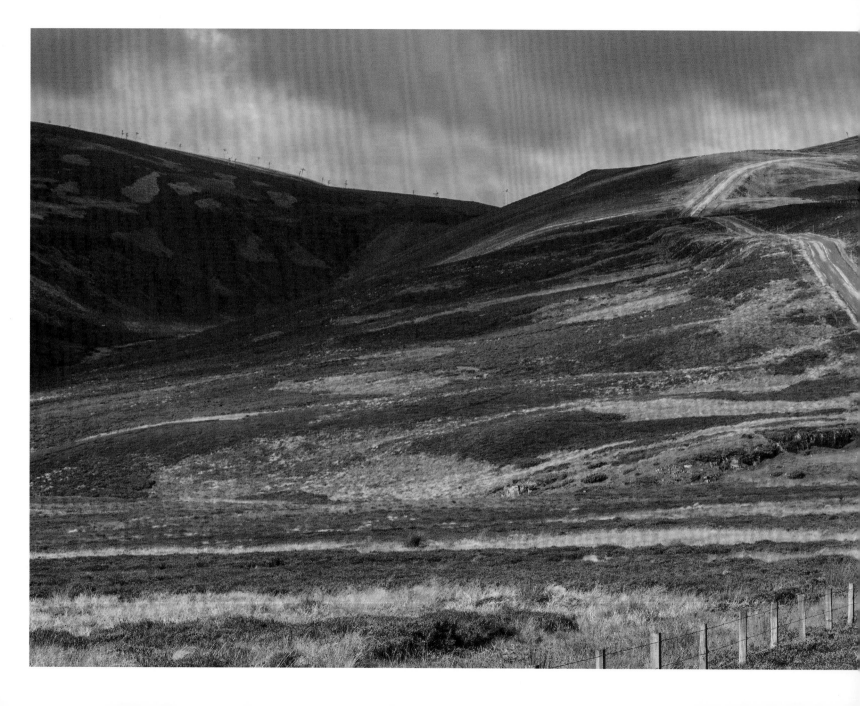

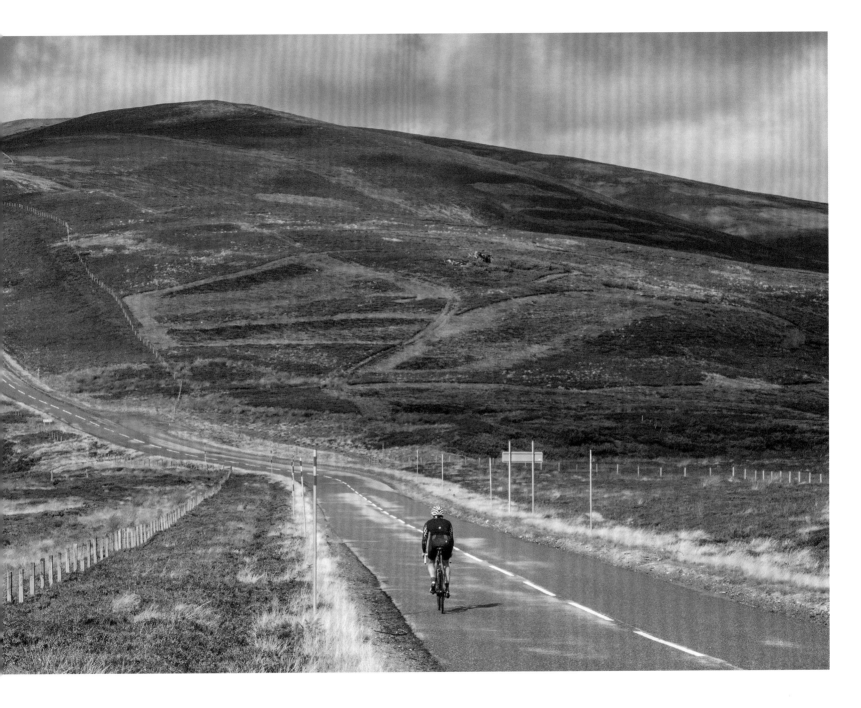

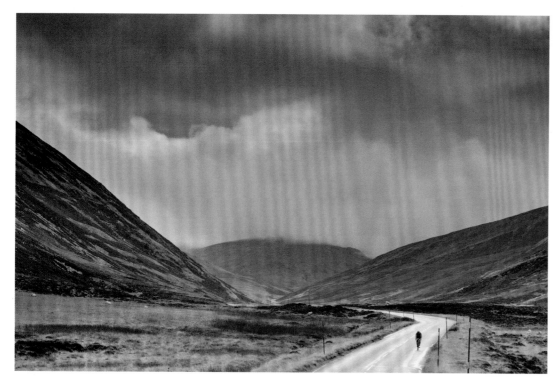

ride at Nethy Bridge, via two more testing lumps, before you drop all the way down through the Boat of Garten and on to Coylumbridge, just south of Aviemore.

Here is where, if you are splitting the ride in two, you can head into town for the night or, if you are doing the 'Full Monty', turn left to seek out your third ski station of the day, lying in the shadow of Cairn Gorm itself. This is Scotland's best appropriation of a European Alpine summit finish, a snaking road with a couple of classic hairpins that ends at the top of a mountain, where people can get their kicks throwing

themselves down snow-covered banks at speed. At 5.5 kilometres it is only about half the length of your standard Tour de France ascent, but still it's well worth the detour, before starting the west side of the loop back home.

It's true this route is somewhat front-loaded with climbs and drama, and you could argue the rest of the ride is simply about completing the circle and getting back to base, and in many ways you'd be correct – but that is the challenge. The primary goal of the project was to build a ride that ringed the mountains and crossed the Lecht; the next task was to get back to Pitlochry

while avoiding the A9 trunk road.

The first 25 kilometres are simple, as you shadow it to the south sticking to the B970, passing through the string of villages all the way to the A86 at Kingussie. Following the A86 briefly, you arrive in Newtonmore, where you head south and momentarily join the cycle path before exiting to continue on the minor road into Dalwhinnie, home to the distillery of the same name. The tiny settlement that lies just south of the home of the famously smooth single malt is the last outpost of any description for quite some time, as you head once more into the sparsity of the mountains across the wide base of Glen Truim.

You could if you liked stick to the A9, and it would speed up your progress, but I would strongly advise against this, so instead turn onto the bespoke bike lane that accompanies the road south. As you leave Dalwhinnie you will see a large sign on your right marking the start of the path to Pitlochry, which ensures you don't miss the turning just before you reach the main road. Made up of old roads and purpose-built paths, it's an amalgamation of surfaces old and new, narrow and wide, that allows you to safely span the vast Pass of Drumochter through the exceedingly spartan landscape. After close to 30 kilometres of traffic-free bliss you then re-join the roads at Calvine for the final few kilometres via Blair Atholl and Killiecrankie, all the way to the finish in Pitlochry. Here you'll end what can only be described as a truly *epic* adventure though true mountain territory, and hopefully a day you'll never forget.

ABOVE *Dwarfed by the Scottish drama.*

RIDE 26 SCOTLAND

CAIRNGORMS

DISTANCE 274KM

CLIMBING +3,497M

DIFFICULTY 10/10

FOOD & WATER | BRAEMAR / TOMINTOUL / KINGUSSIE / DALWHINNIE

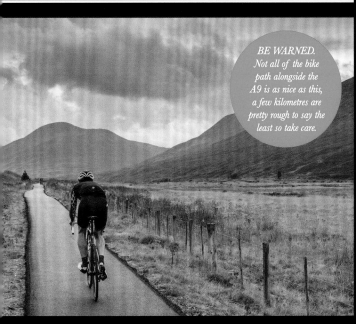

> *BE WARNED.*
> *Not all of the bike*
> *path alongside the*
> *A9 is as nice as this,*
> *a few kilometres are*
> *pretty rough to say the*
> *least so take care.*

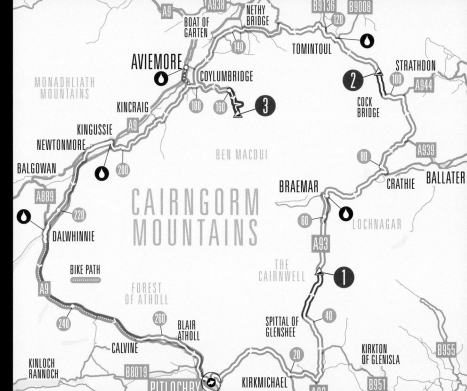

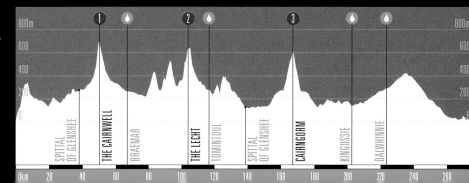

KEY CLIMBS

1 THE CAIRNWELL
8,175m +349m

The first 6 kilometres of The
Cairnwell are very gentle
and you'll hardly notice the
gradient which explains why
its total average is just 4%.
The final 2 kilometres, though,
are hard work with ramps
as steep as 12% so keep
your powder dry for the long
sweeping bend to the top.

2 THE LECHT
4,196m +250m

The Lecht is a true monster
which is tackled in two parts,
both as hard as each other. First
you kick up from Cock Bridge
on the 20% gradient through
the forest, then, just when you
think the worst is over you
catch sight of the enormity of
the second half to the summit
which stops you in your tracks.

3 CAIRN GORM
5,491m +297m

Mimicking the great Alpine
climbs by rising to a dead
end at a ski station the Cairn
Gorm climb is tougher down
the bottom where you'll find
the steepest gradients. With a
5% average the higher reaches
are much kinder to the legs
as they sweep round hairpins
classic mountain style.

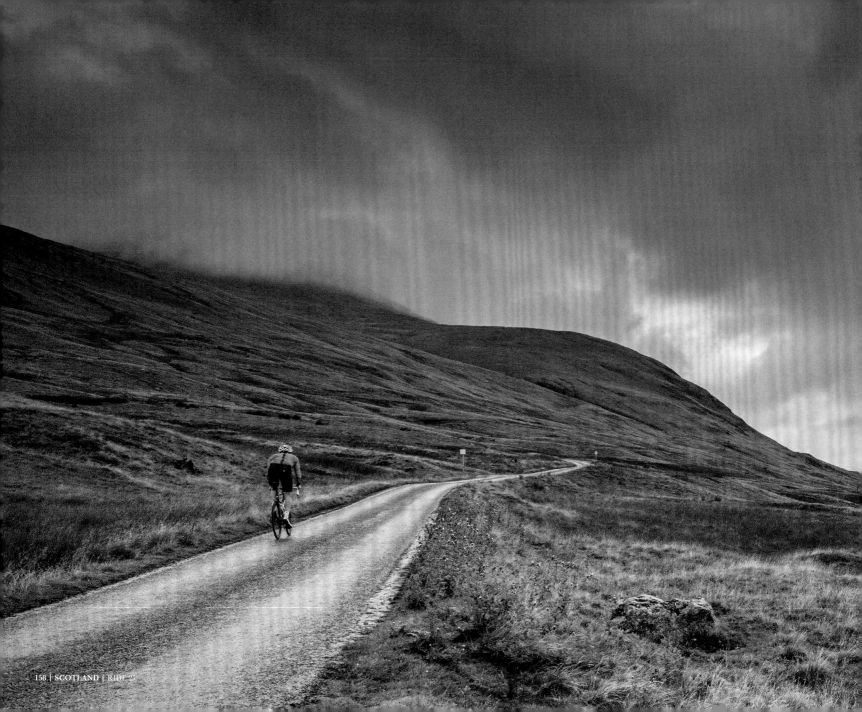

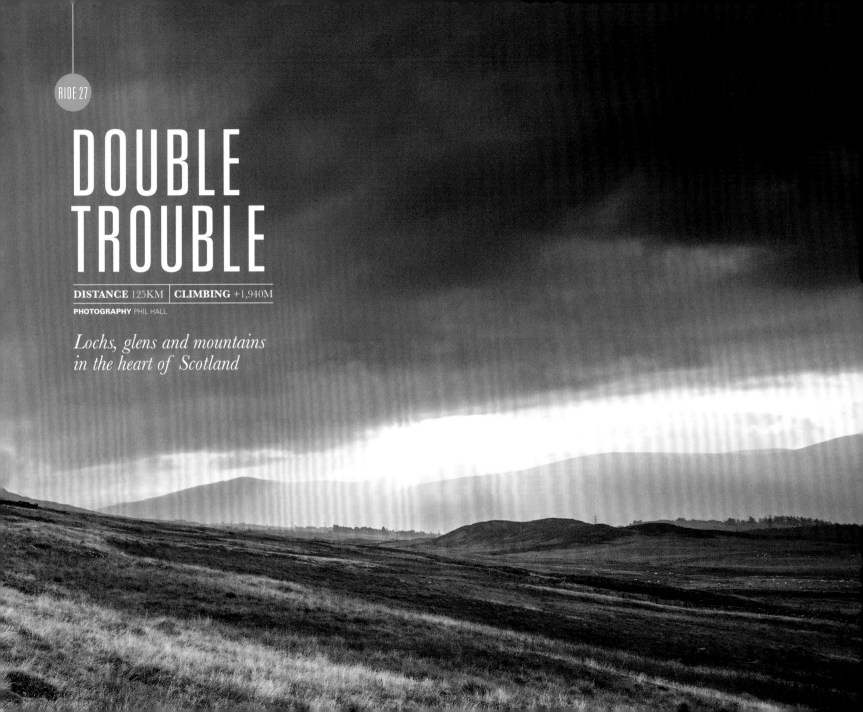

DOUBLE TROUBLE

DISTANCE 125KM | **CLIMBING** +1,940M

PHOTOGRAPHY PHIL HALL

Lochs, glens and mountains
in the heart of Scotland

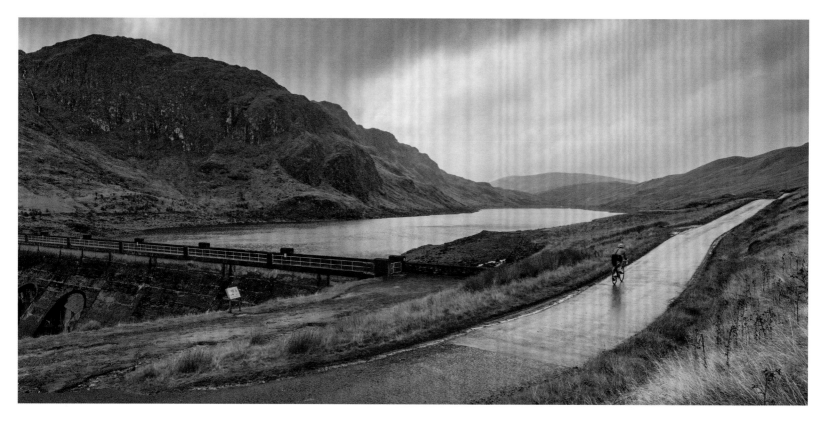

Looking to base a ride in south or central Scotland, I was torn between a number of locations. Initially I was drawn to the Trossachs and Loch Lomond, or further south in Fife, but I just couldn't put together what I wanted, until I settled on this loop around Loch Tay. It is in fact two loops, a contorted figure of eight, centred on the town of Kenmore, yet starting and finishing in Aberfeldy.

The two points of focus are Ben Lawers in the west and Kenmore Hill in the east, and it's the huge Ben Lawers that is tackled first, albeit after a lengthy amble to get there. Leaving the base in Aberfeldy, don't take the A827, which is the direct route: head north out of town on Poplar Avenue, and cross the River Tay to turn left at the T-junction and continue west. These first 7 kilometres are pan-flat as they cross the river basin but, turning south, over the narrow iron bridge, the first bumps soon arrive. Across the Strath of Appin, take the minor road to skirt along the edge of Tay Forest Park to join the A827 in Kenmore. This is the first of two journeys through Kenmore, so keep your eyes open for potential café stops for next time when your reserves will be considerably depleted. Heading south on the main road, cross Kenmore Old Bridge at the head of the loch, then, at the first junction the other side, turn west to follow its shores towards Acharn.

Hugging the water's edge to begin with, then rising slightly up the bank, the narrow road undulates continually though Ardtalnaig,

ABOVE *Passing Lochan na Làirige heading towards the summit of Ben Lawers.*

Ardeonaig and Auchmore to arrive in Killin. After 30 kilometres of heading west, you will have noticed, through breaks in the trees, looming over your right shoulder and monitoring your progress, the giant mass of Ben Lawers. Standing at 1,214 metres above sea level, this is the 10th-highest mountain in the British Isles, and offers a formidable test for your climbing legs, which will be begging to get stuck in.

Turning back east in Killin, you have to take the A827 along the north shore of the loch for 6 more flat kilometres before the wait is finally over. Now, the road doesn't climb all the way up to the 1,214-metre-high summit – we're not in the Alps – but it does get to about half way, to top out at a satisfactory 549 metres. The base of the ascent is well marked, with a sign to the Bridge of Balgie, and the badge of honour all the best roads wear, warning caravans, buses and HGVs to STAY AWAY. This simple advice, of course, attracts cyclists like moths to a flame, because it means there will be a) less traffic and b) twisting tight corners, narrow roads and, best of all, steep gradients.

Both sides of the climb up Ben Lawers are spectacular, both are over 7 kilometres long, but this side is a little gentler on the legs, which is out of character of me to include, I know, but I'm being kind on this ride. The toughest climbing is lower down – in fact, it kicks up viciously from the base, before winding through the small wood onto the open hillside. Following the predominantly horizontal nature of the profile

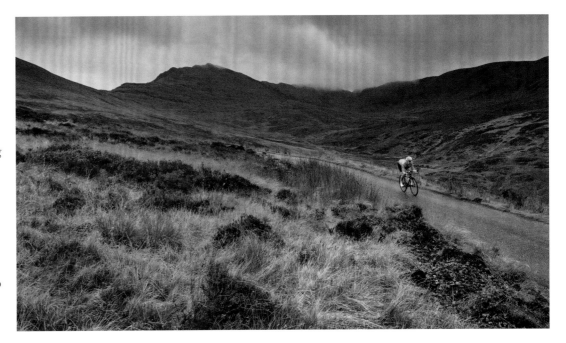

so far, this will be a gigantic shock to the legs, so don't be alarmed if they begin to moan a little at first. With the peak of the mountain dead ahead, make your way across the barren tundra, climbing high above the glistening waters of the loch below into the magic of the mountains. (Oh, the waters may not be glistening – in fact, it's more likely you'll not even see them for driving rain, but you never know.)

Across the Burn of Edramucky the narrow road heads north-west, as you rise to the culmination of the hard climbing at the colossal wall of the Ben Lawers Dam. A stunning, brutal, piece of industrial architecture, it spans the valley like two giant arms protruding from its central towers, braced to hold the might of

the water behind. With its dark stone and bold shapes, what should be an eyesore, and in many people's eyes probably is, to me fits right in with the drama of the surrounding hills. Once past this imposing sight, the slope abates, and the remaining journey to the summit is nice and steady along the side of the murky water, reflecting the dark rock of the mountainside above. On your left, jagged peaks, on your right, towering grassy banks, this valley in the sky is simply magnificent, and gently directs you to the peak, following a final short spike, to finish with a flourish. With this giant climb under your belt, it's now time to reap your reward in the shape of the descent, through the equally magnificent scenery the other side, to the base of Glen Lyon.

ABOVE *Plummeting down from Ben Lawers into the shelter of Glen Lyon.*

Carrying on to the Bridge of Balgie, you turn east to follow the fast and gradually falling road all the way back, eventually to Kenmore. Losing just 100 metres of elevation in 25 kilometres, it's hardly a ski ramp, but the continual downward trajectory will put a spring in your step as you pass through Innerwick, Camusvrachan and Invervar back to the B846, churning that big ring over and eating up the kilometres.

Following the second time through Kenmore and, if you like, a diversion to sample the local produce, you line up for the next killer climb, shorter than Ben Lawers, but a fair bit harder. From the junction at the base and past the narrow-road sign, you rise immediately into a series of frenetic switchbacks, on a slope that approaches 20% at times. Searching out a line to minimise the effect of the steep twisting corners, drag yourself through the forest in search of the shallower gradients further on. If you're going for a KOM attempt on this hill there are big gains to be made on the vicious lower section, but they can also cause great damage, so don't throw the kitchen sink at it too soon. At about the midway point you pass a small house: this is where the forest ends. Soon you'll be on the tops and, after a couple more bends, you'll be able to look behind you across the valley, before pressing on up to a tiny reservoir. This landmark signals the third distinct change in the pitch of the slope, and the climbing becomes a degree easier still as you continue to search for the summit.

Your surroundings are rough and rugged,

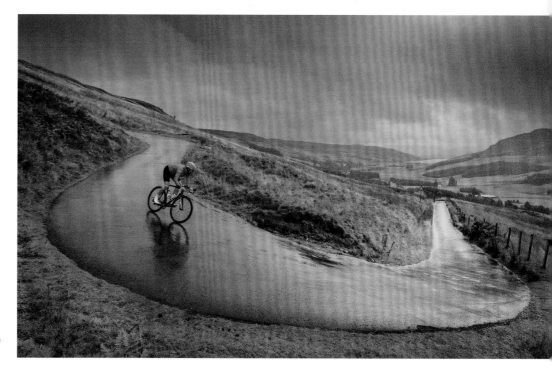

but lacking the drama of high peaks; they have a more Yorkshire Dales feel than Scotland as you approach the next treat this ride has up its sleeve. Once you've finished across the moors and turned westward slightly the road falls away, to open up monumental views down into Glen Quaich. Leaving the high ground behind, and dropping like a stone, you arrive at a brace of hairpins that could have been plucked right out of the Tour de France. As you plunge into them, let your imagination transport you to the end of a mountain stage: you've broken away from the field and, closing in on the finish, you swirl effortlessly round the corners in your search for

victory. (Without hitting an oncoming car or ending up in the ditch, though.)

Still heading down, past Loch Freuchie, then flat all the way to Ballinreigh and – yes, I know I said there were only two climbs on this route. There are only two really big climbs: the next one, back over to Aberfeldy, isn't that bad, honest. As the only way to return is via the A826, this is the road you must take through Glen Cochill, in and out of the intermittent forest, up to the perfect, mirror-flat waters of the tiny Loch na Creige. The finish comes in the shape of a fast 5-kilometre drop back into Aberfeldy, to complete this wonderful Loch Tay figure of eight.

ABOVE *Descending into Glen Quaich whilst dreaming of riding the Tour de France.*

RIDE 27 SCOTLAND

LOCH TAY

DISTANCE	125KM
CLIMBING	+1,940M
DIFFICULTY	5/10

FOOD & WATER | KILLIN / KENMORE

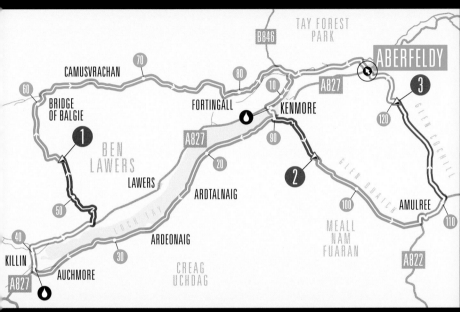

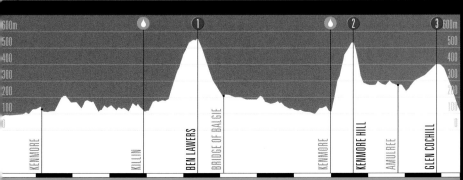

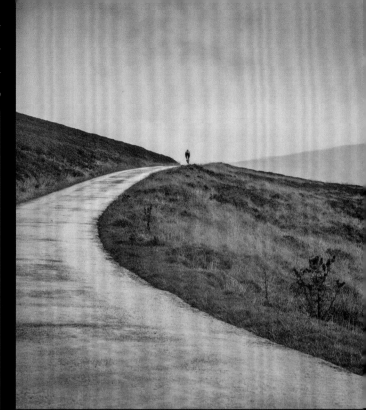

KEY CLIMBS

1 BEN LAWERS
7,361m +361m

Although not quite as tough as the north flank of the pass this side still packs in some serious climbing, most of which comes in the first 5 kilometres up to the dam wall. Averaging close to 7% to this point the rest of the climb is much easier past the reservoir (oh – apart from the final kick to the summit).

2 KENMORE HILL
5,222m +415m

A climb of two halves. The first sheltered in the forest twists back and forth flirting with 20% gradients and navigating hairpin bends. The second lines out on a much shallower pitch but across open moors which on a blustery day will make it feel just as hard.

3 GLEN COCHILL
7,912m +165m

Nowhere near as tough as the previous two climbs, this 8-kilometre ascent only has an average gradient of 2%. It is a little steeper in the lower slopes through the slight deviations in direction but there is nothing that should put the legs in any degree of trouble all the way to the top.

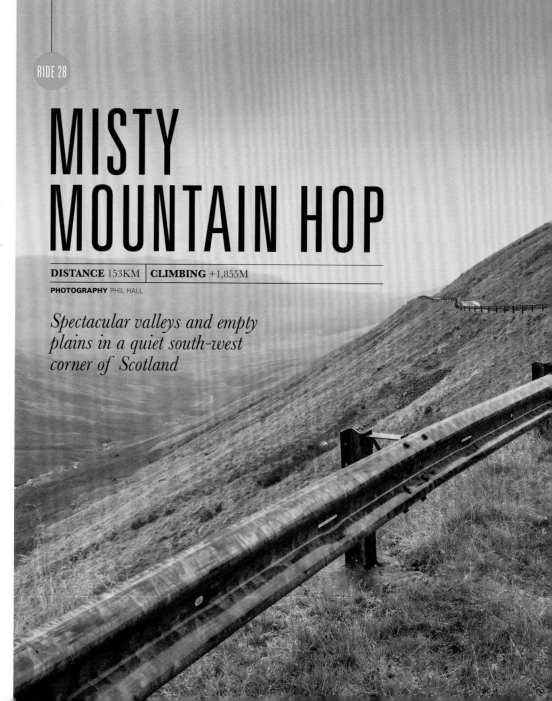

The Girvan three-day cycle race, or just 'the Girvan', was a mainstay of the British domestic racing calendar for over forty years until its demise in 2009. Raced on the tough roads of Ayrshire and Dumfries and Galloway, it attracted the best riders in the country to do battle in the beautiful and, of course challenging, scenery in this south-west corner of Scotland. Starting and finishing in Girvan, the big climbs on this route are packed into its first half, spread out over 50 kilometres, to climax in the real star of the show, the 'Nick of the Balloch'.

Begin by heading east on the B734 for a couple of gentle kilometres. Then, where the road bends south in Old Dailly, start to gain some altitude. This, the first of four large peaks to cross, is composed of 4.5 kilometres of moderate gradient that gets wilder as it climbs. Starting between neat fields and passing through the few houses that form the village of Penkill, it reaches its summit at the head of the Penwhapple Reservoir in the shadow of Green Hill. Exposed but not devoid of life, the top lies surrounded by low, rolling hills adorned with lines of the soon-to-be-very-familiar wind turbines. Rolling over the top, descend into the village of Barr, then leave the B734 to turn left, then left again, and follow the valley for a brief while to the foot of the next climb.

Shorter than the previous ascent, but a degree steeper, this one kicks off as you take the left turn over the River Stinchar, heading back north. With a 6% average, and passing through land

MISTY MOUNTAIN HOP

DISTANCE 153KM | **CLIMBING** +1,855M

PHOTOGRAPHY PHIL HALL

Spectacular valleys and empty plains in a quiet south-west corner of Scotland

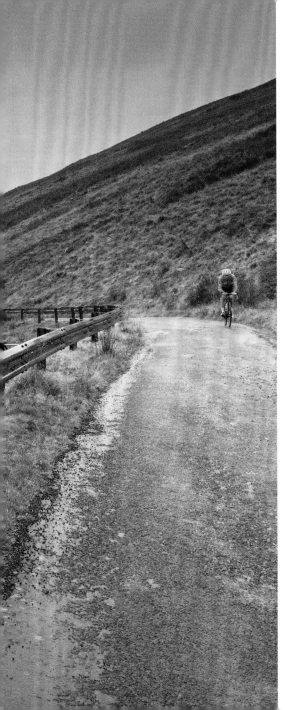

LEFT *In better weather this is one of the best views in Britain.*

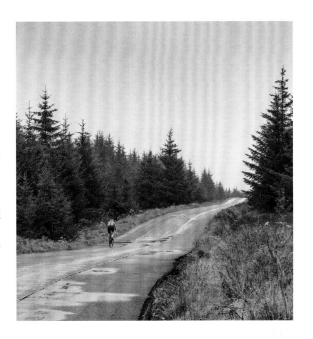

with far less evidence of human activity, this is where this route really comes alive. At just over 2.5 kilometres long, through many twists and turns, it leads the way over the barren hills to the top in the midst of the wind farm. In between patches of forest the road reaches its summit in the pass between Delamford Hill and Hadyard Hill, before descending through equally beautiful scenery the other side. This long, fast drop takes you all the way through the low, wide valley from the desolate upper slopes to the farms and fields lower down, to join with the B7035 just east of Dailly. Turn right here for a relaxing passage along the valley floor, then, at the triangular junction, turn right, following the sign for the Welland Garden Campsite.

Upon reaching a T-junction, turn right and head south into the longest climb of the day, up to the wonderfully named Black Hill of Garleffin. As with the previous two ascents, the road transitions from agricultural land to open moor as it gains altitude on its narrow lonely path south. It's not totally empty, though: small patches of conifers in various stages of growth punctuate the gentle, rolling hills as you pass the Diel's Elbow. With little variation in terrain over the final few kilometres, and on a slope that is kind to the legs, roll over the sparse summit, then take the short descent back to the twin settlements of North and South Balloch. Here, starting from the junction of the River Stinchar and Balloch Burn, is one of my favourite corners of Scotland: the Nick of the Balloch. A more

perfect climb you will be hard pressed to find. Steep, but not too steep, long but not too long, it meanders a little as it hugs the hillside heading upwards. As you wind south, with a small barrier protecting you from the fall into the gully below, the surrounding hillsides, adorned with rocky outcrops, frame the most magnificent valley you can imagine. It's one of those places that forces you to stop to take a photo, and you'll find yourself rooted to the spot, unable to tear yourself away from its pure, elemental beauty.

Move on you must, though, and, after you reach the summit and the high point of the day, it's time for one hell of a descent down the other side. For close to 20 kilometres you'll fall before you face anything that will require more than gentle pressure on the pedals. All the way through

ABOVE *There are times on this ride when you can feel like the only person alive.*

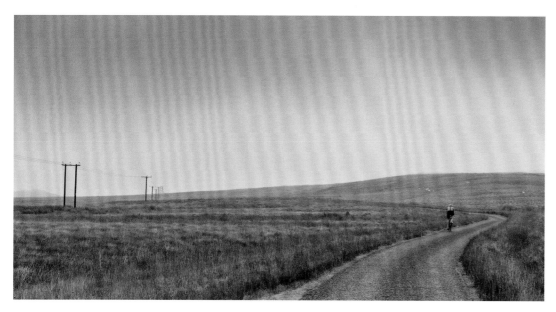

but, fear not, they soon vanish, and it's back to the epic nothingness that so blesses this corner of Scotland. Endless straight roads, featureless horizons and big skies are in store across the moors as you join paths with the Cross Water of Luce. From here the scenery is a little more varied, the river has cut a slight cleft in the land, and the tiny road follows its snaking path north. Gently rising and falling, framed intermittently by low stone walls, and still far from the chaos of modern life, ascend all the way to the high point of this road at Chirmorie Cairn.

This cycling nirvana ends at the village of Barrhill where, unfortunately, you must join the potentially busy A714 for a short while into Pinwherry. All downhill, you turn left in the village onto the B734, then, a short while later, take the right turn towards Lendalfoot. The last climb of the day offers a last taste of the empty grassland, as the single-track road picks its way to the base of Knockormal Hill. The ascent is about half the length of the descent, which will please you at this stage of the ride, and, after crossing the summit, it's time to drop down to the coast and one last treat before the route ends.

Turning right in Lendalfoot, you'll find the last 10 kilometres utterly pan-flat and sitting right on the very edge of the coast looking out to sea. Regardless of any traffic the Ayrshire Coastal Path may attract, it is more than worth it for the pleasure of hugging the coast (unless there is a strong wind coming in off the sea), and a perfectly serene end to an amazing ride.

the Glentrool Forest, it goes, until you take the left turn in Glentrool Village, then go left again, to keep falling and falling all the way to Newton Stewart. As the only settlement of any note, this makes the perfect place, with 75 kilometres in the can, to refill your bottles before embarking on the journey back north. With all the big climbs behind you, the remainder of this ride is more rolling: never flat, just lightly undulating through the sparse plains and eerie forests. Yes, eerie. This is a fantastically quiet part of the world as, bar the forestation, there is very little else going on, so it's just perfect for bike riding.

Taking first the A714, then turning left onto the B7027, head east into the back of beyond. Turn left off the B-road at the sign that points to a hotel 7 miles away and, crossing the Glassoch Bridge, ride east through 20 kilometres of blissful

silence. With just one junction to negotiate, where you take the right to New Luce, there is little if anything to distract you from the simple art of pedalling your bicycle as fast or slowly as you like. After the turn, where the scenery gets even better, even more featureless, this is real Wild West country: an endless, flat horizon broken only by the sweeping blades of yet another wind farm and the odd patch of pine forest. Exiting the great plains, enter the small village of New Luce, which has a hotel and shop if you need it, then head north.

I promised no more 'proper' climbs in the second part of the ride, but there is still a substantial amount of elevation to be gained and lost; just not all in one go, or on anything that could classically be regarded as a climb. There are more signs of farming around the village

ABOVE *Crossing the empty plains between New Luce and Barrhill.*

RIDE 28 — SCOTLAND

AYRSHIRE AND GALLOWAY

DISTANCE 153KM

CLIMBING +1,855M

DIFFICULTY 5/10

FOOD & WATER | NEWTON STEWART / BARRHILL

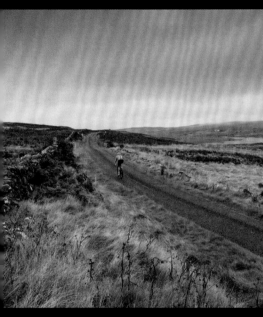

KEY CLIMBS

1 GREEN HILL
4,280m +185m

This climb is nothing to be afraid of with an overall average of just 4.3% but that doesn't mean it is a total walk in the park. The upper slopes towards the summit at the Penwhapple Reservoir do ramp up quite sharp.

2 BLACK HILL OF GARLEFFIN
9,350m +324m

The climb essentially starts as you cross the Water of Girvan heading east although the first 2.5 kilometres are very shallow. The bulk of the stiff climbing comes between kilometre 3 and 6, then it eases back again and also drops slightly before the final kick to the top.

3 NICK OF THE BALLOCH
3,858m +248m

The standout climb in the area this road is a pure gem and worth the journey to deepest Ayrshire alone. With a 6% average and stretches of 10% it won't break your legs but the scenery will blow your mind.

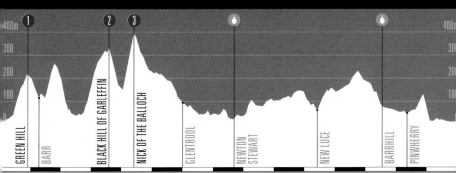

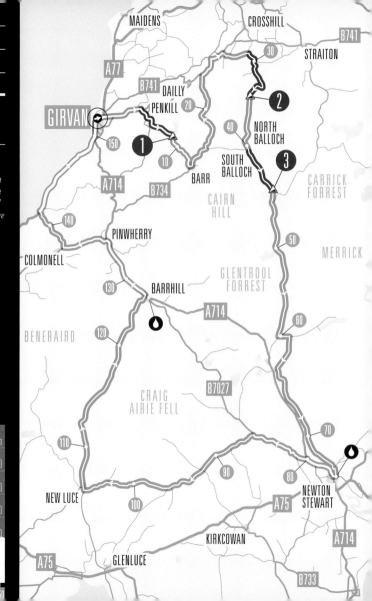

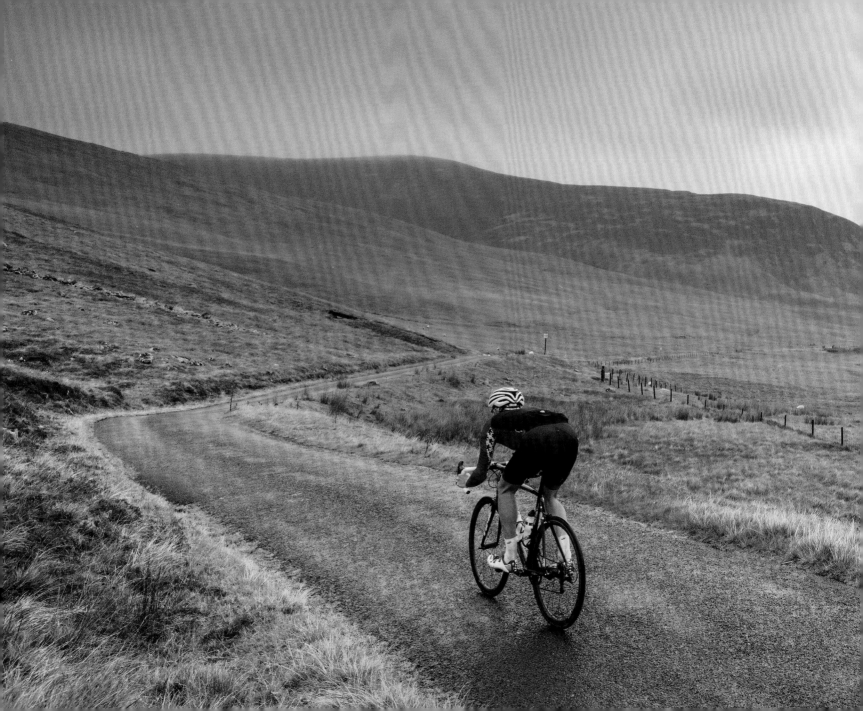

HEAVEN IS A PLACE ON EARTH

DISTANCE 174KM | **CLIMBING** +2,317M

PHOTOGRAPHY PHIL HALL

A spellbinding trip around Scotland's Southern Uplands

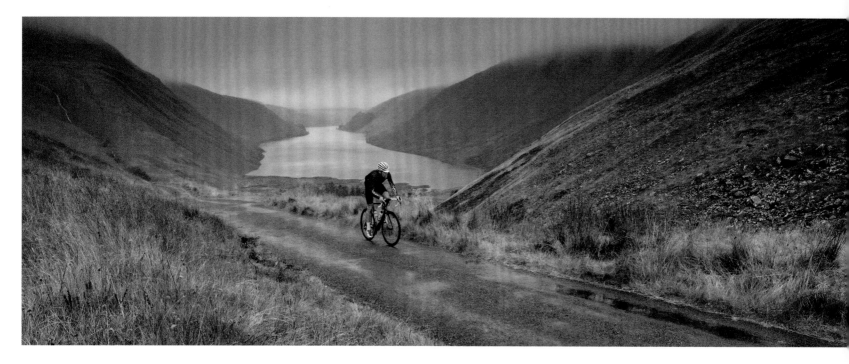

The mountains of Scotland are roughly grouped into three regions: the North-West Highlands, the Grampians and the Southern Uplands. I always assumed the finest scenery and most spectacular views were to be found in the north, hidden far away from us southerners: that was until I visited Lowther Hill. If the sun is shining and the skies are clear what you are treated to from the top of this climb, especially looking north, is a match for anything you'll see in the Highlands. Lowther Hill is therefore the star of this ride, and rightly so, but it has some pretty stiff competition, as you are taken on a journey across passes and through valleys, all of which will leave you awestruck by their beauty.

At over 170 kilometres long this is a serious route, so a decent level of fitness is preferable for an arduous day in the saddle, so get some training in before you set off.

The base is the town of Moffat, just off Junction 15 of the M74, which has all the facilities you needs for the day ahead, and for a pit stop as you pass through at half-distance. The route is made up of two large loops, one to the east and one to the west, and the first challenge kicks up the moment the flag drops, as you ride north to climb the magnificently named Devil's Beef Tub.

The Beef Tub is a 150-metre deep hollow created by four surrounding hills, and this magnificent geographical feature derives its name from being used by the Border Reivers (Middle Ages raiders who took advantage of the instability of the Anglo-Scottish border to pillage and plunder), known locally as 'Devils', to hide their cattle. It's essential you stop at the summit to peer over the edge, as it is quite some sight. However, there is the small matter of 10 kilometres of climbing to contend with first.

Once you've completed the ascent and marvelled at the freakish geography, roll over the top and begin the gentle descent down to Tweedsmuir, where you turn right in the direction of the Talla Reservoir. A short way from the main road there's a slight kick up to the dam wall, which delivers you to the perfectly flat

PREVIOUS PAGE

Heading down the long descent into the Meggett Valley.

ABOVE *Crawling up the Wall of Talla from the shore of the reservoir.*

passage along the water's edge in the direction of the imposing hills. Rolling along this peaceful road, with Garelet Hill on your right reflected in the still waters, all is calm until you catch sight of what lies ahead.

The first time I clocked this road I had to rub my eyes. Seriously? I cried. That cannot be the road – that must be a farmer's track! – it's too steep! It is the road, though, and it is a formidable sight: a single slash of tarmac across the immaculate hillside. You don't need a degree in surveying to work out that it's going to hurt, so take a few deep breaths at the base, turn left, and make the instant transition from billiard-table flat to a wall of asphalt.

The narrow, gnarled road, clinging to the hillside, rockets up without a passing thought for the comfort of your legs, rapidly gaining height above the placid water below. The views behind are simply stupendous, and just get better as you tackle the sections of 20% that twist and kink beneath your wheels as you fight for the momentary refuge of a small bridge. Once over this brief levelling, continue climbing, albeit on a slightly kinder slope to the eventual summit, nestled in the tranquil beauty of Talla Moss, before indulging in the utter pleasure of the descent to the shore of Megget Reservoir.

This perfect road ends as you reach Cappercleuch, and join the A708 at St Mary's Loch, to start the journey back through Moffat Dale to where you set off. This long south-westerly passage begins with a substantial

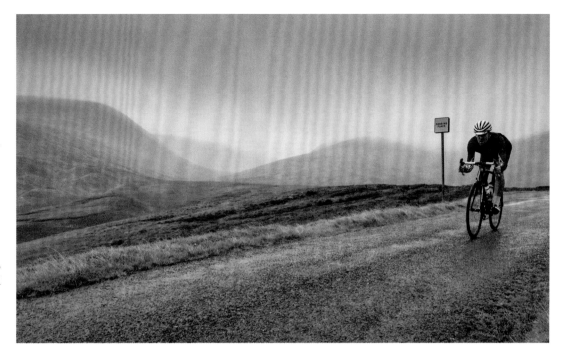

climb, then ends with close to 20 kilometres of downhill, so you can shake the legs out a bit here and allow them plenty of time to recover.

With 70 kilometres in the bank you may choose to stop in Moffatt or press right on; either way, to continue you follow the same route out of town, up the A701, taking in the first 6 kilometres of the Beef Tub to the junction with the B719. After a smidge more elevation drop down into Clydesdale, to then trace the path of the A74M north to the village of Elvanfoot.

It's here that the second loop starts, and one that will deliver you to the finest views in southern Scotland. Linking Clydesdale with Nithsdale, the bottom half of the circuit is played out almost

entirely on the A702, as it rises gently through the rolling hills before dropping rapidly down the Dalveen Pass to join the A76 at Enterkinfoot. Before reaching the head of the pass, and as you approach its summit, if the conditions are favourable you'll notice the white dome of the Lowther Hill radar installation poking out over the horizon. Like its cousin that sits on top of Great Dun Fell, the radar acts as a beacon, calling cyclists from all around, challenging them to reach it – and, yes, this is your next target. First you've the undulating passage of the A76 between Enterkinfoot and Mennock to contend with and – before you take the turn east, and if you're in the need of more supplies – you could divert the 3

ABOVE *The Passing Place sign is as much a part of Scotland as kilts and haggis.*

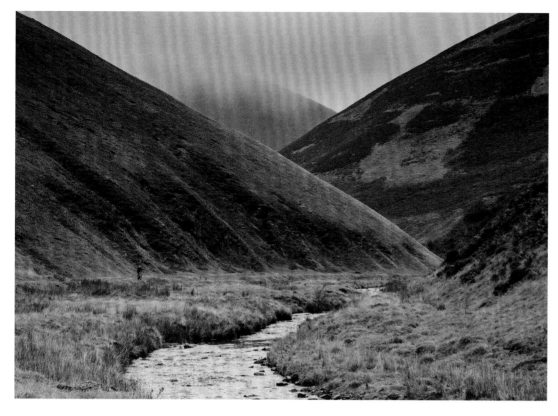

find the entrance to the last part of the climb, up to the radar, just beyond the village.

What lies the other side of a heavily padlocked gate is, without doubt, one of the greatest roads in Britain. Over 4 majestic kilometres it winds round the pristine hills, wide at first, then gradually becoming narrower, then ramping up steeper and steeper. As it twists up to the first clump of radio antennae that protrude from the hillside, you could be on the upper slopes of any giant climb in the Alps or Pyrenees, it is that spectacular. The final push to the summit is also an absolute killer but, once on the plateau, in the shadow of the colossal golf ball of the radar station,, the view in all directions is simply spellbinding, the pristine landscape stretched out as far as the eye can see. What a place, what a climb!

Once you've soaked it in you've still got a ride to finish, and yet more delights await on the journey back to Moffat. Drop back down to Wanlockhead, continue north-east to Leadhills, then take the right-hand turn onto the B7040 to return to Elvanfoot. Predominantly downhill, interrupted just the once by a short, sharp kick up, the rolling valley sides flanking this meandering road are still dazzling – that is, until the huge electric substation looms up to put a damper on things. Retracing the route south through Clydesdale, criss-crossing the A74M, there's one last climb for the legs: the 3 kilometres back to the A701, before the final fast run-in to the finish of what has to be, hands down, one of my favourite rides anywhere in the known Universe.

kilometres north to Sanquar.

The climb to the radar starts with a small, sharp ramp from the main road, which then drops down to enter the wonder of the Mennock Pass. Rising ever so gently, it appears all but flat as you roll along the vast valley floor, dwarfed by the towering hills either side – but trust me: it's climbing. Splitting Auchensow Hill and Brown Hill, Meikle Snout and Wether Hill, the majestic Mennock Pass begins to climb seriously at about 6 kilometres in, and from here the elevation gain

is far more evident, as the interlocking hills part either side of the snaking road. Smothered in heather, they appear to glow purple when it's in flower, which creates the most dazzling backdrop to your ascent into Wanlockhead, the highest village in Scotland.

This is not the summit, though, and if you want to complete the climb of the Mennock Pass before carrying on with the route, you must ride a little way past Wanlockhead before doubling back. To go straight on with the course you'll

ABOVE *Weaving through the interlocking hills on the lower slopes of the Mennock Pass.*

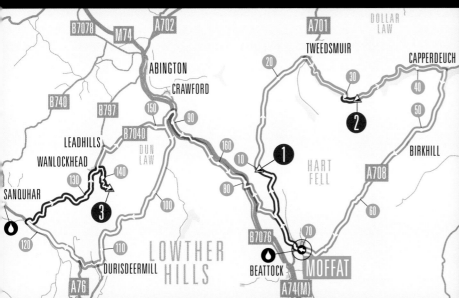

RIDE 29 SCOTLAND

LOWTHER HILS

DISTANCE 174 KM

CLIMBING +2,317M

DIFFICULTY 7/10

FOOD & WATER | MOFFAT / SANQUHAR

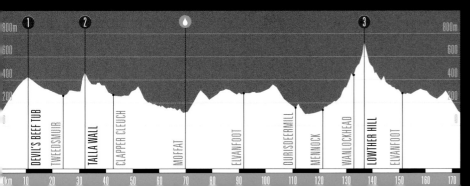

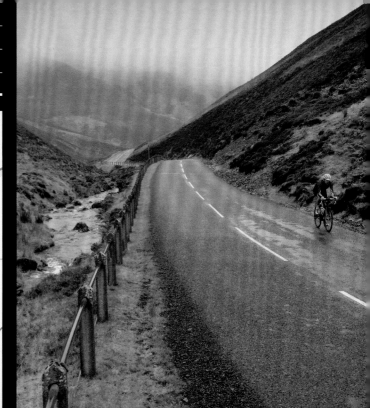

KEY CLIMBS

1 DEVIL'S BEEF TUB

10,323m +300m

Ten kilometres of climbing delight set on a near perfectly consistent slope from start to finish. There are a couple of slight peaks and troughs and it does reach 10% at one point but on the whole it's a climb to be tackled sat down tapping out a steady rhythm.

2 THE WALL OF TALLA

1,902m +158m

In this case the word wall is no understatement, as approaching from the shore of the reservoir that is exactly what it looks like. The first 700 metres are a pure battle over 20% slopes but once past the small bridge the rest of the climb is much steadier.

3 MENNOCK PASS / LOWTHER HILL

14,020m +652m

The first 11 kilometres of this climb from Mennock to Wanlockhead are just the warm up, what you've really come for are the last 4. Turning right onto the service road to the radar at the summit the end of this climb is pure cycling magic.

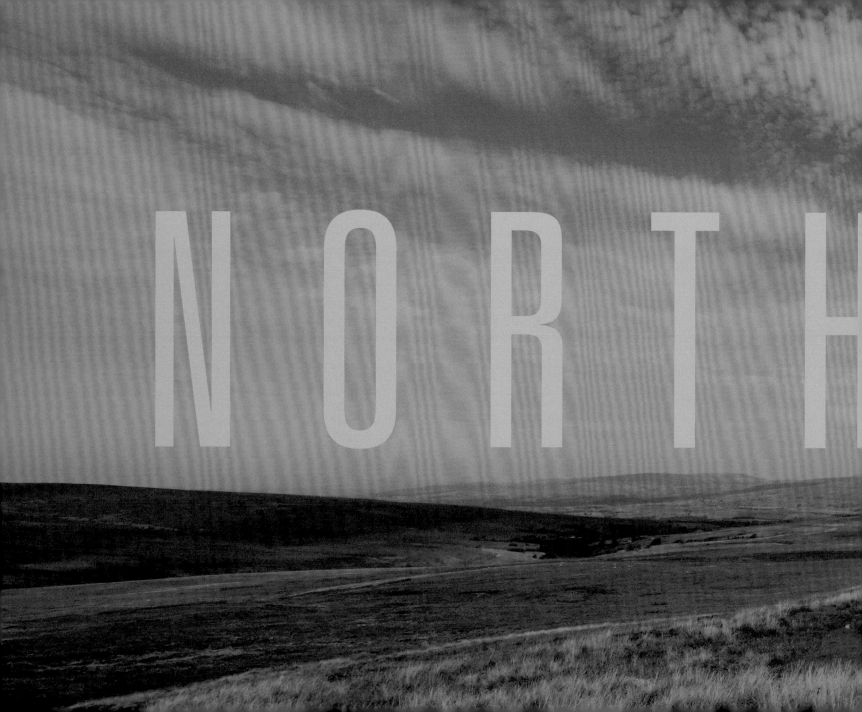

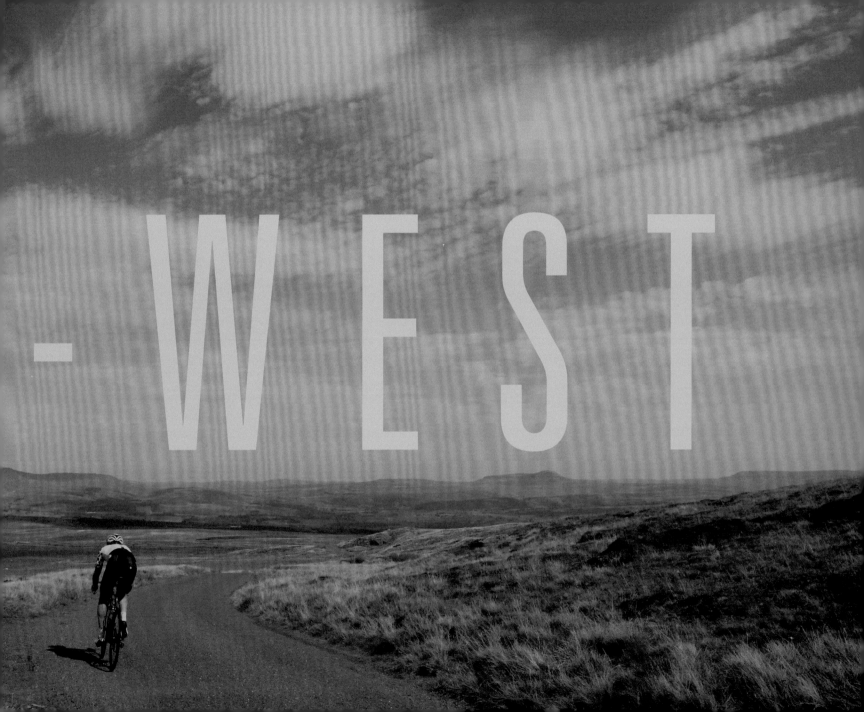

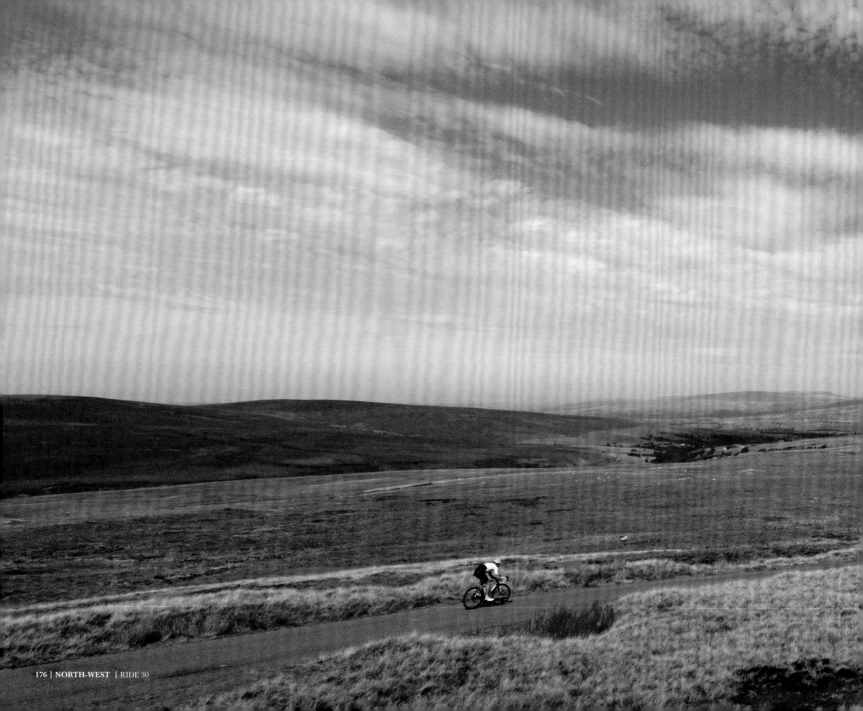

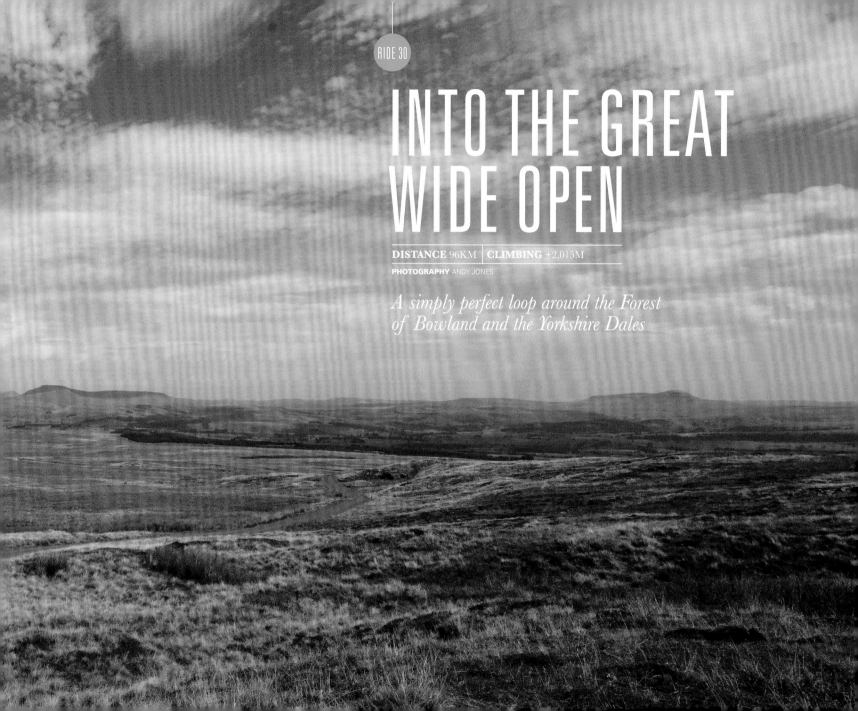

INTO THE GREAT WIDE OPEN

DISTANCE 96KM | **CLIMBING** +2,015M

PHOTOGRAPHY ANDY JONES

A simply perfect loop around the Forest of Bowland and the Yorkshire Dales

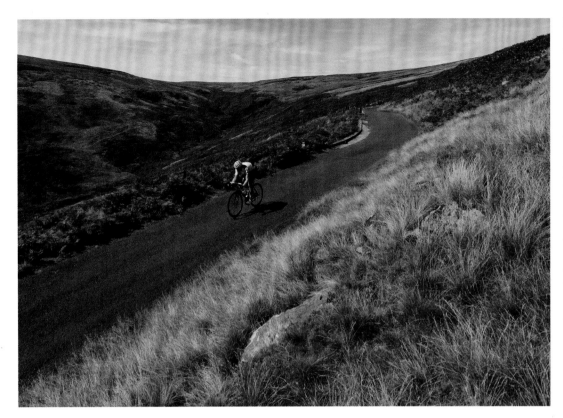

LEFT *The Cross of Greet. Which may or may not have stood at the top of this road.*

Some believe there was never a cross here at all, and that the giant base is in fact a plague stone: the hole in it would be filled with vinegar to allow people to wash money, in the belief that it would prevent the spread of the disease. Anyway, I digress. The journey to where the cross was or wasn't comes in two parts: 5 kilometres altitude gain, followed by 2 lost, then another 3 up to the summit. It's these last 3 that can be classed as the true climb, and it's also here where the toughest slopes are to be found, as the road winds up the valley dividing Lamb Hill Fell and Catlow Fell, teetering on the contours of the hillside.

The summit is always in sight on the horizon, giving you a permanent carrot to chase and, once reached, opens up the grand views out over Lythe Fell and Tatham Fells the other side. The next 20 kilometres are all joyously downhill – well, just about – as you descend to the crossroads to turn west on Mewith Lane all the way to Wennington. Still losing altitude, the route finally bottoms out as you reach the junction of the A683 and A687 on the flat plains surrounding the River Greta. Unfortunately, you must use a stretch of A-road here in order to progress north, up through Tunstall to Nether Burrow, and then very briefly on the A65, which you cross to continue on High Chapel Lane into High Casterton. Once in the next village of Casterton, rejoin the A683 once more for a matter of metres, before forking right to ride through Klondyke Wood and into Barbon.

Riding east out of the village, in the foot

This was the very first route I plotted for this book. It just fell onto the page: a simple loop across four peaks, linking the Forest of Bowland and the Yorkshire Dales, while ticking off Bowland Knotts, White Shaw Moss, Barbondale and the Cross of Greet. My initial plan was to ride it in an anti-clockwise direction, taking on Bowland Knotts first, but then I changed my mind. Not that the route can't be ridden anti-clockwise – it will still take you through the exact same scenery across the exact same roads, and if you have a keen eye you'll see that's the way I'm riding it in the photos; however, I decided on clockwise. Are we all clear? Good, then I'll begin.

Starting in Slaidburn, in the heart of the Forest of Bowland, head north from the village on Lythe Fell Road to instantly start the first climb of the day, up to the Cross of Greet. Dating back to medieval times, all that now remains of the cross is the stone base, marking the border of Whitray Fell and Catlow Fell.

PREVIOUS PAGE *The vast emptiness of Bowland Knotts. It doesn't get much better than this.*

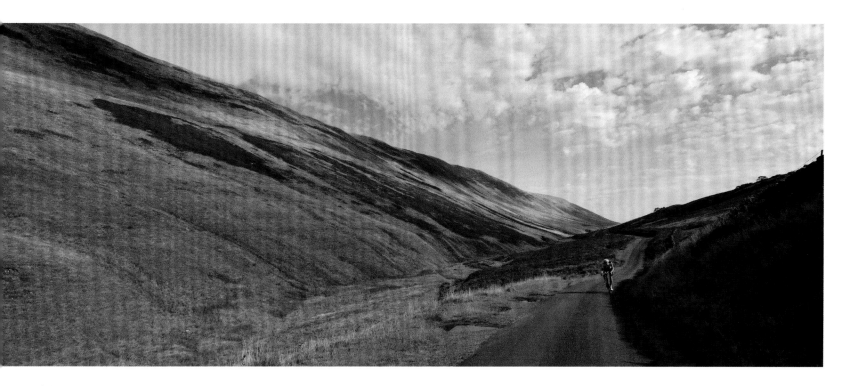

of the valley beside the idyllic Barbon Beck, you approach what is arguably Britain's most beautiful dale, a true wonder of the natural world. Barbondale is peerless on a sunny morning with the sun illuminating the towering wall of grass beside you: it is utterly mesmerising. Linking the peaks of Castle Knott, Calf Top and Combe Top, this magnificent flank of land frames the landscape like no other geographical feature in Britain. For 5 kilometres you climb gently out of the valley, transfixed by your surroundings, oblivious to the gradient being gained or any effort you are expending. As the climb continues, the majesty of the view begins

to eventually fade; then, released from its spell, you plummet down the other side into the small village of Gawthrop. Two 'cols' ticked off, two to go, and up next is a real tough one: the climb of White Shaw Moss.

After navigating the picture-perfect village of Dent, take the left-hand turn onto Deepdale Lane and begin the punishing climb south. Following a multitude of cottages and farms, the congested early slopes squeeze between high hedges and across bridges, passing waterfalls and small caves in the rocks. Following an abrupt right turn, and an even tighter left, you then arrive at a gate which halts your progress, and

marks the end of the cluttered part of the climb. Immediately after the gate, the slope ramps up more steeply, turning right into a brief patch of 20% before backing off to climb, facing Whernside ahead.

This is where this route will start to sting your legs, but you'll not care because, as you climb out of the valley, the views in all directions are simply spectacular on this quiet, forgotten road. It peaks at 468 metres on a sizeable plateau, then the descent the other side is every bit as amazing as the previous ascent, as you follow Kingsdale right the way into Ingleton, perfect for a stop before the last big climb. Take on nutrition here

ABOVE *The magnificence of Barbondale in the sunshine.*

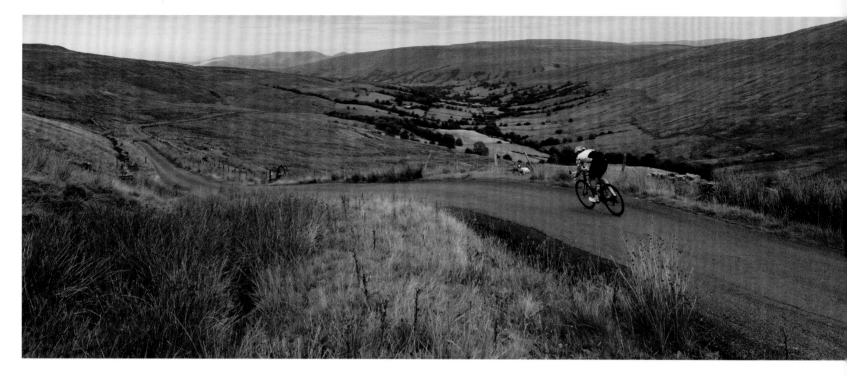

if you wish, then take Clapham Old Road south-eastwards, running parallel to the angle of the hillside to join, then cross, the B6480 and A65. Continue dropping down, through Clapham all the way to the River Wenning, and the base of Bowland Knotts.

A firm favourite of mine, Bowland Knotts will blow your mind – what's left of it, that is, after riding though Barbondale earlier. To me it evokes images of the Wild West: the endless, rolling, grass-covered hills under the vast skies – in fact, all it lacks are herds of buffalo. Oh, and maybe the odd cactus here and there. This long yet shallow climb rises for 7.5 kilometres all told

and, even though it does touch 10% briefly, it will never put your legs in too much difficulty. The Knotts themselves are a series of jagged gritstone outcrops that line the horizon, making the border between Yorkshire and Lancashire, and visible from a long way off to give you something to aim for as you ride. The final part of the climb passes through Clapham Common which, in this incarnation, is about as far removed from the better-known Clapham Common in south London as you could possibly get. The scenery is simply immense in every direction, as will be the effort needed to climb if the wind isn't in your favour, so fingers crossed.

ABOVE *'Descending' the climb of White Shaw Moss above the fields in Dentdale.*

With Bowland Knotts bagged, that's the four giant peaks covered, and now it's time to close the loop by dropping though the Gisburn Forest to the edge of Stocks Reservoir. Far from being a gentle run in, the ride has one more surprise in its locker as, once past the large lake, it kicks up through the trees into 4 final kilometres of climbing, split across Hole House Lane, Dugdale Lane and the B6478. Empty the tanks on the main road up to the final brow, and then sit back to enjoy the last 3 kilometres of this outrageously beautiful ride back into Slaidburn. Then, after a big lunch, maybe head back out to ride it in the opposite direction? I'll leave that with you.

RIDE 30

NORTH-WEST

FOREST OF BOWLAND AND YORKSHIRE DALES

DISTANCE 96KM	
CLIMBING +2,015M	
DIFFICULTY 6/10	

FOOD & WATER | BARBON / DENT / INGLETON / CLAPHAM

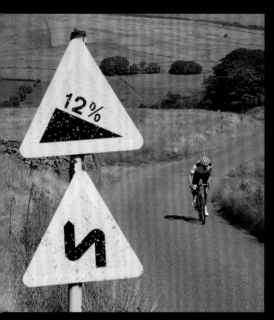

KEY CLIMBS

1 CROSS OF GREET

2,932m +183m

With a 6% average this is a fairly stiff opponent to begin the ride with. The toughest climbing comes at the start and towards the summit where the slope will reach a modest 13% in places.

2 WHITE SHAW MOSS

2,189m +227m

Starting in Deepdale this impeccably quiet road rises gradually at first then as the tight bends arrive ramps up much steeper. There
is a gate that splits these 20% slopes then another further up which break your rhythm or give you a rest from climbing depending how you feel.*

3 BOWLAND KNOTTS

7,446m +297m

A lovely steady climb which has a 4% average so your only real foe will be the wind if there is any. It rolls up and down slightly to begin with and along the way there are a couple of false summits which when crossed reveal yet more glorious climbing.

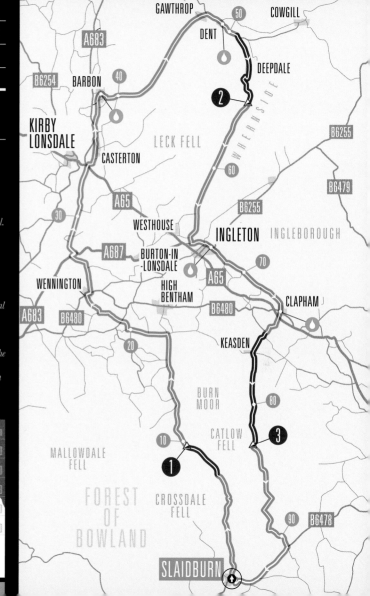

FOR THOSE ABOUT TO CLIMB . . .

DISTANCE 162KM | **CLIMBING** +3,130M

PHOTOGRAPHY PHIL HALL

*A hundred miles bagging the
big beasts of the North Lakes*

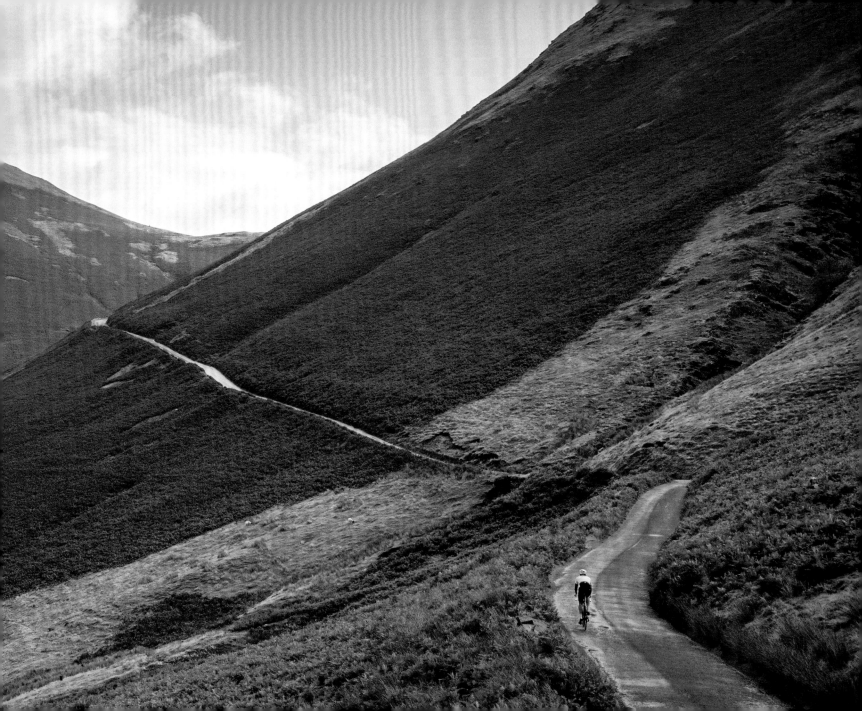

Although it is possible to cross all the great Cumbrian passes on one route (the Fred Whitton sportive does – see page 197), I've shared them out across two rides in a sort of north–south divide. Choosing which to allocate to which (albeit governed slightly by location) was reminiscent of picking a football team in the school playground. Imagine the two ride captains one side and all the climbs lined out in front of them: whoever had first choice would have to pick Hardkott Pass first – which comes as a pair with Wrynose, because Wrynose can't be on the opposite team to its buddy. To counter this choice, the other captain would go for the next strongest player, in this case Honister Pass, which links up well with Newlands Pass, so that's two stars for each team. Back and forth the process goes until our current ride, or team, finished its line-up with Whinlatter, Red Bank and the infamous Struggle.

Starting in Keswick, you'll be pleased to see the first 10 or so kilometres heading south past Derwent Water through Borrowdale are reasonably flat, allowing you to digest your Cumbrian sausage (vegetarian/vegan options may also be available), before arriving at the foot of the team's star player, Honister. This is the slightly easier of the two ways to the top, as the steepest slopes come right at the bottom, unlike the north face, which gets tougher the higher it climbs. Arriving in Seatoller, surrounded by fells on all sides and approaching what appears to be a dead end, you just know there's only one way out (unless someone builds a tunnel) – and that is up and over.

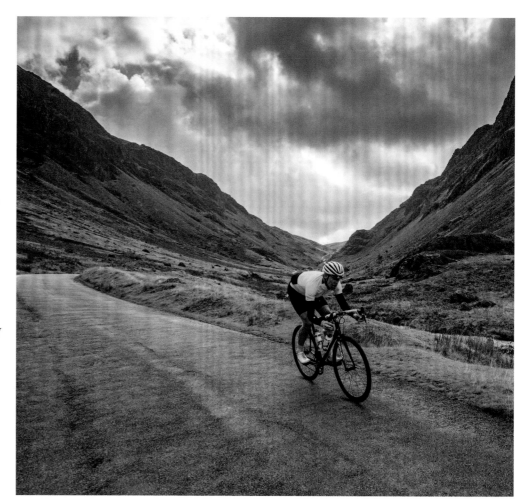

ABOVE *Hurtling down the precipitous slopes of Honister Pass towards Buttermere.*

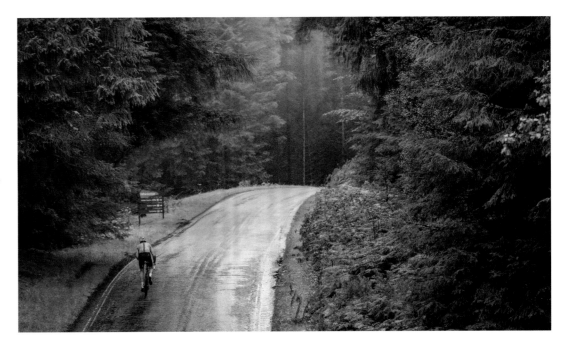

Honister starts with a punch to the guts and straight away the slope, bending left, rockets up to 20%, then gets steeper. It's oh, so beautiful, though, and you'll have all the time in the world to take in the scenery as you rise, at a snail's pace, away from the gushing stream in the valley towards the open slopes above. The temptation to put a foot down will be strong here, and I've experienced it many times, but don't give in! Don't listen to those evil voices in your head! Just keep your eye on the horizon where the tree cover breaks, because you can and will make it. At this point the gradient backs off and you will see the rest of the road, framed by the magnificence of the surrounding peaks, snake towards the summit outside the slate mine.

Passing the mine, you reach the huge stone walls at the top of the north face, which stand like ancient posts that once held a giant gate guarding the magical realm beyond. The following descent is perilous in the dry, and can leave you in need of a change of shorts in the wet, so TAKE CARE, especially on the tight changes of direction near the top. After the short run along the side of Buttermere it's then time to take on my favourite climb in the UK: Newlands Pass.

From my very first visit I knew I'd not see better. The pure simplicity of this road, the isolated sliver of asphalt cutting its line across the hillside surrounded by towering hills on all sides, is cycling heaven. If heaven involves slogging away up long periods of double-digit gradient and a nasty 20% final right-hand bend, that is.

Two big climbs ticked off, and it's time for the third, Whinlatter Pass, which, although still a serious challenge, is a degree kinder than those you have just crossed. Up through the conifers, like the lower slopes of an Alpine mountain, Whinlatter flirts between stretches of 17% slope and periods of relative levelling, all the way to the café and adventure centre at the top. Until now the route has traced the classic 'Fred' route but, instead of breaking left towards Cold Fell, I'm routeing north into the upper reaches of the Lakes to uncover some delights off the beaten track.

Heading through Lorton Vale towards Cockermouth on the B5292, turn right on Hundith Hill Road, and cross the A66 into Lambfoot to climb through Bully Wood. Crossing the top of

Bassenthwaite Lake and into Bassenthwaite, the road then heads east up North Row to Horsemoor Hills and Orthwaite. Obviously overlooked for the lack of vicious climbs and stunning valleys, this part of Cumbria still has much to offer, including, thankfully a bit of a rest. Skirting around the edge of the Uldale Fells and Caldbeck Fells, through Longlands and Hesket Newmarket, there is nothing on your right-hand side apart from uninterrupted scenery. It's more agricultural than the National Park, but with fewer tourists. You loop north, then back south, climb up West Fell for close to 3 kilometres, before meandering gradually downwards to meet the A66.

On the way to Threlkeld I've done the best I can to avoid the A66, which, although plenty

ABOVE *Deep in the forest, the final tough kick to the summit of Whinlatter Pass.*

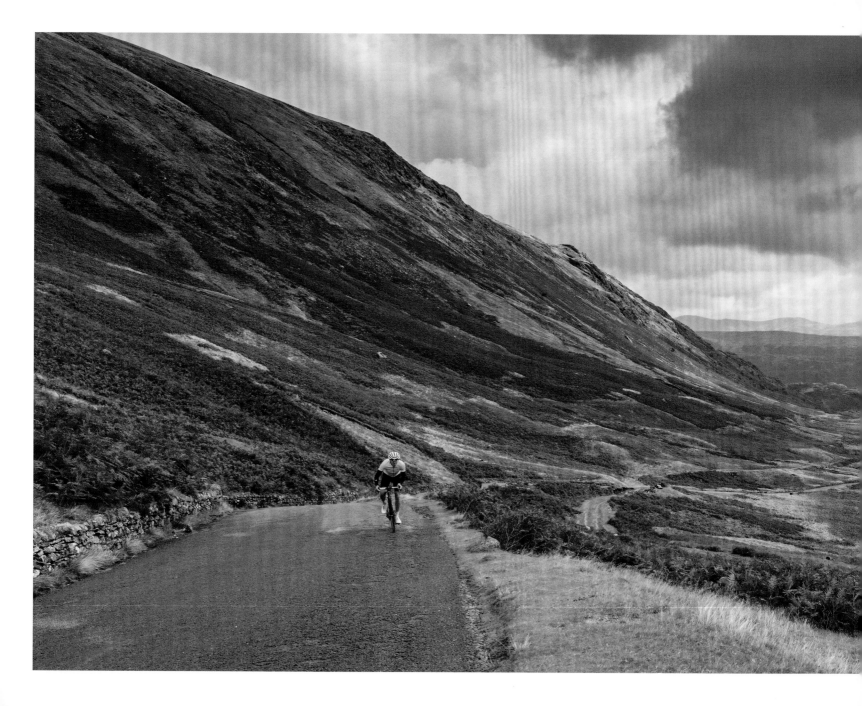

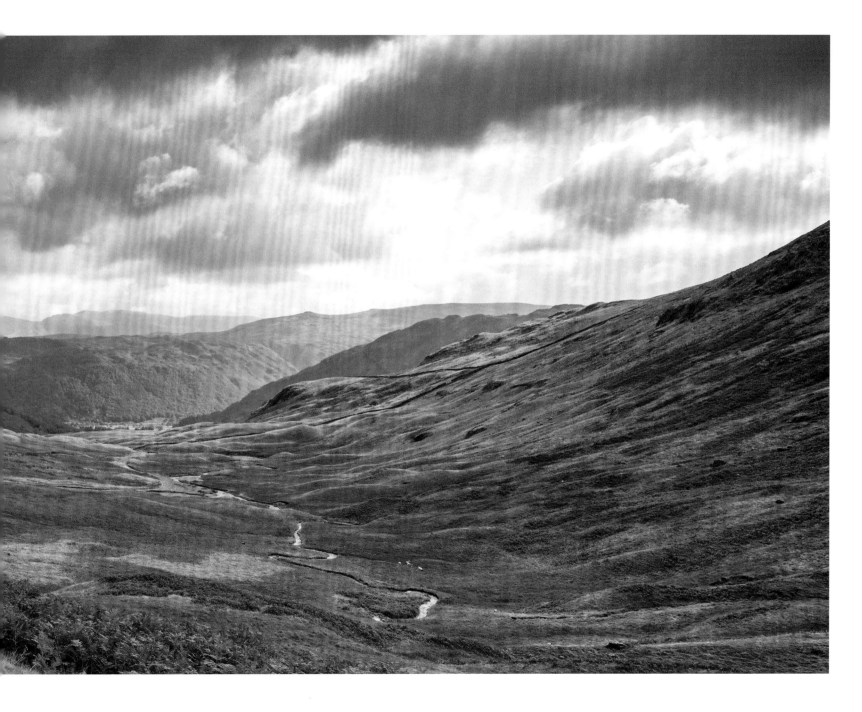

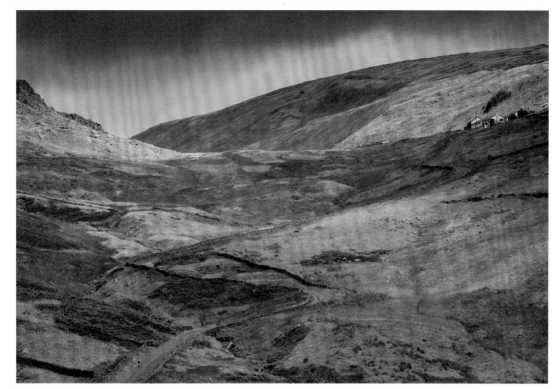

PREVIOUS PAGE *The higher slopes of Honister Pass will leave you speechless.*

and bends at the finale, but this climb is so much more than that. To forget about the pull out of town is to forget just how hard The Struggle is, and it's the first 4 kilometres that really do the damage. Leaving the relative comfort of Ambleside behind, push up through the 20% corners via Kirkstone Road, in and out of trees, past houses and farms, in search of the midway interval, which arrives not at the midway point but at four-fifths distance. I'd go so far as to say that if you actually want to enjoy The Struggle – and of course you do – then do all you can to preserve energy lower down and, as you crest the last fake brow, erase all memory of it before tucking into the glorious finish to the top. Famous for forcing the legendary Bradley Wiggins off his bike during the Tour of Britain, this is by far the best way to climb up to the famous Kirkstone Inn and the peak of the highest pass in the Lakes.

Up next is one of the great descents in Britain (someone should write a book), but also another that can have you a little nervous at the top, as it switches right and left, so keep an eye on your speed, but enjoy the thrill of plummeting down to the shores of Ullswater, which you follow to the final climb of the day, Matterdale. It's a mere blip compared to some of the giants you have tackled but, as you close in on 100 miles in the saddle, it is sure to hammer the legs. Continuing north, all that then remains is to head back into Keswick, once again trying to avoid the dreaded A66, to finish a stupendous day in the Lake District hills.

wide enough for any traffic to pass safely, always seems to suck the life out of my legs when I ride it. Turning south after Threlkeld, therefore, take the B5322 through St John's in the Vale to Legburthwaite, cross the main road, then follow the shores of Thirlmere beneath Helvellyn Screes all the way down to Wythburn. Heading south between the towering fells, the route does all it can to avoid contact with the A591, but where no other option is available it does briefly venture onto the main road, so take care. You've no option but to mix in with the traffic for a short while until

you reach Town Head, where you leave the main road to round the back of Grasmere, in order to come at Ambleside from below.

This route also allows me to sneak in an extra bit of climbing as you rise up the back of Red Bank, before dropping to Skelwith Bridge, then through Clappersgate, and at last into Ambleside. This would be a good place to stop for fuel, or maybe even take something for your nerves, because you have a right to be nervous, as next up is the most perfectly named road in the land: The Struggle.

The title is attributed to the jumble of twists

ABOVE *The final bends of The Struggle, really are A STRUGGLE.*

RIDE 31

NORTH-WEST
NORTH LAKE DISTRICT

DISTANCE 162KM

CLIMBING +3,130M

DIFFICULTY 9/10

FOOD & WATER | BASSENTHWAITE / AMBLESIDE

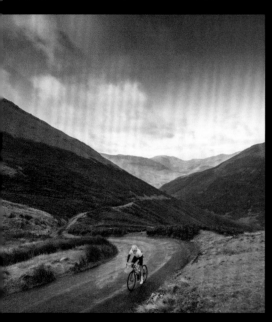

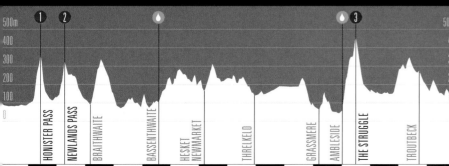

KEY CLIMBS

1 HONISTER PASS

2,375m +246m

For just about all of the first kilometre from Seatoller you'll have no need for your saddle as it's all pretty much 25%. Then breaking out of the trees the second part of the climb is much kinder.

2 NEWLANDS PASS

1,883m +215m

Just because it's beautiful doesn't mean it doesn't bite. After kicking up from the shores of Buttermere through a few gentle turns you then see the rest of the climb ahead. After a brief lull the gradient is consistently hard and ends with a 25% corner to the summit.

3 THE STRUGGLE

4,603m +379m

The Struggle comes in three parts. First the struggle out of Ambleside which goes on forever. Then the struggle to recover on the easier mid section. Then lastly the struggle through the 20% switchbacks to the Kirkstone Inn.

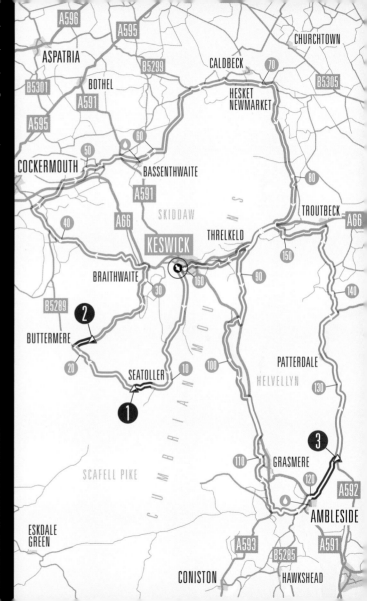

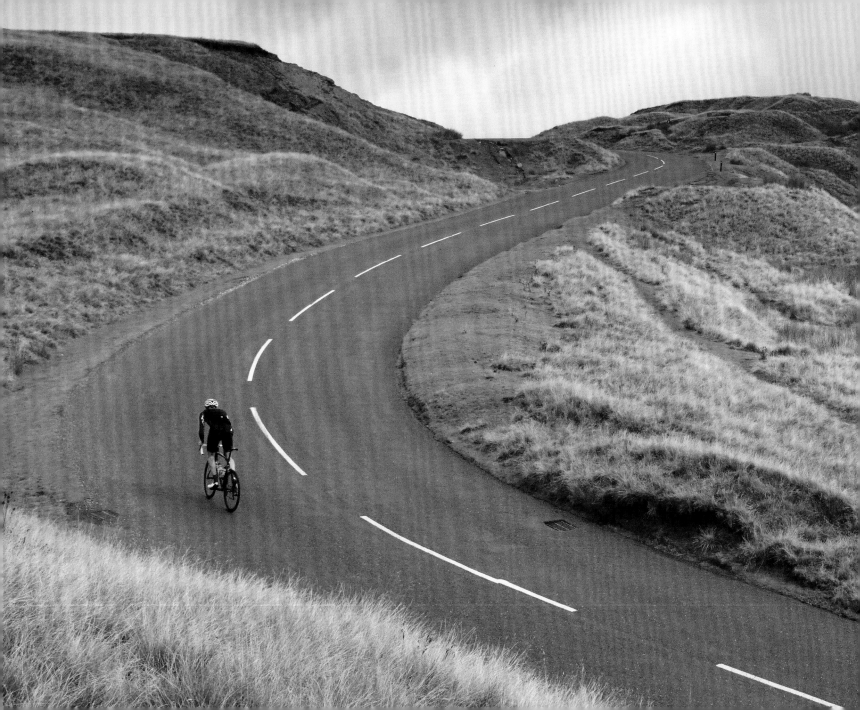

HIDDEN TREASURE

DISTANCE 107KM | **CLIMBING** +2,258M

PHOTOGRAPHY ANDY JONES

*A journey through the wonder
of the Trough of Bowland
and Pendle hills*

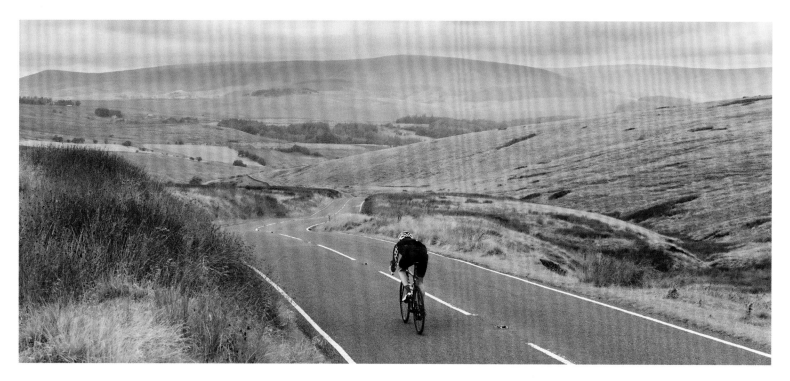

discovered the Forest of Bowland on my first visit to its showpiece climb, the Trough of Bowland, and I fell in love right away. Tucked away to the south-west of the Yorkshire Dales, this oasis of solitude has long been a favourite cycling destination. Comprised of two loops with an interconnecting passage, this route does a pretty good job of ticking off a good proportion of the killer hills in the vicinity, as well as its most beautiful roads.

Leaving Clitheroe, the ride wastes no time in gaining altitude as straight away it heads for the high point of the route on top of Newton Fells. With barely a couple of kilometres' 'warm-up',

it's time to dig out the climbing legs to get stuck into almost 5 kilometres of steady incline out of the Ribble Valley. This side of the climb is far more agricultural than the northern side, and it's only really when you reach the summit that you're truly on open ground and within the boundaries of the Forest. I say 'forest', but it's more barren fells than thick trees: in fact, there is very little left of the ancient woodland that would once have smothered the entire region. Heading down the other side, the descent is fast, very fast, as it weaves through beautiful sweeping corners, so keep an eye on your speed and that of other road users, as the temptation to test the limits of their

vehicles will lead some to act like proper idiots.

Arriving in Newton, it's now time to head into the solitude and make your way to the exquisite Trough of Bowland. Turning left in the small town, follow the signs to Dunsop Bridge along the narrow lane set on the steeply sloping hillside, trapped between intermittent stone walls. Take the right turn at the junction in Dunsop Bridge to follow the course of Langden Brook and, after a few kilometres of very gentle downhill, it's time to start heading up again. Now on the Trough Road, which, as you may have guessed, lies at the base of the valley, you ride north-east in search of the sumptuous

PREVIOUS PAGE *Approaching the top of Nick O' Pendle, this is hallowed ground for hill climbers.*

ABOVE *You will pay good money at a theme park for the same thrill you get descending Newton Fell.*

climb that will lead you out at the other end. As you pass the hamlet of Sykes the valley walls begin to close in further, signs of farming and general human activity fade, and ahead you'll see the wall of hills you must cross. There's nothing to fear about the Trough of Bowland climb, though: its gradient is never too harsh, its corners flow like the curves of the body, and it's so beautiful it could never hurt the legs.

Once over the summit, drop down the other side and, tracing exactly the path of the gushing stream on your left, make your way eastwards. It's so calm here, so quiet, it's simply a delight to ride this road. Past Marshaw you carry on round to the right, then take the left turn to head through Abbeystead, all the way to Lower Green Bank. Hugging the edge of the Forest boundary, turn north towards Quernmore to reach the turn. The purpose of arriving in Quernmore is to reach the right turn which marks the foot of the climb up to Jubilee Tower.

Standing high on Hare Appletree Fell, and built to commemorate Queen Victoria's Jubilee, not only does the tower offer outstanding views out over the fells, it's also a perfect carrot to chase as you toil away on the long climb to its base. Used for generations as a venue for races, you'll find its slopes being pounded by local Lancastrians heading off into the Forest beyond or just looking for an escape from the town below. High up on the fells the scenery is sublime, the views are massive.

Once you're over the top it's time to retrace

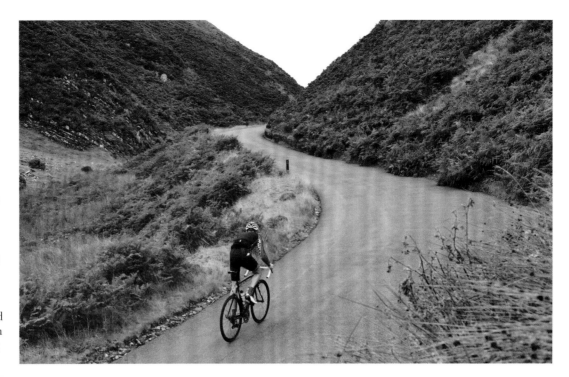

your steps back through the Trough. This is a road so perfect it's never a chore to ride twice, and this time you'll get to enjoy it from the opposite perspective. The climb between the valleys is a little kinder from the west, although it does ramp up a bit towards the top. Then, as you rattle over the final cattle grid, you get to soak up the legendary views down the neat little valley. With the Trough of Bowland well and truly ticked off, it's time for some more climbing, and there are four sharp ascents left, including one absolute beauty. On your return to Dunsop Bridge turn right to head south, down along the flat valley floor to Whitewell, then in the village,

take the abrupt left turn to face up to Hall Hill.

If the first part of this ride was all about flowing hills and steady inclines, the second is quite the opposite, to which this kilometre of almost constant 10% gradient is ample testament. Once over Hall Hill, drop down to Cow Ark, turn right and continue almost due south in the direction of Longridge Fell, a playground for local cyclists and boasting a multitude of different ascents, including the much-feared Birdy Brow.

The climb you are heading for is Jeffrey Hill, with 20% gradients and a fantastic switchback corner. The rapid gain in elevation opens up

ABOVE *The perfect curves of the climb through the Trough of Bowland.*

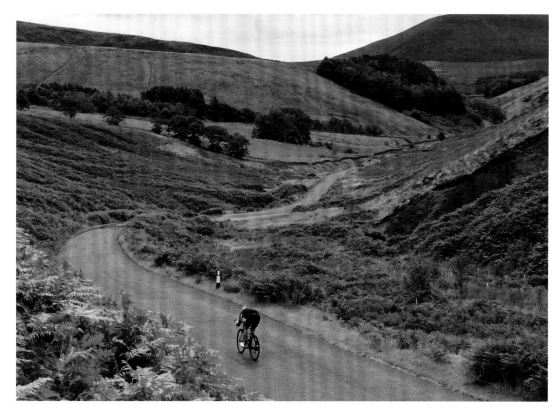

the University Hill Climb Championship in 1994. Our ramshackle university cycling team hired a Transit van, stuck a sofa in the back and, together with our bikes and a few bottles of homemade wine, headed west. I knew all about the road I was going to face: it's where Malcolm Elliot won the National Championship in 1980 and where Chris Boardman took his first title in 1988. It's a perfect climb for a race, with the most amazing natural amphitheatre for spectators surrounding its final testing bends at the top. My performance, if we can call it that, was not spectacular, somewhat due to poor preparation – oh, and the homemade wine (we had to drink out of Coke cans because no booze was allowed in the youth hostel). Still, it was one hell of a fun trip.

As you turn left in Sabden the climb hits you right away, and assumes its 16% incline all the way to the brow ahead. This part is a real grind. Then, once you cross the cattle grid, the scenery opens up, the slope backs off a smidgen, and the pitch becomes more agreeable. Ahead you'll see the flowing hills, carpeted in grass, the road winding between them to the summit. Towards the top the slope bites a bit more, but throw everything you have at it, because once you crest the summit you're done for the day, as all you have left is the rapid descent back into Clitheroe. If you have time and the legs, I'd recommend exploring more of the Pendle hills but, after all you've already climbed, you'll probably leave that for another day.

more tremendous views, the horizon lined with the tops of the surrounding fells. Heading over the summit, turn left along the Old Clitheroe Road, then right to drop down the other side of the fell through Great Mitton and into Whalley, to conclude the ride with a classic double whammy.

Entering Whalley on Station Road, turn right onto King Street. The other side of the River Calder, you reach the base of the first of the two remaining climbs. Whalley Nab is an evil little road with a 25% corner right at the bottom, and

a gradient that offers scant relief all the way to the top. Over the crest carry on south all the way to the edge of Great Harwood, take the B6535 to ride east to briefly join the A680 north, cross the River Calder again, and join the A671 towards Sabden.

It would have been nice to include a few of the Pendle hills, but I didn't want either the distance or climbing to get out of hand, so I've just included one, the Big One: Nick O' Pendle. The first time I rode this hill was at

ABOVE *The second passage of the Trough of Bowland is a little easier.*

RIDE 32

NORTH-WEST	**DISTANCE** 107KM	
	CLIMBING +2,258M	
FOREST OF BOWLAND	**DIFFICULTY** 6/10	

FOOD & WATER | WHALLEY

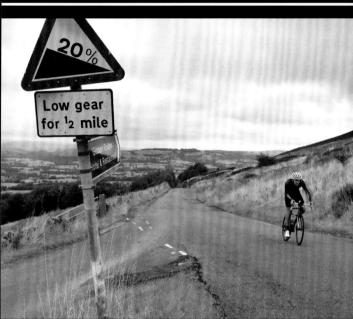

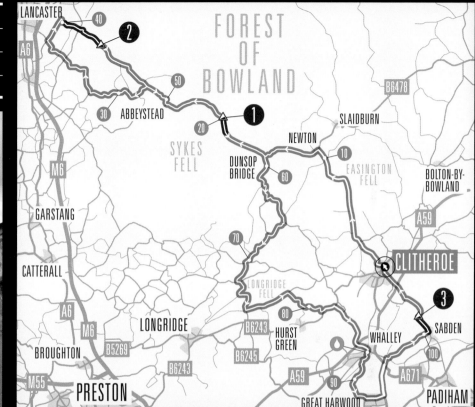

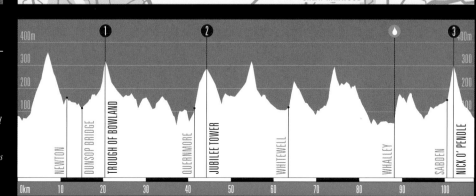

KEY CLIMBS

1 TROUGH OF BOWLAND
2,285m +144m

This climb starts ever so gently so as not to shock the body then assumes its moderately steep gradient which hardly changes all the way to the top. With an average of 6.5% it's no killer, just hard enough to make you sweat while you round its sweeping bends.

2 JUBILEE TOWER
4,145m +230m

A pretty long climb all in all it starts where you cross the River Conder with the first stretch taking you to the crossroads. From here the next part is the hardest, bending right then heading straight up the bank before easing for the long steady drag to the finish alongside the Tower.

3 NICK O' PENDLE
1,300m +145m

The worst bit of this climb is the first half out of Sabden up to the cattle grid. It's consistently around 16%, dead straight and the scenery offers very little. Once you cross the cattle grid though the pitch eases (briefly) and you get to ride through the wonderful grass-covered hillocks.

DESTROY ALL MONSTERS

DISTANCE 121KM | **CLIMBING** +2,932M

PHOTOGRAPHY ANDY JONES

Crossing the legendary climbs
of the southern Lake District

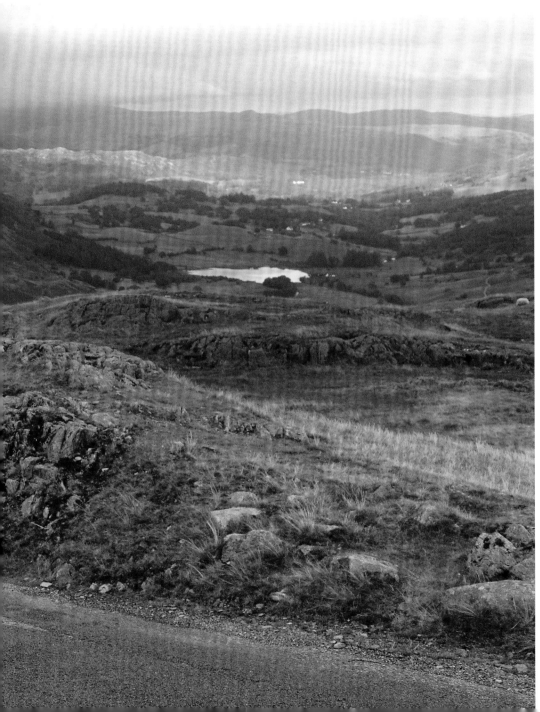

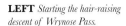

If I think of the Lake District I think of the Fred Whitton sportive – the annual 112-mile challenge that crosses all the giant Cumbrian passes in one ride – and if I think of the Fred Whitton sportive I break out in a sweat and my palms start to clam up. I'm taken back to the top of Hardknott Pass in the early stages of a snowstorm, facing the prospect of arguably the most technical descent in the UK, on a road that is fast turning white. Too cold to stop, hands so numb they could no longer change gear – to this day I still have no idea how I made it down on two wheels, never mind how I managed to also get up and over the following Wrynose Pass in one piece.

That was my first 'Fred' and, as soon as I finished, with frostbite setting in, I said categorically, NEVER, EVER AGAIN. Trouble is, I had secretly fallen in love with this ride, so of course I went back the following year, and the one after that, and every time it rained so much I would have gone faster in a canoe. Three years of pure suffering. My fortitude had been tested, and that was it for the Fred and me. I couldn't put myself through it any more.

Naturally, in subsequent years the sun shone and everyone got burnt to a cinder so, after a substantial sabbatical, I decided to give it one more shot to try and break my curse.

In May 2018 my prayers were finally answered. I woke to glorious sunshine, and what a difference it made to ride those oh-so-special roads under clear blue skies! That year was utterly perfect: I finished a wreck, but not a single second of it had

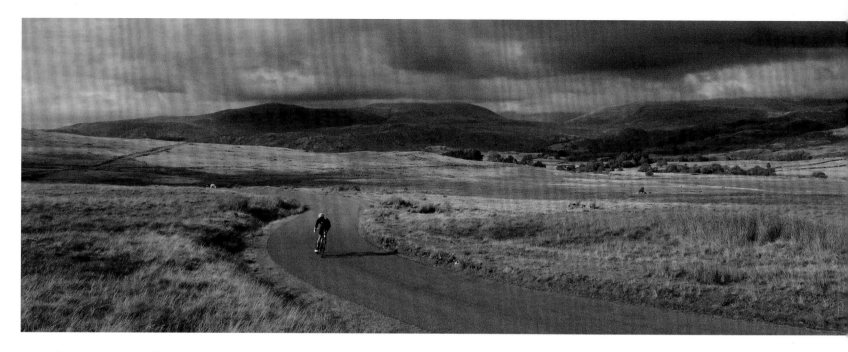

been an ordeal, and for once I'd been able to soak in the views without picking grit out of my eyes or dodging piles of snow.

It would be easy for me to simply reproduce the Fred route here, but that belongs to Fred, and besides there's far more to the Lakes, so I've split the giant passes that populate the infamous sportive across two rides to squeeze in a few more of my favourite roads.

The first Lakes ride starts in Ambleside, by heading south-west out of the busy tourist hub on the A593 before departing left at Clappersgate, dropping into the gully, then continuing on the B5286 for a short while heading towards Hawkshead Hill. Turning right from the B road the route undulates through the woods,

gaining elevation in stages, punctuated by short descents and plateaux. This road, a mix-match of gradients and never too steep reaches its peak at Hawkshead Hill where you re-join the B5286 then descend to the shores of Coniston Water to enjoy a period of calm on the main road.

The peace is shattered, though, by the arrival of the Old Rake: a narrow, arrow-straight climb that veers off the main road with such ferocity it's like riding into a sand trap. Fingers crossed you'll still have fresh legs, so can hit it with force. When the body has recovered from the initial shock, it will relish getting stuck into the 20% slopes which rise to reveal the tremendous views out over the Irish Sea.

With the first serious climb done, roll along the

top, drop down into Broughton Mills, then line up immediately for the next, Kiln Bank Cross. Not as stiff a challenge as the route from the north, and with a gate to negotiate midway, the beauty of this road is to be found on its upper slopes, set amongst the dramatic rocky outcrops of Stickle Pike.

Falling down into Dunnerdale, there are no giant climbs for the next 35 kilometres, but there is a barrage of little spikes to keep you busy. Heading further south-east, it's time to venture into the lesser-visited part of the Lake District – in fact, you leave the confines of the National Park after passing through Ulpha and Stonestar to cross the river at Duddon Bridge. Nip onto the A595, then, avoiding the climb up through Beckman Brow Wood, turn onto Lady Hall Lane

ABOVE *Crossing the high plains of Birker Fell.*

to skirt along the edge of the plains surrounding Duddon Sands. Passing through Lady Hall and Hallthwaites, across the A5093, you then face Lowscales Bank, before rejoining the A595 to follow the peninsula round to eventually find the base of Corney Fell. Now at roughly half distance, you will have climbed 1,250 metres to this point, and if you subtract from the final total of 2,950, you don't need to be a genius to work out that the second half is going to be substantially tougher.

Ahead of you lie, one after another, seven immense climbs, kicking off with the giant Corney Fell. Six-and-a-half kilometres, with an average gradient of 6% and a couple of patches of 15%, this climb, in the far south-west corner of the Lakes, is often regrettably overlooked as riders stick to the more famous roads to the north. Starting in the forest, yet finishing on the wide expanse of the fell, it has a cheeky fake brow that tricks you into thinking you're at the top, only to reveal the true summit considerably further in the distance.

Up next is a real treat, a place so beautiful it hurts as, after returning to Ulpha via the rapid descent of Bobbin Mill Hill, it's time to witness the majesty of Birker Fell. The first time I was here, on a cold February morning, I was blown away: I thought I'd seen all the Lake District had to show me, but I was so wrong. From the top of the climb, looking north-east out over Scafell and Great Gable, topped that day with a light dusting of snow, it was nirvana. If it hadn't been so bitterly cold I'd have stood there for hours, in

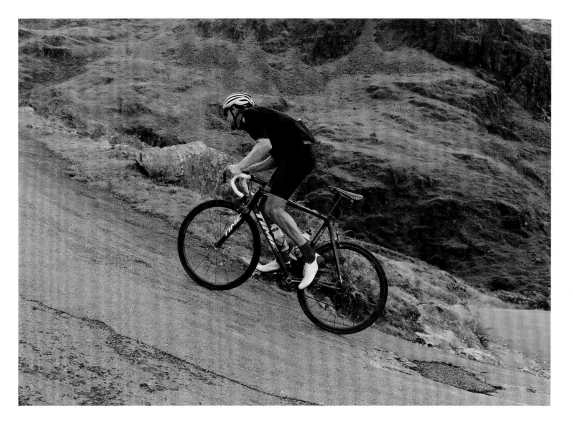

awe of the scenery, and since then I try to return whenever I can.

Although the route descends the 'tough' side of Birker Fell, it's necessary to ride the climb this way to deliver you to the obvious star attractions of any ride in the Lakes, the stupendous double act of Hardknott and Wrynose. What can I write that hasn't already been written about these roads? I've been obsessed by these roads since I first saw them on an old OS map in the 1980s. Looking like the twin prongs of Barad-dûr on the ride profile,

smothered with severe gradient chevrons – so many that they obliterate the road – these are the Holy Grail for anyone addicted to savage climbs.

It was many years, though, between scanning a road atlas and arriving at the base, and in fact the first time I rode them was during that dreaded Fred Whitton in the snow. With cold and battered legs I cramped on Hardknott, forcing me to fall sideways from the bike, clutching my hamstring and wailing in agony, before dragging myself up to hobble forwards on foot. As soon as 33%

ABOVE *NO I haven't tilted the picture. YES it is that steep at the top of Hardknott Pass!*

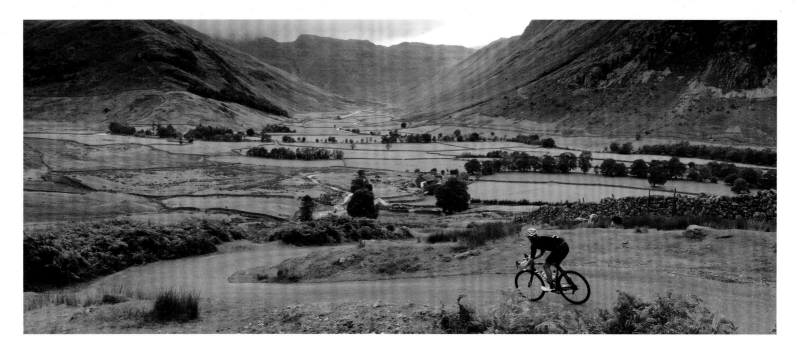

turned to 20% I re-mounted, and gingerly began to pedal forwards until the pain disappeared. Gutted that I'd not made it up, I went back the next day before heading home, took the bike out at the base and smashed it up, just to make sure I returned to the south with my pride intact.

The first sight of Hardknott simply takes your breath away. It's just crazy – but that's why we love it: it's such a fantastic challenge. There are always people sitting at the side of the road on the upper slopes looking broken, having a 'quiet moment' to themselves before trying to press on. There are countless stories of failure, followed by triumphant returns, because if you don't make it first time you must go back: everyone must conquer Hardknott at least once.

Once over and down the perilous descent the other side, you cross the exquisite Wrynose Bottom, then climb once more. If taken in isolation Wrynose would be the star on any ride but, due to its proximity, it always plays second fiddle to Hardknott, as it's just that degree more manageable. By this point, however, your legs may beg to differ.

With the twin peaks conquered, or not, as may be the case, the temptation would be to head right back to the main road and home, but to do that misses out on another wonder of the Lakes: Great Langdale. Almost immediately after what I consider the most terrifying descent anywhere in the world, off the top of Wrynose, a few hundred metres along the flat valley floor turn left, for

another healthy dose of 20% up to Blea Tarn. The gradient sign may fill your tired legs with dread but, fear not, it's only a short climb, and the reward at the top is yet another colossal view, this time out over Langdale Fell. Snake down the sumptuous curves the other side, then race though the valley to Chapel Stile for one last hurrah, Red Bank. A picture-perfect road, lined either side with bracken-covered hills dotted with jagged rocks, it's tough but a breeze compared to what you've already ridden, as you cross the brow past the youth hostel. All that's left is to fall down to Grasmere, then, following a diversion through White Common, join the A591 for the fast run into Ambleside, and the end of an unforgettable journey across these legendary hills.

ABOVE *Snaking down the gorgeous curves from Blea Tarn into Great Langdale.*

RIDE 33 | NORTH-WEST

SOUTH LAKE DISTRICT

DISTANCE 121KM

CLIMBING +2,932M

DIFFICULTY 8/10

FOOD & WATER | CONISTON / BOOTLE

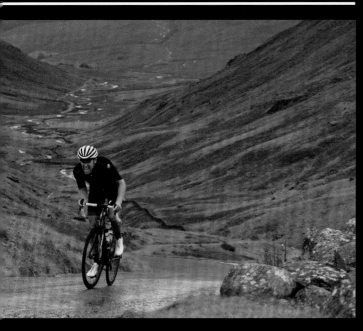

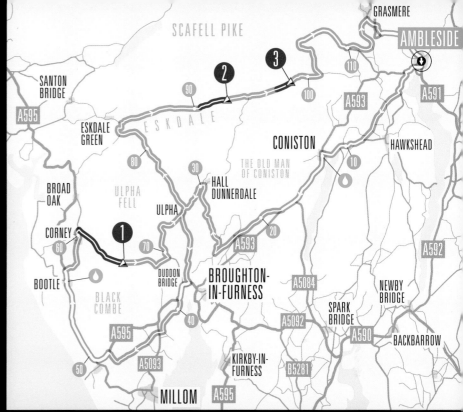

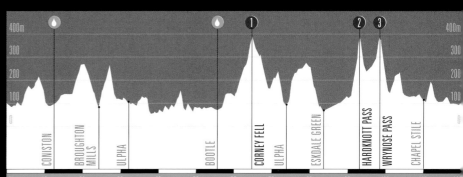

KEY CLIMBS

1 CORNEY FELL
3,930m +286m

After a stiff ramp at the base the first two kilometres of this climb are quite gentle, and are followed by some flat in the middle and a tiny descent across a bridge. Before long though the gradient begins to increase and your progress slows until you hit another *[illegible] batch just before the top*

2 HARDKNOTT PASS
2,203m +293m

Get over this and you can get over anything. Starting as abruptly as it finishes you are forced right away onto 25% slopes and across a cattle grid. Enjoy the break at two-thirds distance then gather all your strength to do battle with the 33% pitch that awaits. Good luck.

3 WRYNOSE PASS
1,790m +146m

Thankfully this is the easy side of Wrynose Pass but with your legs battered from Harknott you won't be complaining. The gradient creeps up on you then before you know it you are battling the 25% slope for almost the whole last 400 metres to the *eventual summit*

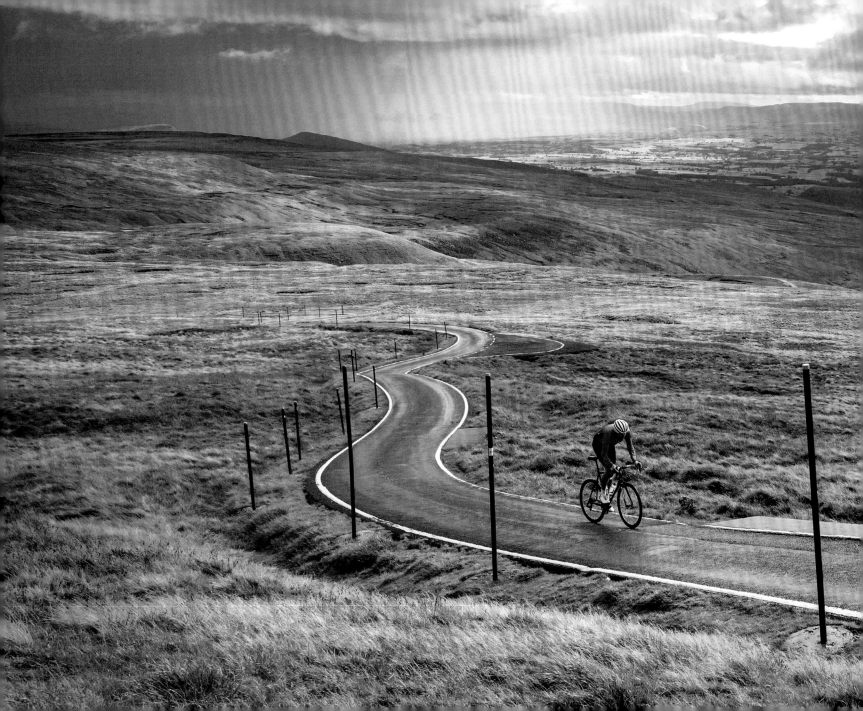

ENGLAND'S MOUNTAIN

DISTANCE 125KM | **CLIMBING** +2,436M

PHOTOGRAPHY PHIL HALL

A Pennine loop with a detour to the top of the world

PREVIOUS PAGE
*The upper slopes of Great
Dun Fell are like nothing
else in Britain.*

The UK government's official definition of a mountain is a summit that lies 610 metres (2,000 feet) above sea level or higher. Great Dun Fell stands at 848 metres, so yes, it is *officially* a mountain. Although not quite as high as its neighbour Cross Fell, which stands at 893 metres, what makes it oh-so-special is that there is a road that goes right to the very summit.

Does a road go right to the top of the 25th-highest point in France?

No.

Italy?

No.

I could go on, but I just want to emphasise how special Great Dun Fell is, and this route, while not being entirely about this mighty road, is at the same time entirely about this mighty road. I've chosen the town of Brough on the A66 as the start–finish point, as it has all the amenities an expedition into the mountains needs for pre- and post-ride fuel and, although this ride is equally as spectacular ridden either clockwise or anti-clockwise, I have gone for the latter, as it saves Great Dun Fell for last. You will be treated to the most spectacular wilderness in England, with hardly a single sign of human habitation inside its boundary, as you circumnavigate the giant fells and rolling hills that collectively form the largest mass of uninhabited land in the country.

Heading north from Brough, the first challenge of the day is the climb of Shot Moss. Six kilometres long and gaining 260 metres in altitude, it sends you across the spine of the mountain

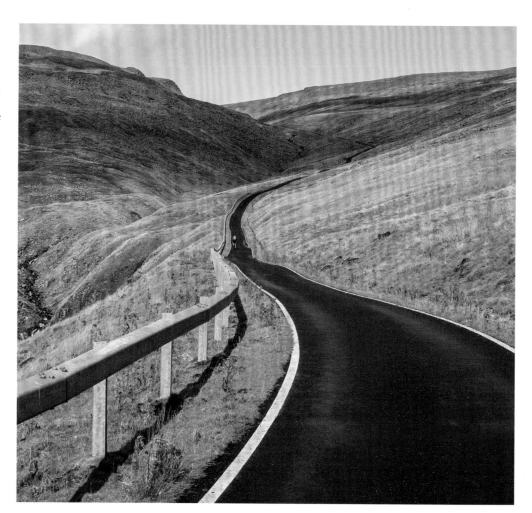

ABOVE *If in doubt, don't look up! It's a long way to the Top of the World.*

range via Grains o' th' Beck, Thringarth and Bowbank, to join the B6277 in Middleton-in-Teesdale. The summit, lying in the shadow of Shot Moss and lined with the soon-to-be-very-familiar snow poles either side, marks the border between Cumbria and County Durham, and the start of the long descent down the other side.

With a taste of the wilderness, you'll be longing for more, and more is what's on the menu after you turn left in Middleton to head towards Alston. Instead of immediately joining the B6227, I've chosen to head up Miry Lane, so you can enjoy the slightly elevated views over Teesdale before plummeting down to meet the main road at Newbiggin. I say main road but, fear not, this isn't the M1: it may be the primary link between Barnard Castle and Alston, but I've never found it to be in the slightest bit busy.

For the next 18 kilometres you gradually climb, following the path of the River Tees, and then, after it flows off to the left, shadowing Harwood Beck all the way to its source further up the valley. Passing though Forest-in-Teesdale and Langdon Beck, and with a few spikes in gradient and kinks in direction, the predominantly straight and steady slope rises north-eastwards into the increasingly sparse landscape.

Glancing left, you'll now have uninhibited views of the fells and, if you are lucky, catch sight of the spherical NATS Radar that marks the peak of Great Dun Fell, your final target of the day. I say if because, statistically, Great Dun Fell is shrouded in cloud for two-thirds of the year,

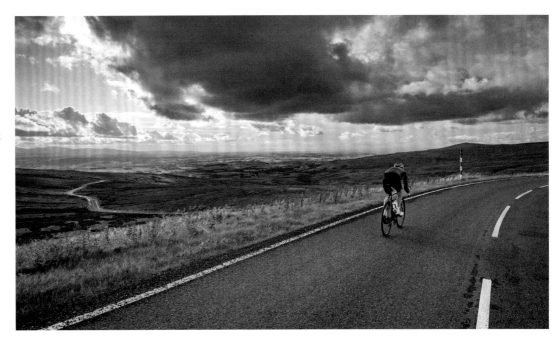

ABOVE *Ready to start the long and fast descent of the Hartside Pass.*

such is its location, so either cross your fingers for clear skies or plan carefully to get the most out of your visit. If indeed the sun is shining on the hills, the huge white sphere, often referred to as a giant golf ball, will shine like a beacon, like a sun as you satellite around it, before pulling out of orbit to make your approach.

There's still plenty more climbing to be done first, though, and the summit of the climb out of Teesdale, which lies at Yad Moss below Burnham Seat, must be reached first. At an altitude of 594 metres, Yad Moss is the highest B-road in England and, to further emphasise its 'extreme' altitude, it's home to one of only a handful of ski stations to be found in the UK. Although small, and never guaranteed snow, it's equipped with all

the paraphernalia of an Alpine slope, and in good conditions provides up to eight runs, so, yes, you are high up, and, yes, you are in the mountains.

Passing the base, and with the 18 kilometres of climbing behind you, cross the border back into Cumbria and start the very welcome descent towards Alston. I've chosen to divert the route around the town rather than cross it, however, to avoid as much human contact as possible. If you feel the need for a pit stop, though, continue straight on the B6277, fuel up, then leave town turning left onto the A686 to tackle the next giant climb of the day, the Hartside Pass.

The best ascent of this climb lies over on the western side but, don't worry, the eastern flank is still a beautiful and challenging climb,

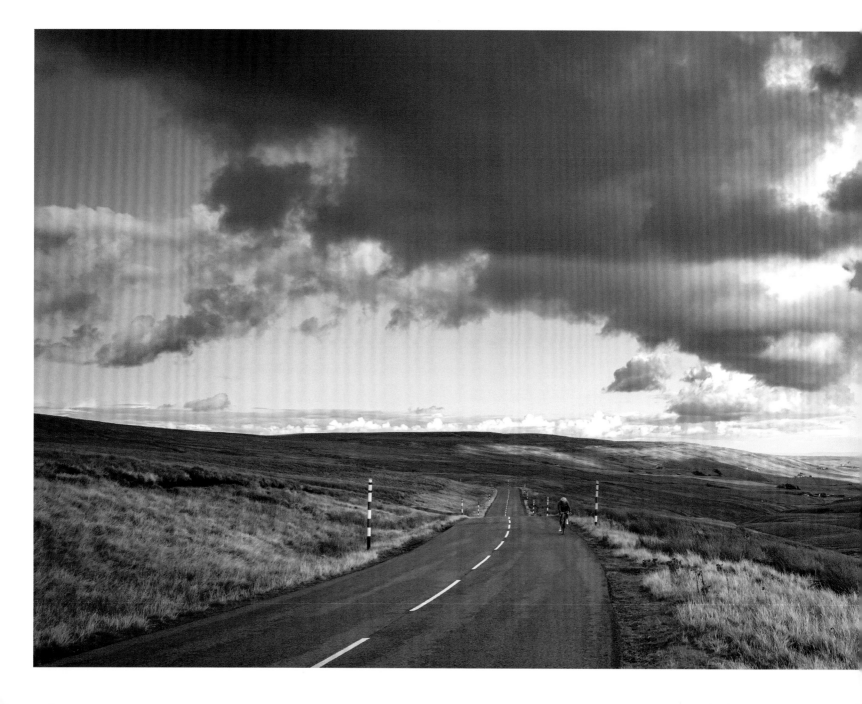

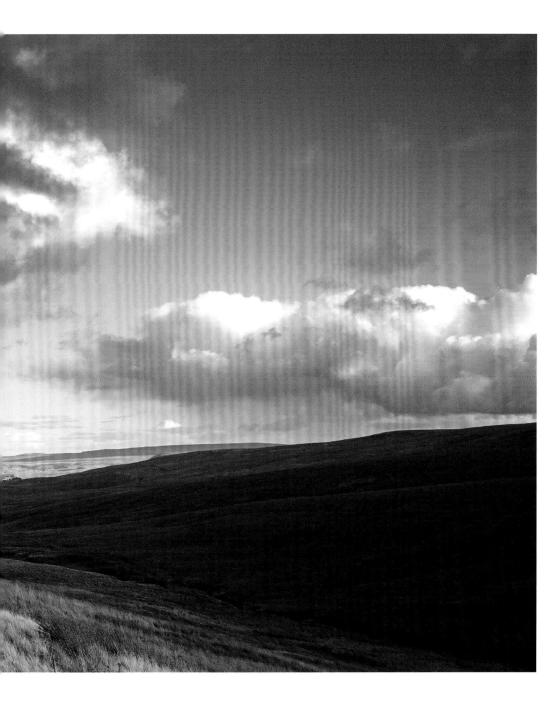

LEFT *The Pennines, home to vast swathes of open land and giant skies.*

which rises for over 7 kilometres before arriving at the summit, where once stood the famous, but now destroyed, café. Up next is one of the best descents in England which, after winding through its initial giant hairpin, hugs the mountainside, a wide smooth road boasting stupendous views out over the Lakeland mountains on the horizon.

Following the 8 kilometres of down, you are rewarded with 15 kilometres in the valley: ample time to stuff down whatever food you have left, shake the legs out and prepare to do battle with the genuine 11/10 climb that awaits. Back on the same side of the Pennines you started – and again, if conditions are favourable, the sparkling white sphere atop Great Dun Fell will be staring down at you as you make your way around the perimeter of the fells. Appearing as little more than a speck in the distance, this physical marker serves to emphasise both the task ahead and the distance, horizontal and vertical, that must be covered to reach it. After turning south in Melmerby and cutting through Ousby, Skirwith, Blencarn and Milburn, you arrive in Knock, and the wait is over. Turn left just before the village, and it's time to face up to the big one.

Between you and the summit lie 7,342 metres of unforgiving tarmac that rise a total of 620 metres in height. Although there are signs along the way to deter motorists, and indeed cyclists, the road is a designated bridleway, so access is not a problem no matter what anyone tells you. Once past the few buildings at the base, the

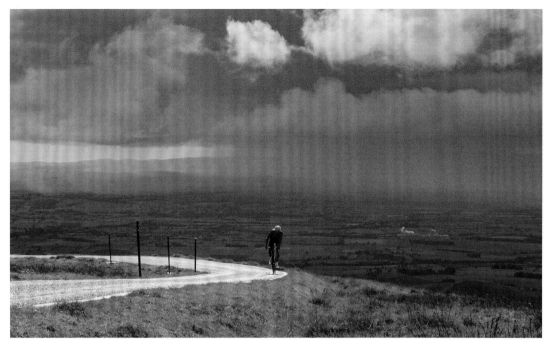

gradient begins to bite, and there's a nasty spike after just 1,500 metres before the slope recedes as you approach and navigate the first of two gates. The ride is now becoming increasingly wild and dramatic with every revolution of the pedals.

The next patch of nasty gradient arrives after 3 kilometres, where the road begins to squirm a little round the shape of the land, before levelling and then dropping at the head of Knock Ore Gill. This cessation in hostilities only serves to amplify the severity of the ramp ahead and, with the golf ball now a little closer, still spying on you from the horizon, it's impossible not to be overwhelmed by the sight of what lies ahead. Surrounded by the rolling hills, take whatever momentum you

can into the next ramp because, for the best part of 1,500 metres, it hovers around the 20% mark, and will chew your legs to bits. Midway up this infernal stretch you reach a minute plateau, which marks the exclusion zone for motor vehicles, and ushers in the final part of the climb.

Up through the towering banks that will be protecting you from the elements, you'll crawl to the horizon to break free of the steep gradient, only to be thrust into whatever weather is present. It's here that Great Dun Fell will remind you of its altitude: in the likelihood of extreme conditions you'll find battling the wind as tough as overcoming the pull of gravity. On the plus side, though – and there are far more positives

to outweigh any negatives – the surface is silky smooth, the scenery epically pristine, and you are also very near the top.

Echoing a true mountain road – narrow, exposed, crossing tundra and lined with snow poles – this final section is all but unique in England, and must be savoured, for it provides a cycling experience only usually found on the continent. Bobbing in and out of view, the radar, with its surrounding collection of antennae, now dominates the skyline, and soon you'll be making the final push to its base. Exhausted, elated and, I do hope, with clear skies, after you've put a warm jacket on, take your time up here to just sit, stand, whatever, and drink it all in. There are only a handful of locations that allow such grand uninterrupted views across England's great fells, and this is the reward for every ounce of effort and drop of sweat shed to get here.

There is still, however, the small matter of finishing the loop, and there comes a time, usually when cloud arrives, to head back down, so take real care on the fast descent, watch out for sheep, and also REMEMBER the gates on your way back to Knock. Heading south-east, you pass through Dufton, gain some height riding through Keisley, then lose it again through Murton and Hilton to reach the A66. To avoid time on the main road I've sent the route straight across into Warcop, then through Great Musgrave, to arrive, after 125 undoubtedly epic kilometres, with the scalp of the giant Great Dun Fell taken, back home in Brough.

ABOVE *Hugging the edge of the mountain high above the world below.*

RIDE 34

NORTH-WEST
NORTH PENNINES

DISTANCE 125KM
CLIMBING +2,436M
DIFFICULTY 7/10

FOOD & WATER | MIDDLETON-IN-TEESDALE / ALSTON / MELMERBY

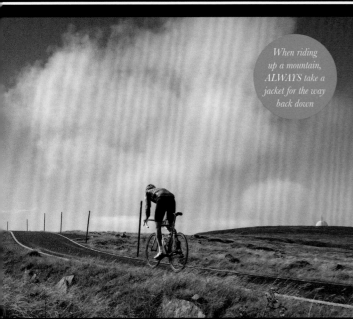

When riding up a mountain, ALWAYS take a jacket for the way back down

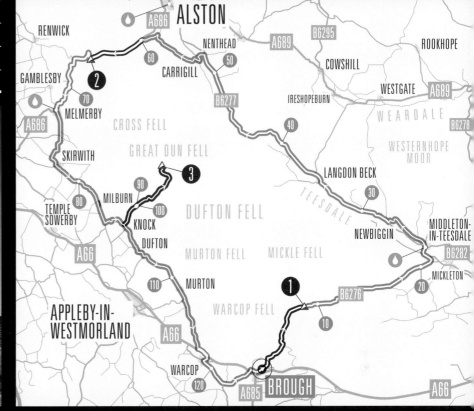

KEY CLIMBS

1 SHOT MOSS
6,119m +260m

A nice long climb on a steady slope that averages 4% across its 6-kilometre journey over the lower fells. Hidden in this ie a few patches of 11% gradient but nothing to hurt the legs too much. There's a bit of a false summit before the actual top so beware if you are *aying down a time*

2 HARTSIDE PASS
6,860m +274m

Starting to rise as it crosses the Black Burn before joining the A686 this is the easier and shorter side of the Hartside Pass. The steepest slopes are lower down, climbing out of the village of Leadgate up to the main road where a gentle 3% gradient takes you to the top.

3 GREAT DUN FELL
7,342m +620m

The peerless Great Dun Fell towers above all other climbs in England and although 'only' averaging 8% it is packed with 25% sectors towards the top. Blessed with silky smooth tarmac, virtually zero traffic, and EPIC views it may take some grunt to get up *but you'll love every minute*

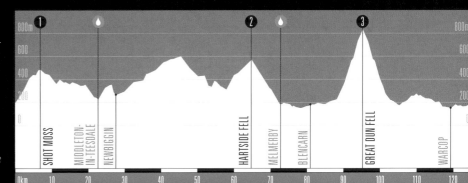

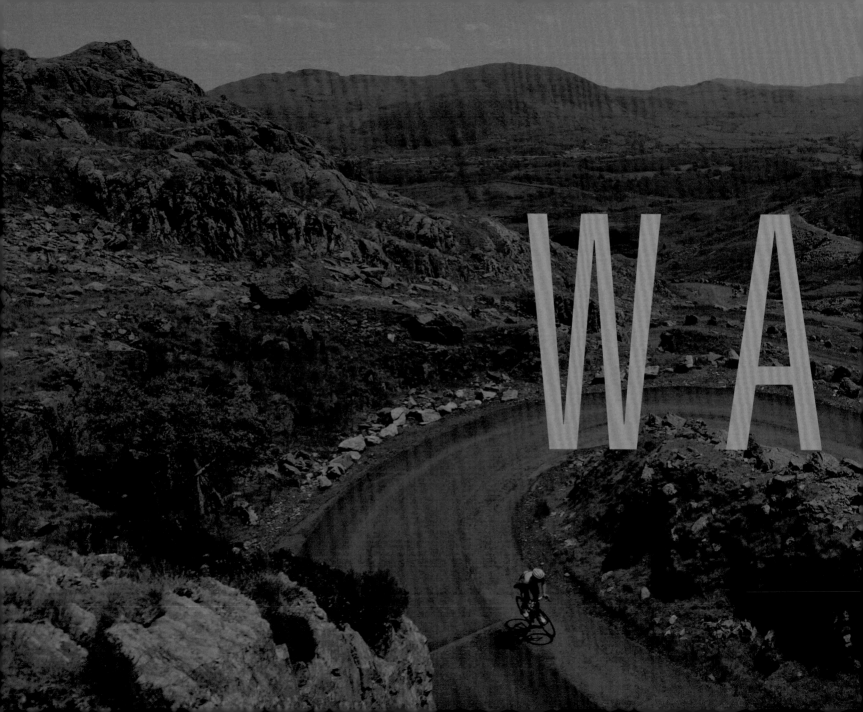

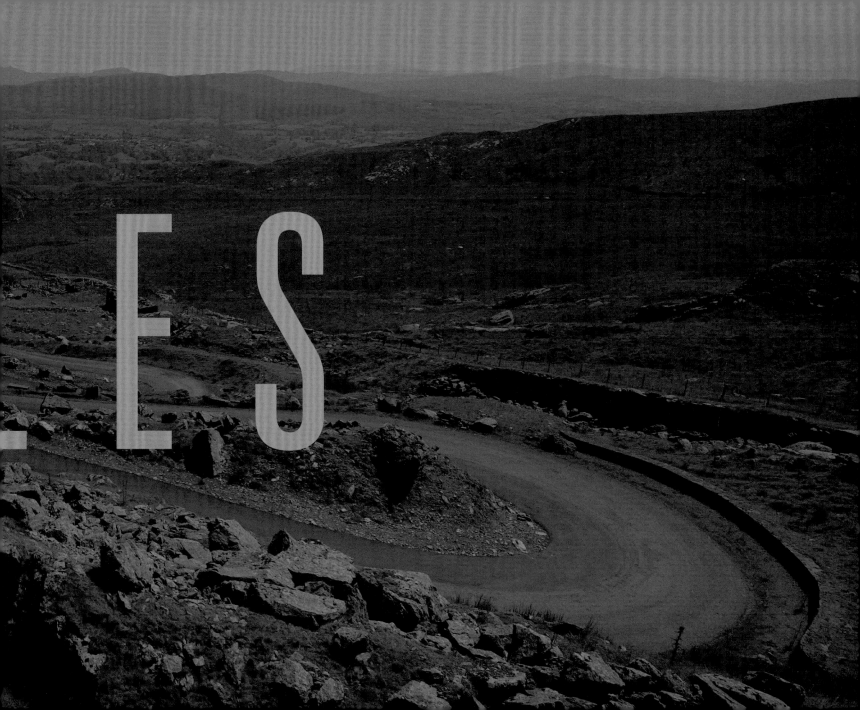

LAKES IN THE SKY

DISTANCE 147KM | **CLIMBING** +3,202M

PHOTOGRAPHY PHIL HALL

A Snowdonian adventure taking you to places you can hardly believe exist

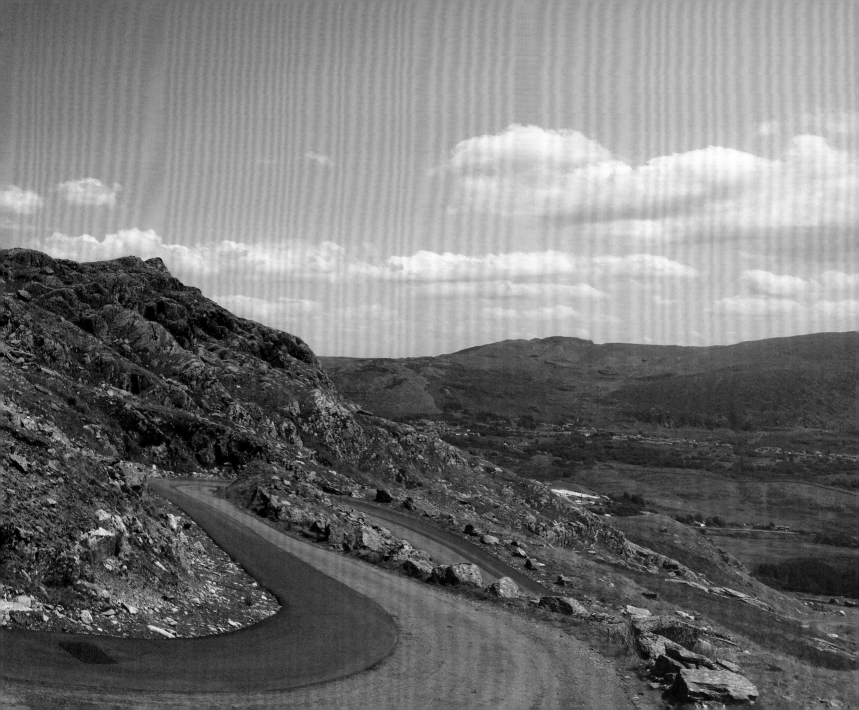

'd had the idea of riding this route some years before I actually got up the courage to attempt it. Having visited the summit of each of its three very special climbs on separate occasions, I just knew one day I'd have to concoct a loop that bagged them all in one go. Coincidentally, the two-time National Hill Climb Champion and local hero Dan Evans had been dreaming of pretty much the same ride, so this was the catalyst for me to take the plunge. A couple of years ago, therefore, we set out together to document it for *Cycling Weekly*. I call it my lakes-in-the-sky ride after the three reservoirs, Llyn Stwlan, Llyn Cowlyd and the Marchlyn Mawr, that lie, hidden high in the Snowdonian mountains, at the top of each of the signature climbs.

You could choose any number of start–finish points, and the first time I rode the route I set off from Llanberis. On reflection, however, I think Betws-y-Coed makes a better base, which is what I have gone with here. This way you get to tackle the hardest climb first, and save the most spectacular for last. Perfect!

From the centre of town roll out north on the B5106, following the River Conwy through the base of the valley, and for about 8 kilometres all is nice and calm. Then you arriving in Trefriw and, like a chest of drawers falling over in the night, or a meteor crashing into your lawn, the calm ends and the chaos begins. Here, rising out of the village and into the mountains, is in my opinion *the* hardest climb in Britain: The

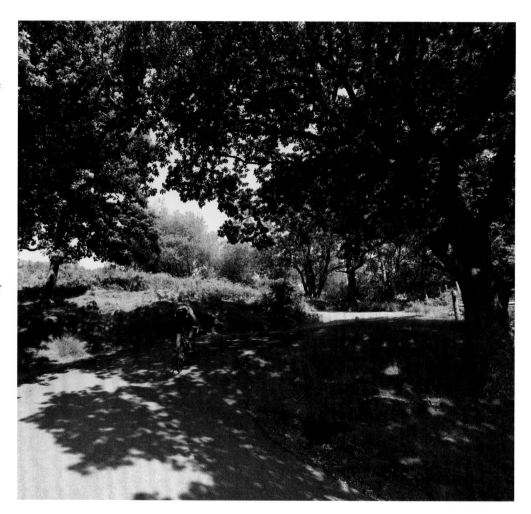

ABOVE *The merciless hairpins of the Cowlyd.*

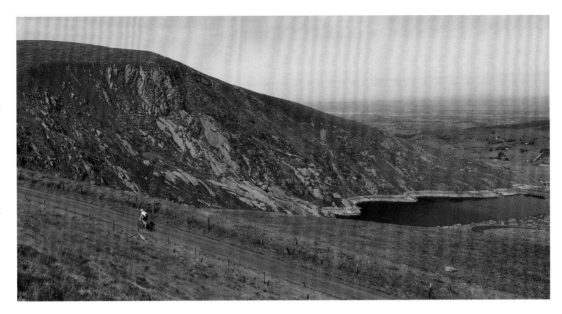

Cowlyd. Forget Hardknott, Rosedale, Great Dun Fell or Bealach na Ba: they are *nothing* compared to this. The sheer amount of 20–25% gradient on this road sets it apart from all others; it borders on the perverse why anyone would want to ride up it. But that's the challenge and all the motivation we need, right?

From almost the moment you turn off Crafnant Road in Trefriw the slope kicks up above 20% and, for close to 3 kilometres, through nine hairpin bends, you'll barely be able to sit down, it's that tough. After first riding it I screamed, '*Never again!*' (probably upsetting a few sheep). But of course I went back. It is simply an amazing piece of tarmac, matched only by the views at its summit. You don't quite reach Llyn Cowlyd (you need a gravel bike for that): all you really have to do is roll over the peak to bag the climb segment, then retrace your steps at a somewhat quicker pace back into Trefriw.

With your legs destroyed, and still 135 kilometres to go, resume your progress north on the valley road, where you have the sedate journey all the way into Conwy to allow your body and mind to recover. In the town turn west and, following a brace of slight lumps, it's time for the next climb on the route, the Sychnant Pass, a mere pimple of a road compared to other beasts along the route, but a beautiful road. Once you've crested the summit, the descent the other side comes with a divine view out to sea.

The next part of the ride is a little complicated, so pay attention. Follow the Conwy Old Road into Dwygyfylchi, turn left and follow it through Penmaenmawr all the way to the A55. Now *don't* join the main road, but instead take to the bike path: just shy of the junction you'll see it marked on your left. You take the bridge over the A55, then follow the path around the cliffs, and leave it to join South Street in Llanfairfechan at the other end. Leave Llanfairfechan on Aber Road to follow another path alongside the A55 before heading back inland. The road from Abergwyngregyn all the way to Bethesda is narrow, twisting and almost continually uphill: not steep – just a steady grind.

It's now time for the second of the day's big three targets: the climb up to the Marchlyn Mawr reservoir, the source of power for the Dinorwig Power Station, which is why in my Welsh climbs guidebook I dumbed it Electric Mountain. Heading west on the B4409 from Bethesda, take the third left via St Ann's Hill to Mynydd Llandegai, then right and left to keep climbing. At the next T-junction turn left and then follow the road upwards, aiming directly for the peaks of Elidir Fawr and Mynydd Perfedd.

Before long you'll see a gate obstructing your passage: you'll need to heave your bike over this, and from then on you'll have the whole road to yourself. And what a road it is, twisting though the immaculate mountain scenery, round bends plucked directly from the Pyrenees – you'll have to pinch yourself. If only it could go on for another 10 kilometres! Alas, all good things come to an end and, when you reach the curved dam wall, so does this road. Soak in the views, then, on the way down, there is the option of taking the detour to climb up to the smaller lake on the mountain, the

ABOVE *Climbing into the hills between the lakes to the Marchlyn Mawr reservoir.*

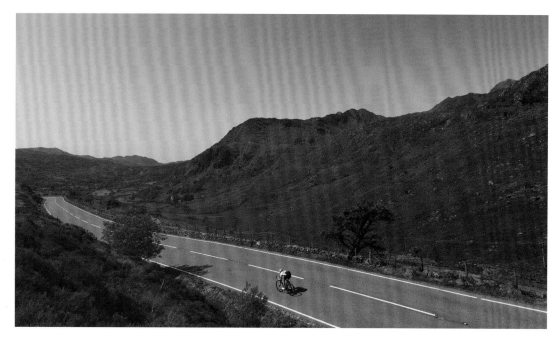

Surge Pool. I'll leave this up to you.

Once over the gate at the bottom, make your way via Deiniolen and Brynrefail to the A4086 to next climb the Llanberis Pass. The location for a thousand photo shoots and TV adverts, the Llanberis Pass rises from Nant Peris, through the gargantuan valley, all the way to the Pen-y-Pass youth hostel at the base of the trails to Snowdon. Blessed with towering rock faces either side, it is without doubt one of the most dramatic roads on this island, yet amazingly it still doesn't make the top three on this ride. Beyond the summit speed down to the junction with the A498 and turn right, to continue the huge descent all the way to Beddgelert, which is the ideal place for a stop. You'll be ready for one.

After refuelling it's time to head onto the final target of the day, and the best road in Wales: the climb up to Llyn Stwlan. To get there continue down to the A498, turn left over Pont Aberglaslyn, then follow the A4085 all the way to Garreg, where you head east on the B4410 to Tan-y-bwlch. Join the A496 briefly, then take the next left to ride the back road through the Vale of Ffestiniog before picking up the main road north towards Blaenau Ffestiniog. You don't ride all the way into town, but take the left turn at Tanygrisiau, following the signs to the Ffestiniog Power Station. Follow this road west to the reservoir, then head back east as it climbs gently to the base of the climb. Just before a small bridge turn left, and roll up to the gate that

prevents traffic going any further.

What lies ahead is almost without comparison in Britain – not in terms of length or height or gradient, but in the sheer number of twisting hairpin bends stacked one on top of each other at the top. A marvel of a road, set in breathtaking surroundings, and yes, to top it off, thanks again to the gate, it's traffic-free. It's almost too good to be true. It's also lucky that it's hidden deep in the Welsh mountains, because if this road was, say, just outside Dorking you'd have to buy a ticket to get up it. Wallow in its splendour, race your mates, dream of the high mountains, of riding the Tour de France, as you throw your bike round the bends and sprint out of each one into the next. Cyclists don't have stadiums, theatres, stages: they have roads like this.

Once you have squeezed every last metre of elevation from the available asphalt, head back down through Tanygrisiau into Blaenau Ffestiniog, to face one more climb before the finish. This one will hurt, I can assure you of that, as, after a huge day in the Welsh mountains, the last thing you need are 3 kilometres of 10% gradient up a straight main road. You'll drag yourself to the top as though stuck in quicksand.

But then it's time to party. With all the climbing now done, what comes next is a proper descent: fast, long and straight – you'll easily hit 80 kph, maybe 90, if you have the courage (warning: take care) – all the way back down the A470 to where the adventure began, what will be many hours ago, in Betws-y-Coed.

ABOVE *Dropping down towards Beddgelert with Snowdon on the horizon.*

RIDE 35 — WALES

NORTH SNOWDONIA

DISTANCE 147KM

CLIMBING +3,202M

DIFFICULTY 10/10

FOOD & WATER | CONWY / LLANBERIS / BEDDGELERT

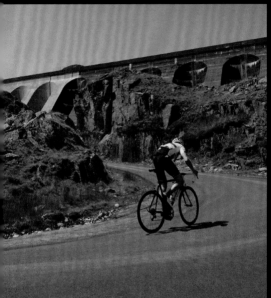

KEY CLIMBS

1 THE COWLYD
2,912m +379m

I rate this the toughest road to ride in Britain because of the sheer volume of slope over 20%: it's enough to make you weep. Packed with hairpins that wind through precipitously steep corners all effort is rewarded with the views that lie at the top.

2 ELECTRIC MOUNTAIN
2,867m +269m

I dubbed this climb Electric Mountain after the hydroelectric plant but it's more commonly known as Marchlyn Mawr. With a 9% average but nothing a whole lot steeper this car-free route into the mountains is heaven on earth.

3 STWLAN DAM
2,787m +265m

Best hairpins in Britain, no question. You'll hardly believe they exist, they are so wonderful. Another traffic-free road, this climb is pretty tough all the way averaging 9% and maxing out at 13%, but it's ALL about those bends.

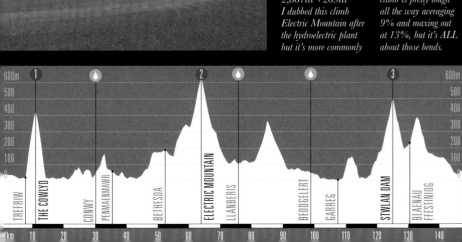

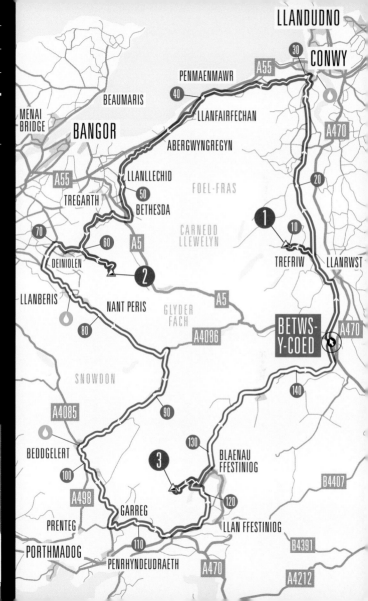

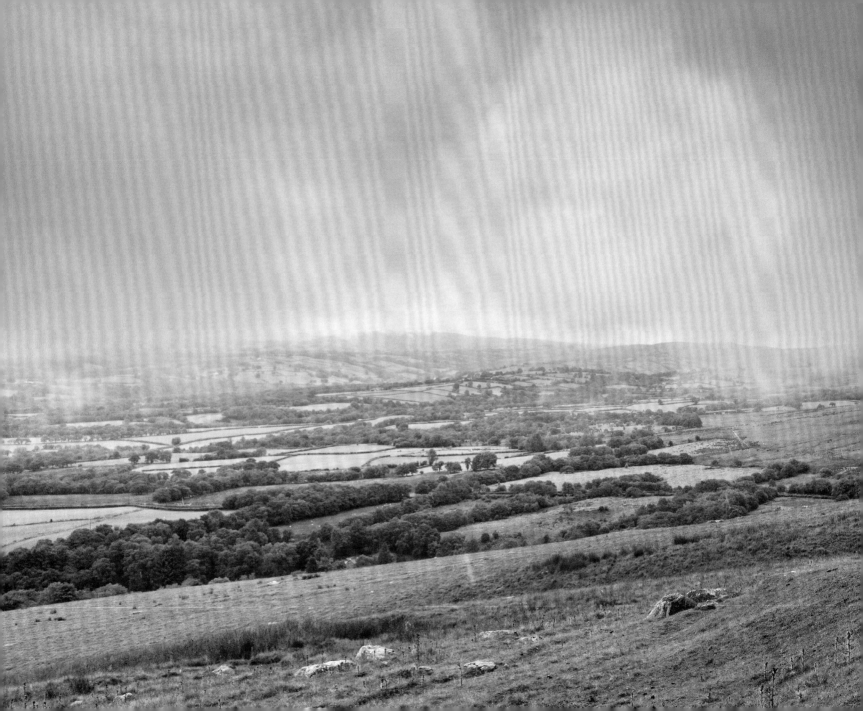

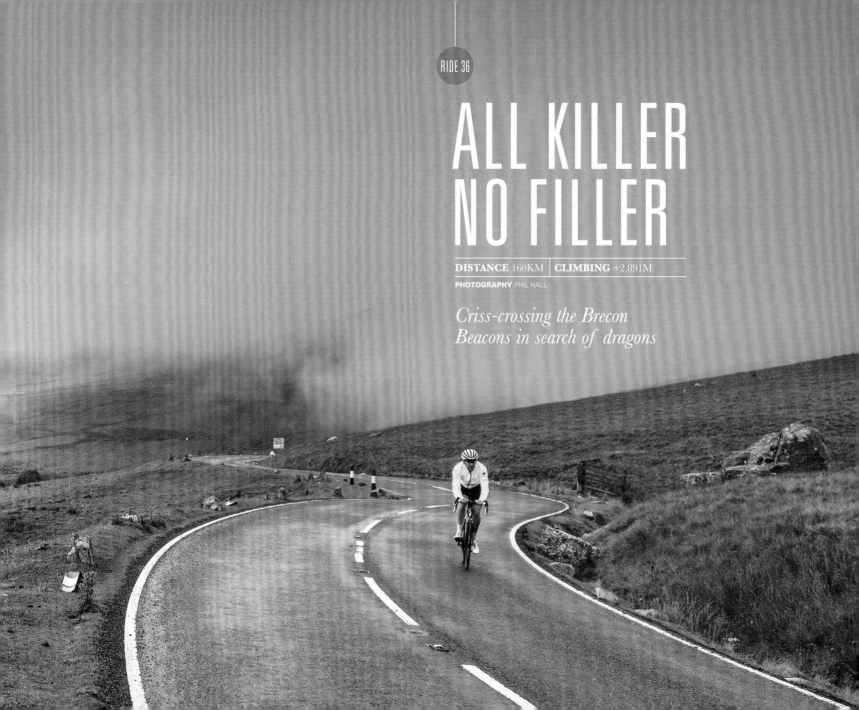

ALL KILLER NO FILLER

DISTANCE 160KM | **CLIMBING** +2,891M

PHOTOGRAPHY PHIL HALL

*Criss-crossing the Brecon
Beacons in search of dragons*

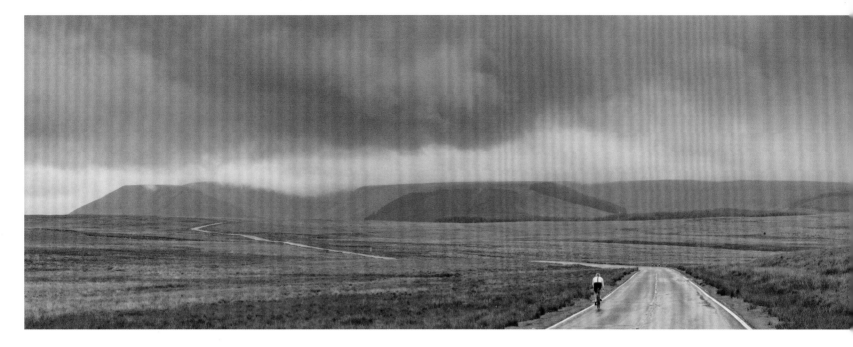

toiled over this route for hours, as there was so much I wanted to squeeze in, without the distance getting out of control or having you spend too long on busy roads or in urban areas. The plan was to include all the big climbs in and around the Brecon Beacons but, each time I plotted it, it turned out too long or too congested. In the end I decided to cast out classic roads such as Llangynidr Mountain and the Bwlch and, choosing quality over quantity, keep the majority of the ride within the sanctuary of the National Park. Anyone who has ridden the Dragon Ride Sportive over the years will notice more than a passing resemblance to its route but, with only a handful of roads crossing the Beacons, this was pretty hard to avoid. I

have chosen Hirwaun as the start–finish point, as it has good transport links, lies at the base of Rhigos, which gives the ride a summit finish, and enables you to start the day with the steadiest passage into the wilderness.

Start the adventure by heading north out of town on the A4059, straight into the heart of the National Park. Passing the Penderyn Distillery (temptation can wait until you have finished), you soon leave the clutter of South Wales behind and enter cycling heaven. My initial journey along this road was on my first Dragon Ride and, having left the group I was riding with, I found myself alone, in the mist, surrounded by nothing but the low, rolling hills. To someone then living in London these were very unfamiliar

surroundings and, although there was an urge to enjoy the scenery, there was a counter-urge to press on, back to signs of life, before the dragons came for me.

At the end of this first passage across the Beacons you meet up with the larger A470 for the thundering descent down the other side. Turning left at the junction, stick it in the big ring and your smallest sprocket, then prepare to make the jump into hyperspace. You'll soon be travelling at the same speed as any traffic, so take care – oh, and make sure you don't miss the left turn onto the A4125, signposted 'Defynnog', or by the time you realise you've gone wrong you'll be several kilometres past it.

Head east, sticking on the A4215 for a while,

PREVIOUS PAGE
*Climbing into the cloud
on Black Mountain.*

ABOVE *Just you, the road
and the huge landscape.*

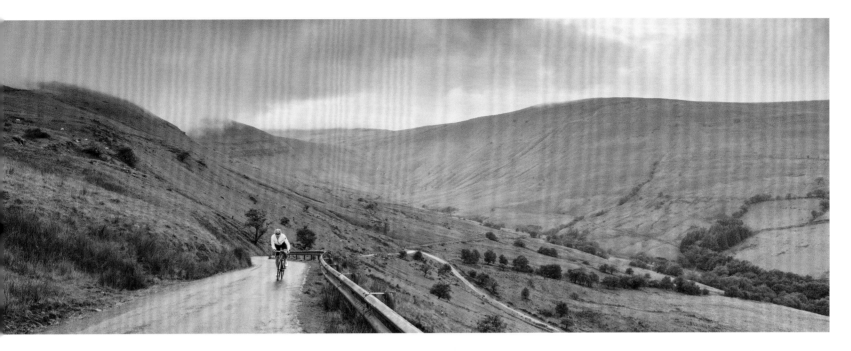

then turn south-west, signposted 'Hoel Senni'. Before arriving in the village take the left turn to Ystradfellte, and follow this road all the way to the only real killer climb on the route, the Devil's Elbow. Not to be confused with the Devil's Staircase further north, the Devil's Elbow is almost as solid a test for man and machine, and from such a fearsome name you'd expect nothing less. Through the gully, dodging sheep (and their business), you'll find the road climbs gradually until the twin hairpins come into view, and it's here that things get tasty.

Deep in the interior of the Beacons, on a rough and rugged track lined with rusty, bent barriers, this beautiful yet punishing road ascends abruptly up the hillside to reveal huge views back up the valley. The summit lies a substantial distance from the second vicious bend so, although the steepest gradients are behind you, there's still a bit of work to do to get to the top. Once the summit is crested, there are nigh-on 15 kilometres of downhill ahead, punctuated with a few undulations, then a short little climb the other side of Ystradfellte to make sure your legs remain primed for battles ahead.

Unfortunately, at the bottom of the descent you have to venture out of the Park briefly, through Pontneddfechan and into Glyn-neath, where you turn right onto the A4109. Rising out of the town, this is a slog of a hill on a pretty ugly road, but it's a necessary bridge to cross in order to reach Abercraf in the adjacent valley.

Up next is my favourite of all the roads that cross the Beacons, Bwlch Cerrig Duon: it is so beautiful, so pure, you just want to bottle it and take it home.

Starting out on the A4067 from Abercraf, first climb on the main road, then, after 7 kilometres, take the turn towards Trecastle and get ready for some real Welsh wonderment. This is a long climb – over 12 kilometres from the base in Abercraf to the summit – but never overly steep; just find a nice gear, set a comfortable rhythm and enjoy the ride. With nothing but grass and rock to your left, and the same on your right, this is the Wales you have been looking for, and you'll never want to leave.

Once you're over the top, the descent is

ABOVE *The sun always shines on TV, but this is Wales.*

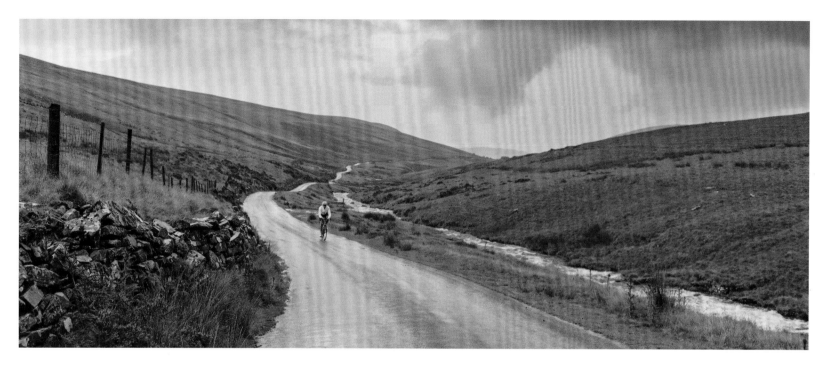

steeper, passing through the Glasfynydd Forest to take you to Pont ar Hydfer, where it's time to turn left. Heading due east, this road will take you, via a series of lumps and bumps, all the way to the base of the giant Black Mountain.

After passing through Twynllanan, you reach the A4069 at Pont-ar-Llechau, where you turn left into 10 solid kilometres of up. Gentle at first, the slope soon assumes its 6–7% pitch, which it hardly wavers from all the way to the top. This is a proper mountain road: a real climber's climb where, if you're carrying a few unwanted kilos, you'll be powerless to stop your skinnier mates disappearing into the distance exploiting their superior power-to-weight ratio. On the increasingly exposed higher reaches and the sweeping, larger-than-life bends, it's more than likely the wind will start to play its part, as you battle through the rugged landscape high above the vast plains below.

The summit lies at the third and smallest of three car parks on the high, barren plateau where, if said skinny friends have raced ahead, you'll find them in the early stages of hypothermia. Once you've regrouped, race down the other side all the way to Brynamman, where you head east on the A4068 to begin the more complicated trek back to base.

I've cut a little loop away from the main road between Cwmllynfell and Cwm-twrch Isaf, which will allow some respite from any traffic. Then once you get to Gurnos, I've sent the route over Rhos Common into the Dulais Valley via a hideous little 20% climb. On reaching the A4109, follow this through Seven Sisters into Glyn-neath, then, after crossing the A465, ride through Pont-Walby on the back road back to Hirwaun.

Now, that's the end of the loop but, if you glance right, you'll see you're at the base of the mighty Rhigos climb and, well, it would be rude – no, downright disrespectful – if you didn't. It's only 5.5 kilometres at an average of 4%, and everyone *loves* a summit finish, don't they? Well, I'll let you decide: the lure of stuffing your face may be too strong, but you know what I'd do.

ABOVE *The clmb up to Bwlch Cerrig Duon: You just want to bottle it and take it home.*

RIDE 36

WALES
BRECON BEACONS

FOOD & WATER | GLYN-NEATH / BRYNAMMAN

DISTANCE 160KM

CLIMBING +2,891M

DIFFICULTY 8/10

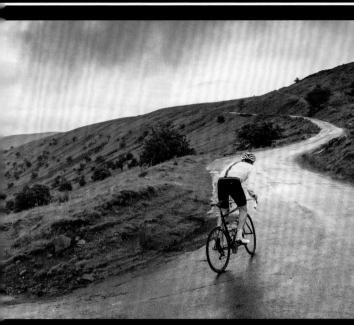

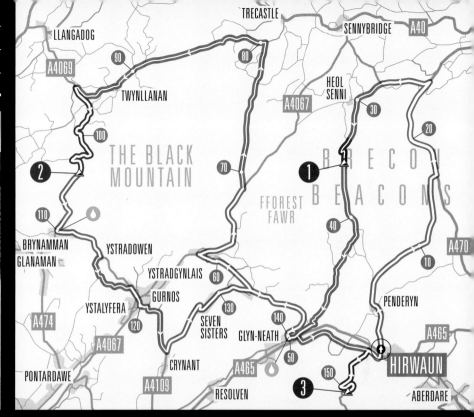

KEY CLIMBS

1 DEVIL'S ELBOW
1,886m +189m

If it has Devil in the name you just know it's going to be brilliant and this climb does not disappoint. Creeping up from the valley the lower slopes are steady but as the first hairpin comes into view you'll need to change down quick because before long you'll be battling a 20% gradient

2 BLACK MOUNTAIN
7,235m +367m

A real favourite of mine, this huge ascent gives you a true appreciation of mountain climbing and packs in some epic views. Although the average is only 5% it is still a proper challenge to reach the windswept summit through its gorgeous sweeping bends

3 RHIGOS
5,622m +283m

To finish the route a Welsh classic, Rhigos. This is the best side to ride in my opinion and having 90 miles in the legs will allow you to really empty the tanks. Boasting only a 4% average and maximum ramps of 7% it's nothing to fear on an ordinary day, but this isn't an ordinary day.

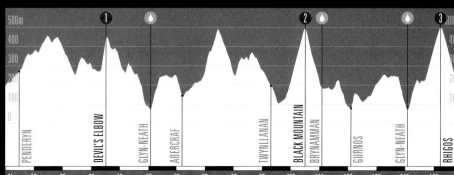

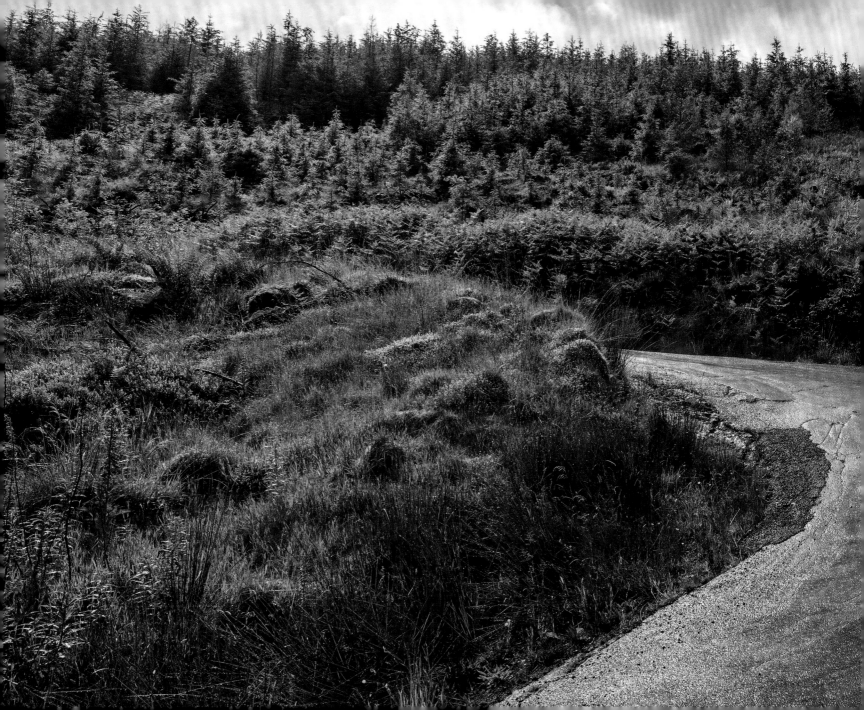

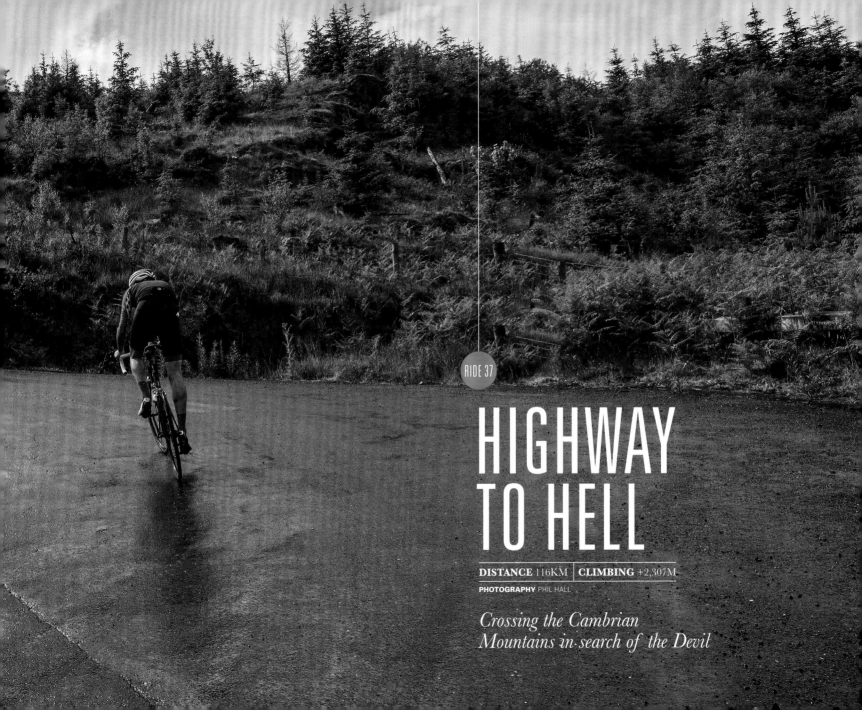

RIDE 37

HIGHWAY TO HELL

DISTANCE 116KM | **CLIMBING** +2,307M

PHOTOGRAPHY PHIL HALL

*Crossing the Cambrian
Mountains in search of the Devil*

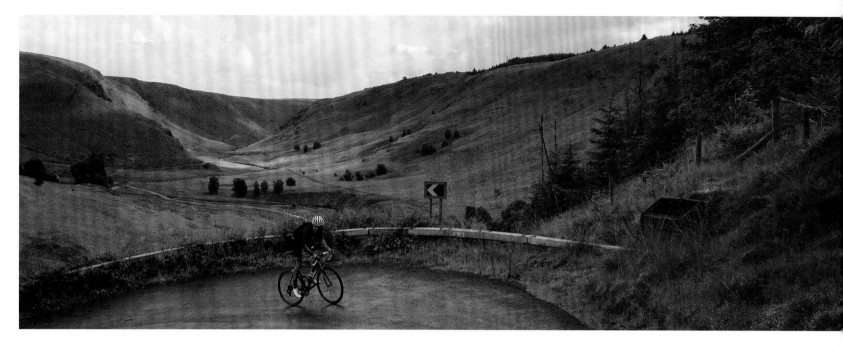

The Devil's Staircase: the very name strikes fear into the heart, makes the legs go limp and beads of sweat form on your brow – a reputation gained over generations, cemented by exploits in the Milk Race and enhanced by every pair of wheels that have ever traversed its harrowing slopes. My first visit to this notorious road saw me more excited than a seven-year-old the night before Christmas.

It was while I was researching my first book. Owing to time constraints that day, I was having to drive the distances between the climbs in order to tick them all off. We left Llanwrtyd Wells and headed west, into the wilderness. About half an hour went by. Then my wife said, 'Where exactly are you taking us?'

'To the Devil's Staircase,' I replied.

'Are you sure we aren't lost? We're in the absolute middle of nowhere!'

She was right. There are very few houses, or people, or anything: this is real *Deliverance* country. Scream, and no one will hear you. Which is exactly why it is such a special place. Once we'd arrived at the base of the climb I unpacked my bike from the boot, and the hairs stood up on the back of my neck in anticipation. Finally, after years of waiting, of watching old race footage and reading reports in magazines, I was (to quote the cycling commentator Phil Liggett) going to 'have a date with the Devil'.

Your date with the Devil comes around the halfway point on this simple mid-Wales loop,

that starts and finishes in Rhayader and begins by going south on the only road out of the town, the A470. For close to 12 kilometres you enjoy some blissful downhill, all the way to Newbridge-on-Wye, where you head east on the B4358. The next stretch all the way to Beulah is spent entirely on this B-road, and during your passage you've five little climbs to cross. Not killers, but the constant undulations that pick their way between the multitude of farms will soften the legs up, ready for bigger challenges ahead.

Once in Beulah, turn right onto the A483, then right again to start your approach to the Devil. As you follow the course of the valley, agricultural land is soon replaced by steep valley sides and thick woodland. Climbing continually,

PREVIOUS PAGE
*A date with the devil
is always fun.*

ABOVE *Rounding the second
of the Devil's vicious bends.*

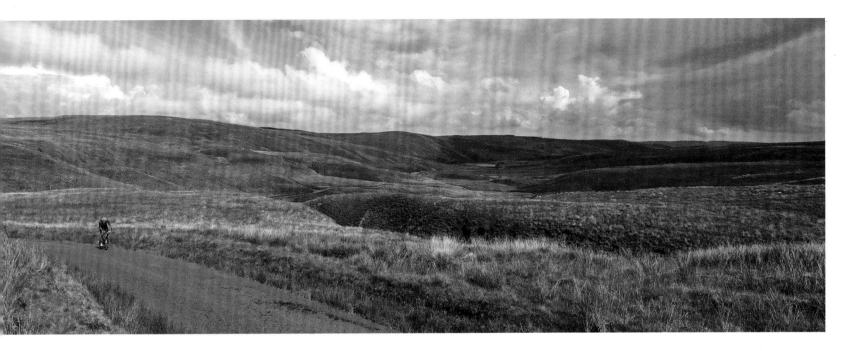

albeit by a steady gradient, this narrow, twisting and gnarled road delivers you to Abergwesyn, the gateway to Hell.

The Devil is a reclusive beast who doesn't like company, which is why he lies deep in the foothills of the Cambrian Mountains, hidden from the world at the end of the remarkably serene Abergwesyn Valley. Leaving the last village for 25 kilometres, you first pick your way through dense woodland, the road seemingly powerless to resist being consumed by the surrounding flora. Engulfed within a cocoon of nature, the road clings to the steep hillside, then exits the tunnel of green into the expanse of the valley. Narrow, claustrophobic, even the tall valley walls, topped with rocky outcrops, close

in around you. Cut off from the modern world, you creep closer to your target, following every kink and bend of the small river beside you. The sign that you're almost there arrives as you cross the first of three small bridges that take the road now on a direct line to your foe. Crossing the third, you climb a little rise, then, as you pass the 25% sign, it's time…

The Devil wastes no time in dishing out the pain. The route ramps up right away, uniformly steep to the first corner, then steeper still up to the next. How they used to race up here on old bikes with highly inappropriate gearing I'll never know. Through the second hairpin – even tougher than the first – grind those pedals over, keep moving forward . . . and at last the slope backs off a little.

But the climb is far from over. The summit lies a further kilometre in the distance, before the road drops like a stone down the other side to cross the River Towy, only to climb again. This next lump is the Gamallt: a climb of two halves, almost as fierce as the Devil in places and just as hard, because your legs will still be throbbing. Climbing across this sparse landscape, still a long way from everywhere, you must cross a third pig of a climb before it's time to return to civilisation via the sumptuous downhill into Tregaron. In your relief to have made it, alive, you may well feel a celebratory pit stop is in order here.

Now you head north-west briefly on the A485, leaving it on a corner next to a small stone barn. Heading north, follow the signs for

ABOVE *Utter perfection of the desolate Welsh interior.*

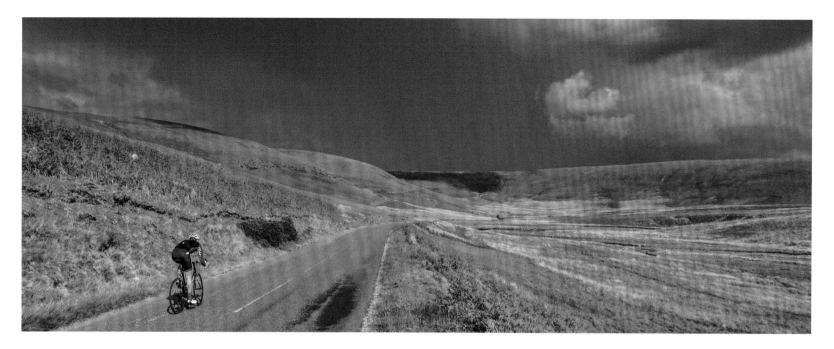

Swyddffynnon and Ystradmeurig. Crossing the B4340, continue north to Ysbyty Ystwyth; then, at the end of a long descent, you arrive in Pont-rhyd-y-groes.

If the first half of this ride was all about the Devil's Staircase, the second is all about the Elan Valley and its collection of reservoirs. The journey there begins as you head east from Pont-rhyd-y-groes up through Coed Lledwenau: 1.65 kilometres at an average of 10% will certainly make you sweat, before you descend gently to Cwmystwyth to begin your passage through the Ystwth Valley. This simple, amazing road, trapped between steep valley walls, peaks at the head of one valley and then falls away into the next. There are no dramatic peaks or troughs, no sudden changes in direction or obstacles: just a serene passage across this pristine (apart from the road) landscape.

Then, at the first junction for 14 kilometres, turn right into what is sometime dubbed the 'Welsh Lake District': the Elan Valley. This chain of man-made lakes was created by the Birmingham Corporation Water Department, by damming the Elan and Claerwen rivers to provide clean drinking water for the West Midlands. Seems a bit cheeky of the English to be taking Welsh water for their own, and I'm sure that argument was had at the time.

There may be no more climbs left on this route as you wind past four of the five reservoirs, but it is drop-dead gorgeous all the same, every single metre of it, as the hills and trees are reflected in the still water of the lakes. At first the scenery remains open and barren, then, as you head further south to the southern shores of the Penygarreg Reservoir, the road delves in and out of forest. Where the Garreg-ddu and Caban-coch reservoirs meet, there is a bridge across them which, though not on the route, is well worth a small detour so you can look out over the water in both directions.

Round the headland and head back northwards, passing the Arts-and-Crafts-style Elan Village, built to house the workers during the reservoirs' construction. Then climb the last few hundred metres to complete the loop and arrive back in Rhayader.

ABOVE *Dropping into the Elan Valley it looks like there may be trouble ahead!*

RIDE **37**

WALES

CAMBRIAN MOUNTAINS

FOOD & WATER | BEULAH / TREGARON

DISTANCE 116KM

CLIMBING +2,307M

DIFFICULTY 5/10

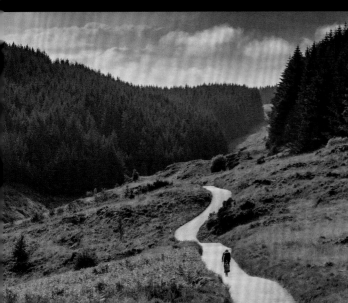

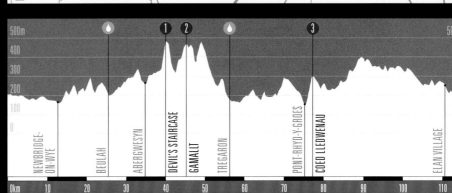

KEY CLIMBS

1 DEVIL'S STAIRCASE
1,148m +137m

A true classic, this road must be close to the top of all British riders' bucket lists. Hidden in the depths of the mountains it takes some endeavour to reach and even more to climb with an average of 12% and slopes that peak some 25%

2 GAMALLT
904m +81m

The first I heard of this climb was on an old Milk Race commentary when Hugh Porter was saying that many riders had been forced to walk; this was all I needed to know. With stretches of 25% you should make it to the top though, unless you are 1980's (42x21) gears that is.

3 COED LLEDWENAU
1,653m +157m

Passing the 16% sign at the base this initially narrow road ramps up into the woods and assumes its punishing gradient. With an average of 9% it isn't 16% the whole way but only starts to relent as you approach the turn from the B4343 onto the B4574.

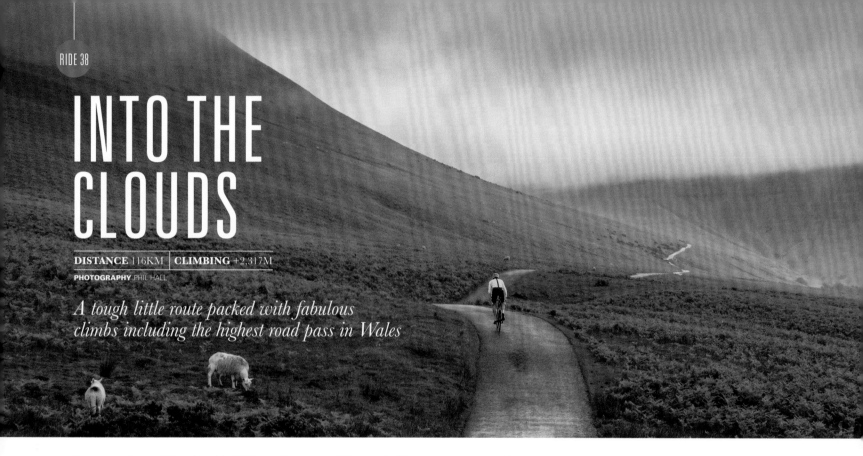

INTO THE CLOUDS

DISTANCE 116KM | **CLIMBING** +2,317M

PHOTOGRAPHY PHIL HALL

A tough little route packed with fabulous climbs including the highest road pass in Wales

I thought about calling this ride 'A Taste of Wales' as this shortish route, straddling the border with England, will certainly give you an idea of the delights this country holds, with four showpiece climbs and kilometre after kilometre of beautiful scenery. There's no escaping the fact that South Wales is a rather congested area but, with a bit of careful planning, you can find empty spaces and quiet lanes, and this ride has plenty of both.

We start in Abergavenny, and the first climb on the menu, while your legs are still sprightly, is one many (if not all) of you will have heard of: The Tumble. It was one of the first on my list when I wrote *100 Greatest Cycling Climbs*, even though I'd never ridden it or really had much idea where it was. Having read cycling magazines for the previous 20 years, though, I knew the name was synonymous with races in Wales. Having played host to the Milk Race, the Tour of Britain and

countless other events and sportives, The Tumble was one climb that had to be on the list.

Head west out of Abergavenny first on the A40, then turn south on the A4143 to head under the A465 and into Llanfoist. To complete your exit from the Usk Valley next follow the B4246 towards Govilon and at the fork in the road turn left, following the sign to Blaenavon. When you arrive at the small stone bridge, this marks the start of the climb, so get ready.

ABOVE *Approaching the summit of the Gospel pass on a Welsh summer's day.*

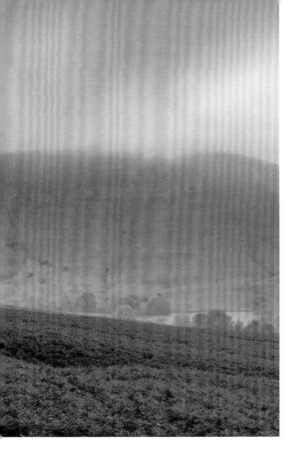

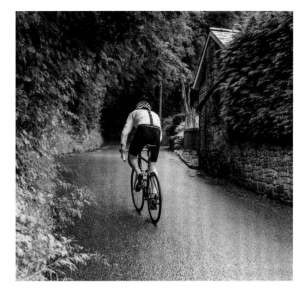

junction on your left, just past Keepers Pond. It's important you roll over the top to 'complete the segment,' but then double back, because the route doesn't head over the hill but takes the road west, signposted Pwll-du.

Now, at time of writing this road did not have the best surface; in fact, it was in a terrible state of affairs – close to gravel – so watch your speed as you descend across the side of Gilwern Hill back into the valley. There are times up here on the hill it feels like you are a million miles from anywhere, so enjoy the solitude before heading back into a slightly busier part of the ride.

Upon reaching the first junction turn left, then right, then left, to arrive on Station Road, where you take another left turn. Now, heading west, join Brunant Road into the village of Clydach. Arriving at an asphalt clearing, you want to head left here – oh, and get ready for a beating. This is Rhiw Road, a 10/10 climb, and you'll see right away how steep it is by the angle it forms against the houses in front of you. Thrashing this way and that, cutting a tight path between the buildings, it sits on a relentlessly steep 20% slope, which even nudges 25% at times. It's one of the hardest climbs in South Wales, if not the hardest, and the sight of the junction at the top will be a huge relief. But what a challenge, though! and that's two of the day's four beasts ticked off.

Turn right, then immediately left, on an impossibly narrow road, to reach the next junction and turn left once more and make your way to the B4248, which descends into

Brynmawr. Negotiating the town (yes, it's too early to stop) and leaving on Intermediate Road over the A465, you roll into 8 blissful kilometres of almost flat riding, following the edge of the hillside that curves north. With a constant, expansive vista to your right, this narrow road is heaven to ride from start to finish. Avoiding the first two right turns, you follow it via a couple of sharp corners to meet the Monmouthshire & Brecon Canal at the bottom. After crossing the water, ride through Llangattock to the B4558, and stick to this road all the way to the village of Llangynidr. Up next is climb three of four: the marvellously named, Llangynidr Mountain.

Yes, Mountain. Fear not: it's not as tough as Rhiw Road or The Tumble, but it does have tight hairpins and epic views, just like a mountain road should. A wide road set on a steady 7% gradient, it climbs for almost 6

It kicks up sharply right away into the first of its two tight corners, bending left and then, a short while later, right. After this second bend it's a straight line to the summit, the pitch undulating slightly, but always a tough challenge. As you cross the cattle grid, the scenery opens up, and this is what you came for: empty hills, giant views out to the right, and a huge climb to take on. All told, The Tumble is close to 5 kilometres long, and the summit lies at the

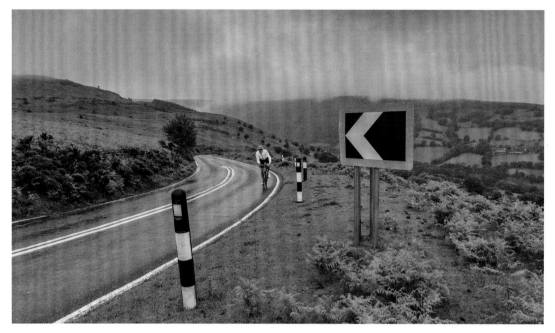

kilometres if you go right to the summit; alas, though, the route diverts east before you get there, but feel free to add on a bit extra to properly bag the climb. Much like the upper reaches of The Tumble, the landscape at the top is barren, windswept and gorgeous. Before you reach the true summit, in a brief hiatus in the climbing, you need to turn left to plummet back into Llangattock, across the River Usk and into Crickhowell.

Now, at 50 kilometres it is probably time for a stop and, as there is little else on offer for the remainder of the ride, I'd take it to grab anything you may need and fill your bottles. Leaving the village, there is a short, (relatively) sharp (definitely) climb up Bellfountain Road to

negotiate, then a considerable period of calm through the quiet country lanes following Grwyne Fawr, past a multitude of farms scattering the valley to Llanvihangel Crucorney. Don't enter the village, but stick to the minor road; then head north, hugging the inside of the Welsh border, before crossing into England to reach the village of Clodock. With the Black Mountains on your left, continue north into Longtown, then, after crossing the River Monnow, climb all the way back into Wales. You'll be heading upwards, gradually but nonetheless continually gaining altitude, for close to 8 kilometres before, just shy of the border, shedding some on the way to the base of the final big climb: the Gospel Pass.

In common with the majority of passes,

there are two ways to climb and descend, and this orientation of the Gospel Pass is by far my preferred route. By riding north to south you get a) the steepest ascent and, b) the longest descent – which, at close to 20 whole kilometres, might just be the biggest in Britain (I haven't compiled a list of descents yet). Turning left at a small triangulation of roads, begin the passage up through the woods on a slope that is as harsh as 17% at its steepest. Once free of Tack Wood, the pitch subsides to a more agreeable degree, and climbs steadily along the quite frankly amazing flanks of the Black Mountains.

With the whole of Wales out to your right, and the towering grass banks on your left, this road is up there with the best. Ahead, you'll see the summit in the distance, where the snaking climb divides the interlocking hillsides, and this gives you, dwarfed by the majestic surroundings, a continuous point of focus to aid your progress. Not that for a moment climbing this amazing road is ever a chore: every pedal rev, every centimetre, is to be relished – and, yes, once you're over the top the descent is off the scale.

There may be a couple of slight interruptions to the perpetual loss in altitude as you pass through Capel-y-ffin and Llanthony between the steep valley walls either side, but nothing to upset the apple cart. It's only when you finish your passage through the Vale of Ewyas, and take the turn just shy of Llanvihangel Crucorney, that you're in for a final few lumpy kilometres to complete the circuit back to Abergavenny.

ABOVE *Just a couple of bends left to the summit of Llangynidr Mountian.*

RIDE 38 WALES

BLACK MOUNTAINS

FOOD & WATER | BRYNMAWR / CRICKHOWELL

DISTANCE 116KM
CLIMBING +2,317M
DIFFICULTY 8/10

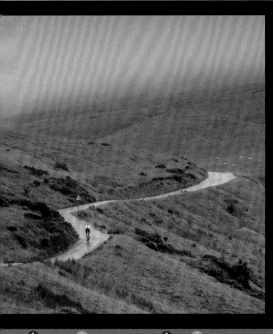

KEY CLIMBS

1 THE TUMBLE
4,979m +362m
Leaving Govilon The Tumble soon ramps up and passes through a brace of tight bends in the lower wooded section. Crossing the cattle grid the complexion of the climb changes in an instant and on the way to the top you'll be treated to slopes as steep as 16%.

2 LLANGYNIDR MOUNTAIN
5,800m +383m
Worthy of its name this climb has a real feel of a mountain road with its sweeping hairpins,
its 7% average gradient and ramps that approach 14%. Note, if you want to climb the full height you need to deviate from the route slightly then double back.

3 GOSPEL PASS
4,719m +278m
Long and stunning the climbing on this road is split into two distinct parts. Steep at the bottom up through the woods then much shallower as it crosses the empty hillside in search of the summit which lies at the gap on the horizon.

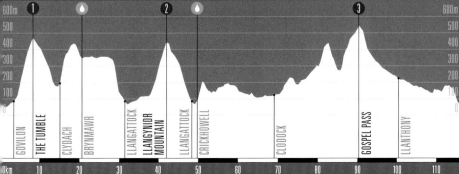

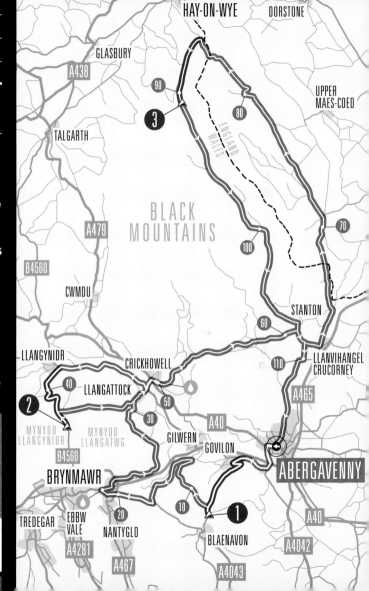

THE GOD OF HELLFIRE

DISTANCE 142KM | **CLIMBING** +2,973M

PHOTOGRAPHY PHIL HALL

Traversing southern Snowdonia
and taking on the infamous
Bwlch-y-Groes

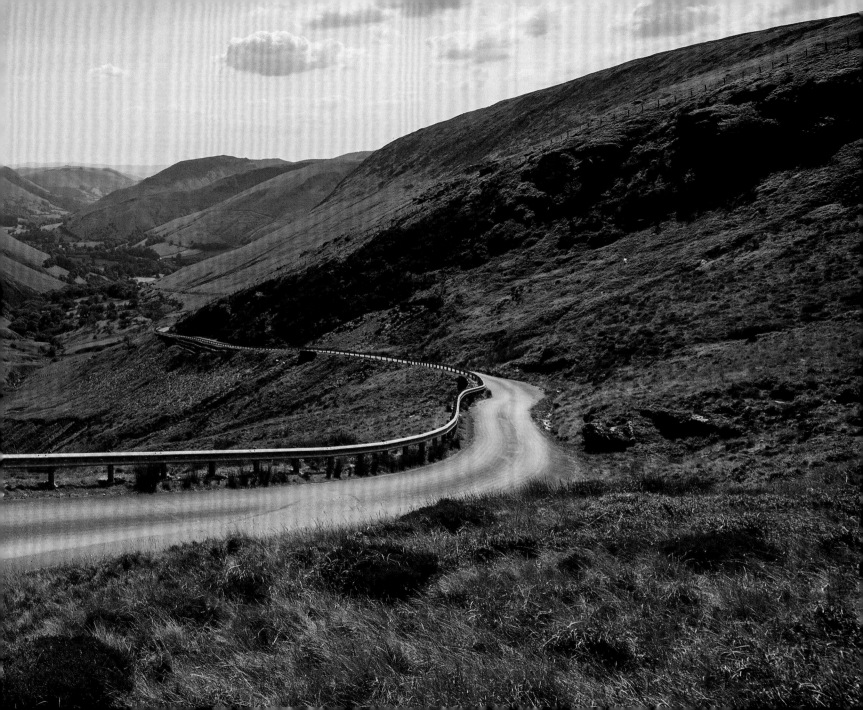

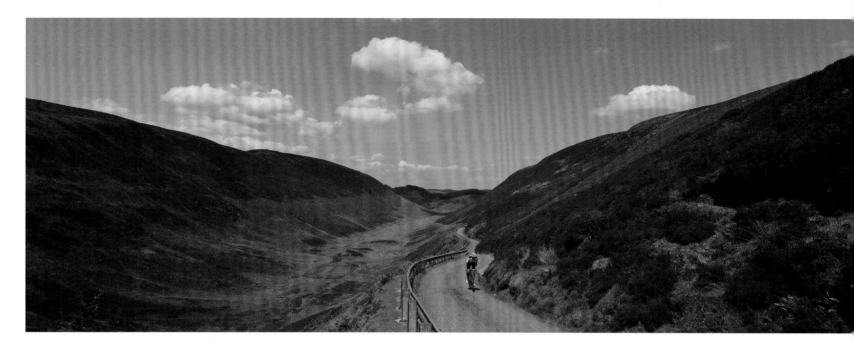

After surviving my first Fred Whitton Sportive back in 2009, I foolishly decided to go looking for a bigger test: something *longer, harder,* more *stupid* – and what I found was the Dave Lloyd Mega Challenge. Dave, an ex-professional rider renowned for his huge training rides in the Welsh mountains, had created an event in his own image which, at 145 miles long and with 5,500 metres of climbing, promised to be the toughest in Britain. It was insane. In fact, after three years it ceased to exist, because people were so scared that no one entered.

Well, almost no one. I rode two of the three incarnations. However, at my first attempt I had a bit of a wobble. Feeling far from my best upon reaching a split in the routes, I had 'a moment',

and had to sit at the side of the road to call my wife to tell her I couldn't go on. I'd never not finished an event before but, presented with the option to take the 'medium' route home, I bottled it and wimped out. Do you know why?

Because, regardless of not feeling on top form, I was scared of riding up the Bwlch-y-Groes. I'd never shied away from a climb before but, in a weakened mental and physical state, at the thought of this legendary foe, not to mention the significant distance needed to get to it, I bailed. Now, before you panic, this route doesn't trace the course of the Mega Challenge, so you can relax, but it does go up the Bwlch-y-Groes, oh yes, and it's *one hell* of a road.

Base for the day is Bala, and the ride begins by

heading to the marvellous climb of the Hirnant Pass. Starting on the B4391, you head south across a small bridge, then take the right-hand turn towards Rhos-y-gwaliau and Lake Vyrnwy. There is a sharp kick up after the junction, then, as soon as you're past Rhos-y-gwaliau and following the River Hirnant, the progress up the wooded valley is gentle for about 7 kilometres. Once free from the forest, and with spectacular views ahead, the slope begins to bite now and, for the final 2 kilometres, sits on an average gradient of 8%. Climbing between smooth, sloping banks either side, the narrow road crawls its way to the summit at the head of this simply impeccable valley. Lined with battered old barriers, the tarmac weaves a little, and the slope

PREVIOUS PAGE
Shock and Awe. Bwlch-y-Groes has it in spades.

ABOVE *Climbing the Hirnant Pass from of the immaculate valley below.*

spikes at close to 20% near the summit, so be prepared to put some proper effort in here.

Beyond the top it's time to drop down to the shores of Lake Vyrnwy, and start the first of two ascents to the top of the Bwlch-y-Groes. Named the Hellfire Pass by the English, the Bwlch-y-Groes is the second-highest pass in Wales – but no need to panic yet: this side is the easiest by far of the three routes to the top. Ride along the western edge of Lake Vyrnwy for a short while, then take the right-hand turn following the sign to Dinas Mawddwy. Heading west and deep into the forest, follow the River Eunant to escape onto the sparse higher ground. Surrounded in all directions by empty rolling hills devoid of anything taller than a sheep, the scenery is sublime and the gradient shallow.

Before long, you'll arrive at the junction where you'll join up with the true Bwlch-y-Groes from the left – but don't look down: it will only scare you. You want to head right on the now much tougher gradient (a taste of things to come), to progress much more slowly to the summit. Over the top, the descent is ferocious, as it twists down the side of the mountain, clinging to the edge of a perilous drop to oblivion. For 10 kilometres you'll plummet down all the way to Llanuwchllyn on the A494, so hold on tight and stay safe.

Here starts a transition period of the route, and unfortunately you'll have to take the A-road because, well, it's the only road. It's not terrible but, be warned, traffic flow may be high at peak times. After roughly 10 dead-straight kilometres,

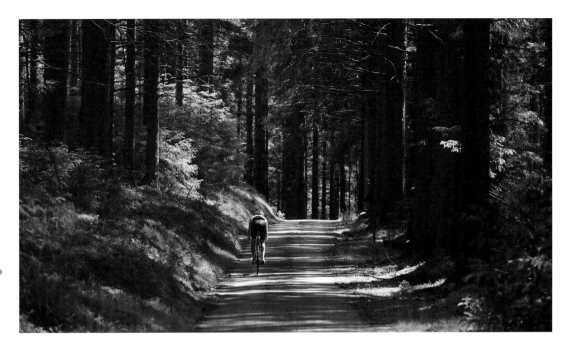

take the left turn towards Drws-y-Nant to continue south-west on the back roads. At the next junction turn left, and then head up and over a sharp little climb to join the B4416, which will take you to the A470. After climbing briefly on this road, you take the right at the junction, to join the A487 due south and continue to climb.

The road rises all the way to the top of Bwlch Llyn Bach, and the views over the other side will blow you away. Part of what is known as the Mach Loop, where the RAF trains pilots in low-level flying, this is where photographers and people who love fast jets camp out to catch a glimpse of the machines of war up close. If you're not expecting them, let me tell you from experience, they come out of absolutely

nowhere, and can have you jumping out of your skin, such is the sudden noise, so be warned. Drop down to the shores of Tal-y-llyn, then continue over another strength-sapping climb to the town of Corris, where you leave the A-roads behind. Heading north-east, your next destination is the Dyfi Forest, a place so quiet and seemingly cut off from the world you can imagine getting lost in it and never being found.

It's not the first time in this book I've referenced the film *Deliverance*, and both have been on routes in Wales, which isn't an accident. If you're at all adverse to being alone in the middle of nowhere, then I'd not recommend you ride this road alone. If, on the other hand, you relish that experience then you'll love it. Oh,

ABOVE *Heading down to Lake Vyrnwy between the towering conifers.*

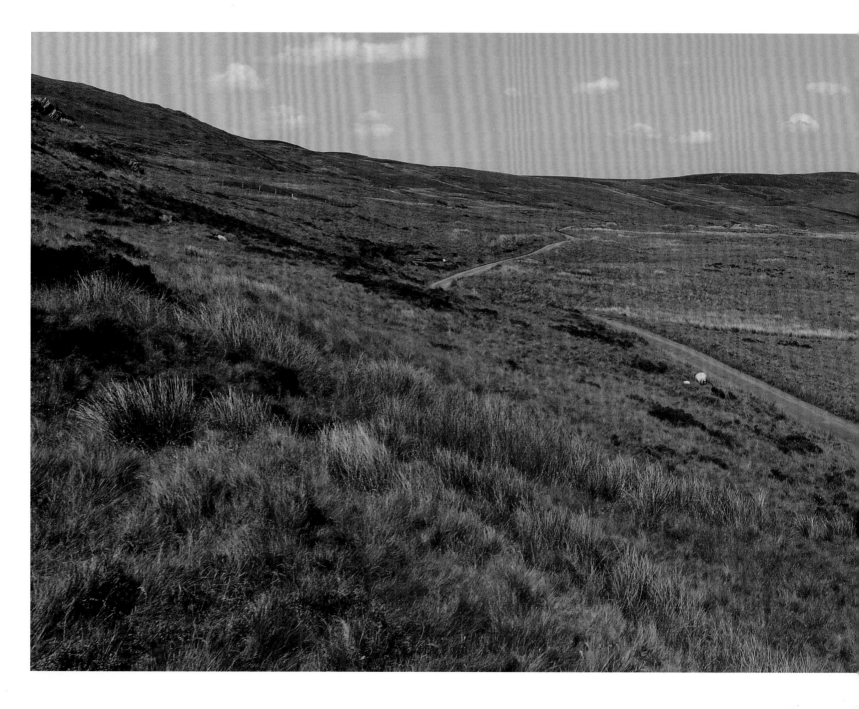

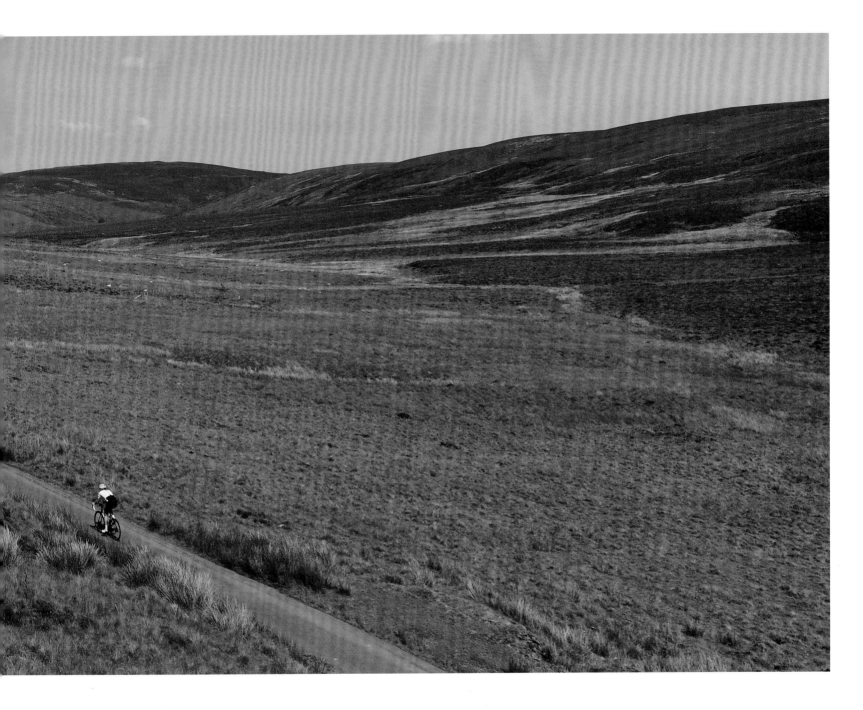

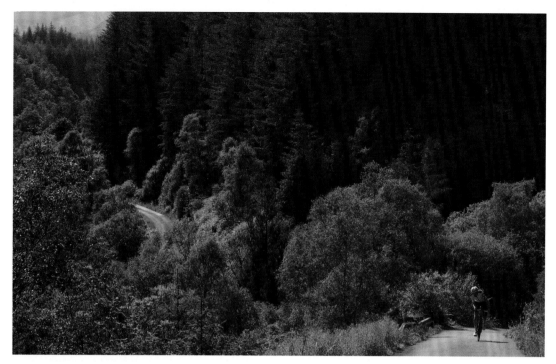

PREVIOUS PAGE
*Are these the empty roads you
have been looking for?*

you'll have passed through some hours earlier, the route does actually turn right, *but* you must first continue to the summit to complete the full climb before looping back to then continue east.

Up next is the long descent back to Lake Vyrnwy, where you can recover somewhat as you leave the exposed high ground and return to the shelter of the forest. At the junction on the shore, turn right, and follow the western edge of the lake all the way to Llanwddyn, then continue on the B4396 to Abertridwr all the way through Hirnant to Penybontfawr. With 120 kilometres covered, you're now just 20 from home, 6 of which are uphill, mind. Turning left in the village, head north on the B4391, through the Tanat Valley to Llangynog, then strap on your climbing legs for one final climb up yet another magnificent valley.

Wooded at first, then opening up to rise beneath the shards of rock that protrude from the hillside, it is spectacularly perfect in every way. The view back down behind you could not have been created better in Hollywood. As this route draws to a close, the scenery is every bit as wonderful as it opened with. Then, with just a short passage over the barren plateau at the top, you leave the high ground for good, and it's time to buckle up for the drop back to Bala. Following the B4391, at first on open land and then through the forest via a brace of tasty bends, you'll arrive back at the start, ready to check your diaries to work out when you can do it all over again.

and it's one hell of a climb up through the forest, with multiple 20% ramps and hairpin bends. Once you emerge the other side, just before arriving in the village of Aberangell turn left, and take the minor road that shadows the A470 before joining it at Minllyn, then leaving it at Dinas Mawddwy.

With 80 kilometres in the legs this is a good place to stop: there's a pub, café and shop where you can grab supplies. Have a little rest before facing up to your destiny. The following 8 kilometres are the calmest of the whole route, undulating gently upwards through the valley to Llanymawddwy, but then it's the big one. It's

time at last for the Bwlch-y-Groes.

Now, you may think I have hyped it up a little too much, but, believe me, I haven't. This road grabs your legs tighter than an alligator's jaws and does not let go until you reach the top. A climb dripping in cycling legend, made famous by repeated visits from the Milk Race in the 1970s and 1980s, it is feared by all those who have passed over it. Such is the duration of the consistently steep 17%-plus gradient in the last half it's enough to make you weep. The valley is majestic, though, the views are breathtaking; it's just that the effort required to enjoy them is immense. Upon reaching the same junction

ABOVE *Deep in the
dyfi forest, no one will
hear your legs scream.*

240 | WALES | RIDE 39

RIDE 39

WALES

SOUTH SNOWDONIA

DISTANCE 142KM

CLIMBING +2,973M

DIFFICULTY 8/10

FOOD & WATER | LLANUWCHLLYN / DINAS MAWDDWY

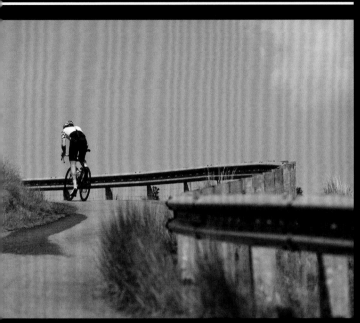

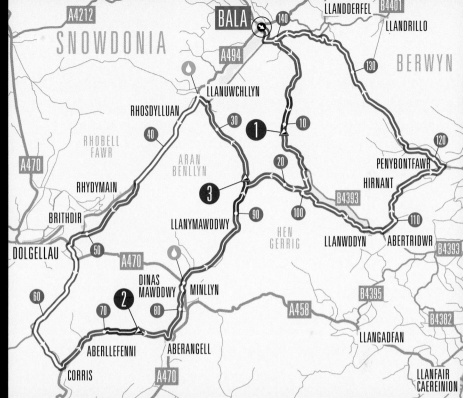

KEY CLIMBS

1 HIRNANT PASS
1,819m +150m

Pure uncomplicated joy is how I first described this climb and that still stands. With the vast open valley and the sheer drop-off from the scree-lined roadside it is pure drama. With an 8% gradient it is a significant challenge to ride especially towards the top where the slope reaches 20%!

2 DYFI FOREST
4,994m +217m

A lonely place, this road linking Corris and Aberangell isn't one continuous ascent but a series of nasty ramps. The first tough stretch is 17% then later there are two much harder 20% sectors to tackle separated by gentle climbing and plateaux all hidden in the detail of the forest.

3 BWLCH-Y-GROES
2,954m +377m

A giant climb with a giant reputation this road really is one of the true monuments of British hill climbing. With an 11% average and slopes as steep as 25% it devours legs for fun, especially the upper section which hovers around the 20% mark for what seems like an eternity.

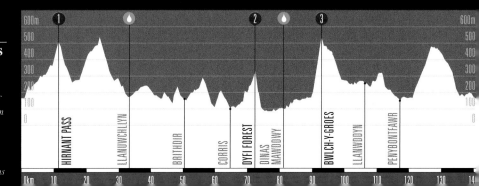

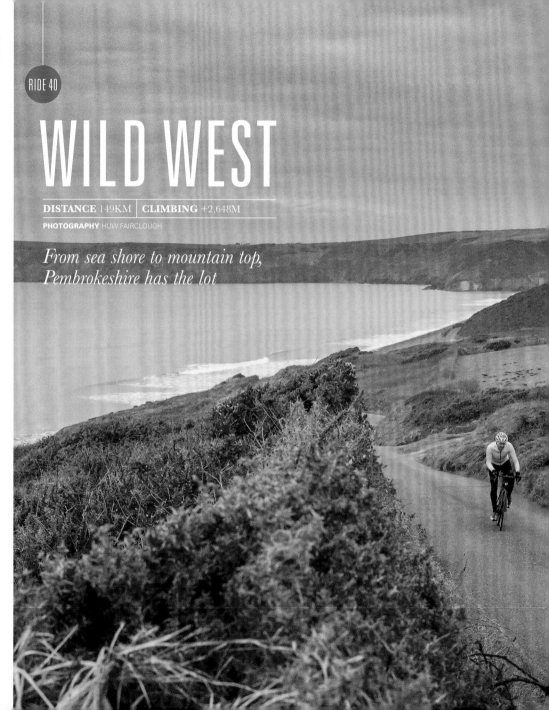

RIDE 40

WILD WEST

DISTANCE 149KM | **CLIMBING** +2,648M

PHOTOGRAPHY HUW FAIRCLOUGH

From sea shore to mountain top, Pembrokeshire has the lot

I'd never been to Pembrokeshire before I started work on my guide to Welsh climbs, which is hardly surprising, as you don't just 'pass through' Pembrokeshire to get anywhere. In fact, it's so tucked away in the far south-west of Wales it almost feels like its own little island. Surrounded on three sides by the Irish Sea, the entire coastline is designated a National Park, and for good reason: it's absolutely stunning. Complete with its own mountain, deathly quiet lanes and a whole host of killer hills, it's a must-ride destination for cycling in Britain, and this route, based loosely on the Tour of Pembrokeshire Sportive route I first rode in 2018, takes you round some of my favourite parts.

I am starting the ride in Fishguard, which seems to be pretty much a day's drive from anywhere else in the world, so allow ample time to get there. Travelling in an anti-clockwise direction, the ride drops out of town, and with breakfast still digesting, ramps up the first of many wicked, steep climbs, hitting 20% from the shoreline into Goodwick. Get ready for a shock: it's like being woken up by a bucket of cold water in the face. Heading west along the protected coastline, ride to Pontiago, then loop around Garn Gilfach rocks, descending towards the coast, then climbing back inland to Trehilyn. Turning right, head south along the rolling, narrow road which, sprinkled with sharp little climbs, keeps going south to meet the A487 at Mathry. Here there's a more significant ramp up into the village, and another when

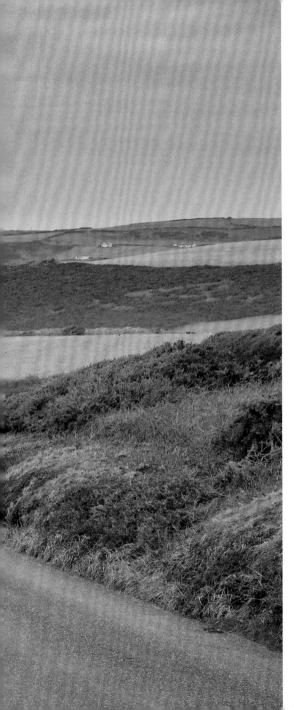

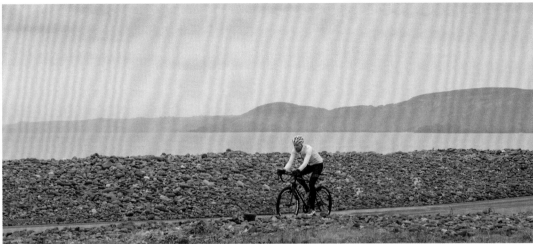

you reach Abercastle, and another just past the village of Trevine. Dipping down to the coast, then climbing rapidly back up again between high hedgerows on impossibly narrow roads, the scenery alternates between neat fields and rugged heathland. Never more than a stone's throw from the shore, continue to head south-west all the way to the town of St Davids, where you make the turn back east. At just 35 kilometres it's a bit early for a stop but, with little other opportunity on the day's route to fill the bottles, it may be wise to.

From St Davids it's time for some real coastal road – I mean, proper amazing: we are talking so beautiful it's hard to ride in a straight line because you can't take your eyes off the water below. And not just that: there's a whole host of little killer hills to entertain you as well on your journey south. From St Davids join the A487 and roll along the tops of the cliffs to Solva, where you drop rapidly to sea level, before crawling back up

the bank the other side of the village. Back on top of the cliffs, although not at the shore just yet, continue to Penycwm, then plummet down the scary fast descent into Newgale to meet the sea. With literally nothing but a couple of metres of gravel piled up on your right protecting you from the onslaught of the waves, the road is utterly flat for a blissful few hundred metres, running directly parallel with Newgale Sands.

Take stock here, then, leaving the A487, it's soon time to start climbing and, as you do, the view just gets better and better. I've never paid too much attention to this climb – yes, it's steep in places, but the view, it's up there with anything in Britain. I love it. Reaching the brow on the top of Black Cliff, you throw all the gained altitude away in an instant to drop like a stone into Nolton Haven, and pass through the tiny village, with its immaculate little bay, to ramp up again. As though this is your own Groundhog Day, the exact same scenario is played out on the

ABOVE *From sea level, the only way is up.*

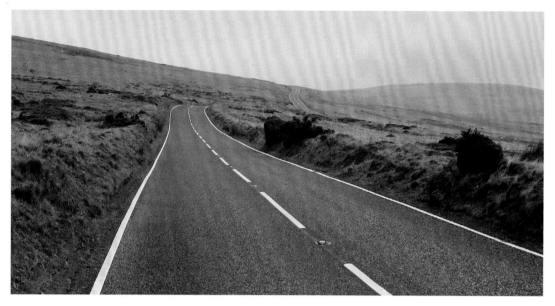

way into Druidston Haven, and a few kilometres further Broad Haven: up and down all the way along the coast, on the most scenic roller coaster you've ever ridden, which, by the time you turn inland in Broad Haven, you'll want to go back and ride all over again, I promise.

From the most southerly point on the route, the climb away from the sea to start the journey inland is a bit of a slog in places, as you head back up to high ground for the most benign section of the ride. Travelling almost due north, you'll reach Simpson Cross on the A487, then Cuffern. Over Cuffern Mountain (don't panic – it's not that bad) and, climbing away from the village, make your way to Hayscastle Cross. Heading west, take time to relax on the stretch of flat land ahead, because there are big climbs on the horizon. Ramping up steadily, you reach

and cross the B4329, then twist down into the valley to the foot of the seriously steep climb of Farthings, which kicks up through and out of the darkness of the woods.

Heading left at the top, ride to Maenclochog then up and down all the way to Mynachlog-ddu and Crymych where, with 100 kilometres covered, you'll be more than ready for a stop and the small town has a few establishments that will cater for your requirements. Refilled and refreshed, it's time to take on the mountain: Preseli Mountain. Heading north-west out of Crymych, make your way via Pontyglasier to Crosswell, then turn left onto the B4329 for this giant of a climb, which adds yet another dimension to Pembrokeshire's scenery. This Goliath of a mound, which has dominated the horizon for half the ride, is finally upon you. With a pitch as harsh as 11%, and at

over 6 kilometres in length, this is some climb up to the wild and exposed summit: a place unique in this corner of Wales, where you can survey the whole county beneath you.

With that in the bag, you are almost home; just a few more treats before you get there. Dropping off the other side, turn right at the junction, then take the next right to make the exquisite journey to Cilgwyn and back through the Gwaun Valley. It's downhill to the turn, then pan-flat on the way back, so get some speed up here, or relax a bit before the final climb of the day, Bedd Morris.

Taking the first right turn out of the valley, following the sign to Dinas Cross, get ready for some classic hairpins. Ramping up from the valley floor into the woods, the first left-hander is an absolute beauty: abrupt, steep and as tight as possible. You swing round and up to the next, legs burning, to drag yourself round. Then, just as the gradient begins to ease, take the left turn instead of continuing to the summit of the climb. From here you are still rising, but more gently now, past Mynydd Melyn, then dropping back to Dinas Cross. At the main road turn left and – I'd like to say it's all downhill into Fishguard, but, sorry – not only is there a sizeable lump on the A487 once you reach the harbour in Lower Town: you also then have the agony of climbing back away from the shore to finish. In fact, this last climb is so nasty that, if you're with mates, I'd be tempted to draw straws and send one person up to fetch the car, so the rest of you can have an ice-cream at the bottom.

ABOVE *No matter where you travel in Wales there's always a mountain to climb.*

DISTANCE 149KM

CLIMBING +2,648M

DIFFICULTY 7/10

FOOD & WATER | BROAD HAVEN / CRYMYCH

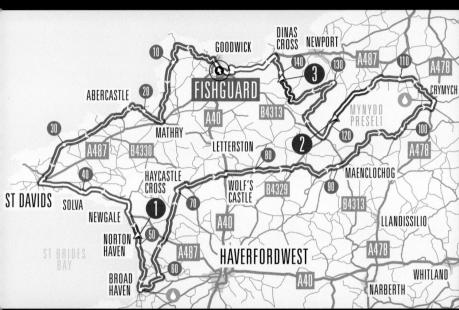

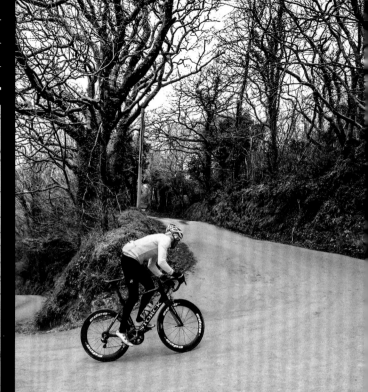

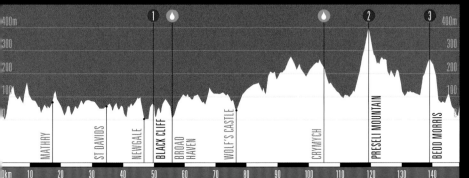

KEY CLIMBS

1 BLACK CLIFF
1,150m +69m

Rising from sea level, snaking slightly and with a multitude of fluctuations in gradient, this climb is set on a slope that while testing is never too harsh as you gradually rise above the waves. With the steepest slopes lower down and an average of 6% you'll be able to stay seated higher up to take in the views

2 PRESELI MOUNTAIN
4,480m +283m

This climb is set on a steady gradient almost all the way up, allowing you to climb comfortably in the saddle and keep the gears spinning. With an average gradient of 6.3% it's not drastically steep, however at almost 5 kilometres long it will wear you down

3 BEDD MORRIS
2,973m +158m

This route only takes in the first part of Bedd Morris but it is the hardest. The start kicks up right from the base where you hit one of the best bends in Wales: a super-sharp left-hand hairpin. With a 20% max it's very hard until the left turn then the rest to the summit is a breeze

INDEX

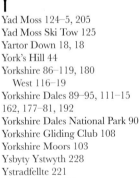

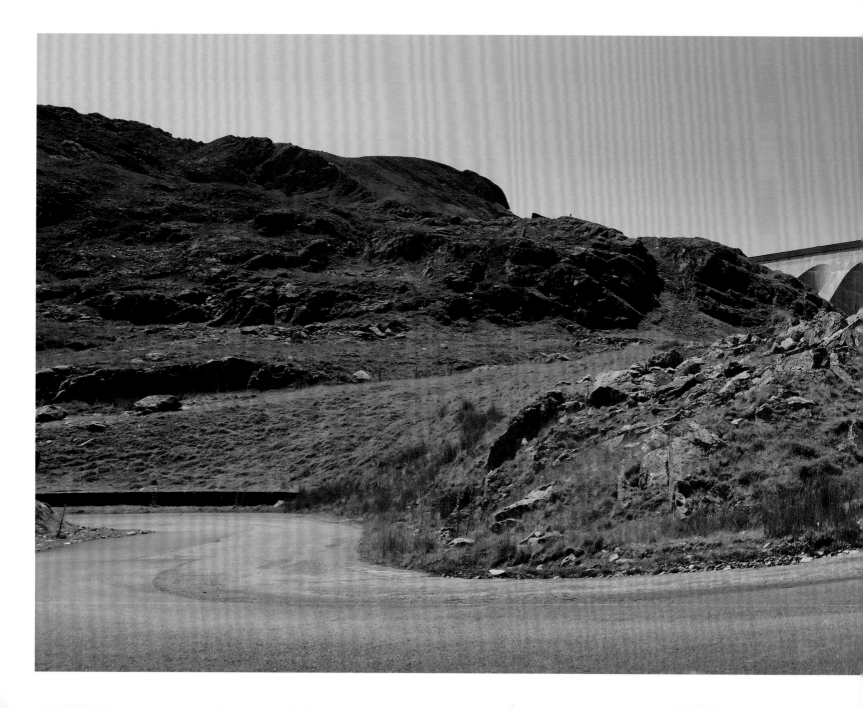

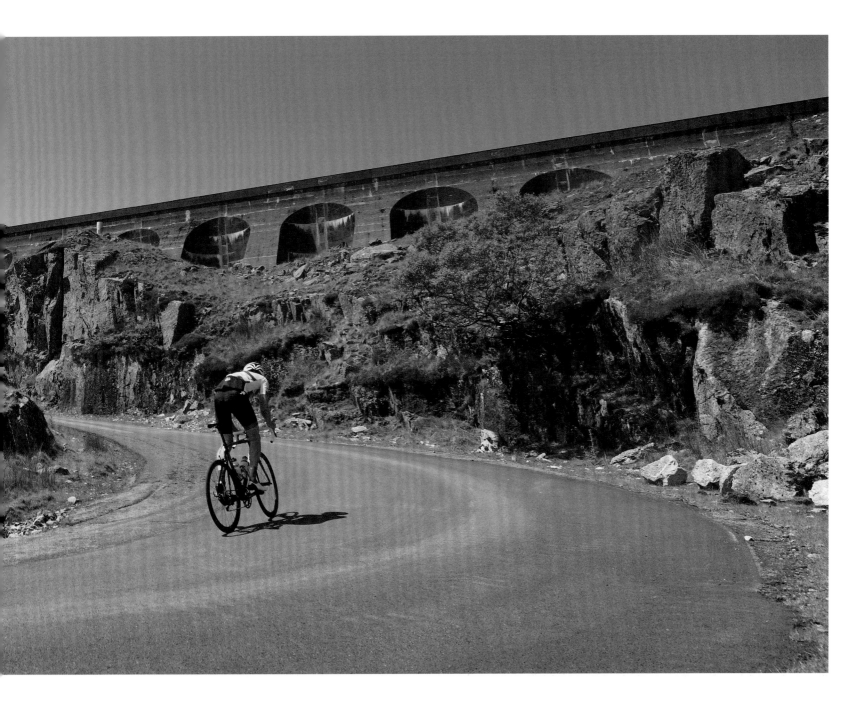

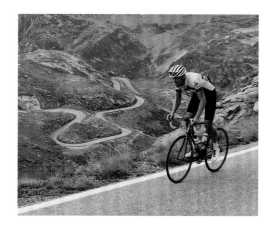

Simon Warren has been obsessed with cycling since the summer of '89, after watching Greg LeMond battle Laurent Fignon in that year's Tour de France. A few weeks later his Uncle David dragged him along to ride his first bike race, a 10-mile time trial on the A1 from Newark to Grantham and back, and he was hooked for life. Although not having what it took to beat the best, he found his forte was racing up hills, and so began his fascination with steep roads. His quest to discover Britain's greatest climbs resulted in the bestselling *100 Greatest Cycling Climbs*, followed to date by 12 more guides to vertical pain, covering Britain, Belgium, France and Italy.

Simon splits his time between working as a graphic designer and running his 100 Climbs brand and lives in hilly Sheffield with his wife and two children.

www.100climbs.co.uk

Also from Robinson by Simon Warren
100 Greatest Cycling Climbs of Italy
Hellingen: The Greatest Cycling Climbs of Belgium